A NEW SHORT TEXTBOOK

CHEMICAL PATHOLOGY

D.N. BARON

Department of Chemical Pathology,
Royal Free Hospital and
School of Medicine, London

J.T. WHICHER and K.E. LEE

Department of Chemical Pathology,
University of Leeds

Edward Arnold

A division of Hodder & Stoughton

LONDON   MELBOURNE   AUCKLAND

NEW SHORT TEXTBOOK SERIES

Some titles in the series
A New Short Textbook of Anaesthetics, Intensive Care and Pain Relief
Jose C. Ponte, David W. Green

A New Short Textbook of Microbial and Parasitic Infection
B.I. Duerden, J.M. Jewsbury, T.M.S. Reid, D.C. Turk

A New Short Textbook of Surgery
Leonard Cotton, Kevin Lafferty

A New Short Textbook of Orthopaedics and Traumatology
Sean Hughes

First published as *Essentials of Chemical Pathology* in Great Britain 1957
Second edition published as *A Short Textbook of Chemical Pathology* 1969
Third edition 1973
Fourth edition 1982
First published as *A New Short Textbook of Chemical Pathology* 1989

British Library Cataloguing in Publication Data
Baron, D.N. (Denis Neville)
   A new short textbook of chemical pathology. — 2nd
   ed.
   1. Medicine. Diagnosis. Chemical analysis
   I. Title II. Whicher, J.T. III. Lee, K.E. IV. Baron,
   D.N. (Denis Neville). Short textbook of chemical
   pathology
616.07′56

   ISBN 0–340–37686–4

Typeset in 11/12 Palatino by
Wearside Tradespools, Fulwell, Sunderland
Printed and bound by Butler and Tanner Ltd, Frome and London
for Edward Arnold, the educational, academic and medical
division of Hodder and Stoughton Limited, 41 Bedford Square,
London WC1B 3DQ

Contents

Preface

The aim of this book is to base chemical pathology firmly on normal physiology and biochemistry. When these are altered, there can be disease: measurement of the alterations can be useful in diagnosis and management. Students need both to understand the biochemical basis of disease, and to learn how to use the laboratory properly in the care of patients. Therefore, as appropriate to the various organs and systems described, normal function is explained in sufficient detail for the student to be able to progress to understanding the changes in disease, and then the appropriate laboratory investigations. This is emphasized by starting each chapter with a serial list of objectives.

The book is designed to meet the needs of medical students, and of doctors in general, for a sound knowledge of the theory and practice of chemical pathology today, and to provide a general basis for the subject for medical and scientific trainees and practitioners of chemical pathology. The material is equally applicable for students of dentistry. It goes part of the way for the needs of the Mastership in Clinical Biochemistry, MSc (Clinical Biochemistry), and Membership of the Royal College of Pathologists, but it is not written on a scale to be a complete reference textbook and candidates will in addition need to consult appropriate large comprehensive texts, monographs, reviews, and original publications. The book should meet the requirements for knowledge of chemical pathology for the MRCP, FRCS, and parallel qualifications, and also for the appropriate examinations of the Institute of Medical Laboratory Sciences.

This is not a textbook of laboratory clinical chemistry, and descriptions of methods are not included. However, the principles of a method for a particular analyte are mentioned when this affects the accuracy or precision of a result. Equally, laboratory management is not discussed, but no textbook of any branch of medicine in the real world can avoid mention of costs. Nor is this a textbook of 'metabolic medicine', but clinical applications are included on topics where the advice of the chemical pathologist is frequently required at the bedside, for example on fluid and electrolyte replacement.

The last edition came out in 1982. Since that time the subject has continued to advance rapidly as a result of developments in the basic sciences, and in their application to medicine. The original author, in conjunction with the publishers, therefore decided early on to invite a younger co-author to join him, and was delighted when Professor D.B. Morgan of Leeds agreed to take part. Many discussions on the nature of the book took place, draft chapters were exchanged – when Brian Morgan's tragically early death halted progress. Many of his ideas have been included and it has been a great pleasure that the Leeds connection has been continued with the new co-authors. This edition is a joint effort. Although different chapters are the responsibility of the different authors, all have been commented on and modified by the other authors.

In the revision the general plan of the previous editions has been maintained. The chapter on the endocrine glands has been divided into four system-related chapters; and plasma enzymes has been separated from plasma proteins. There are new chapters, partly completely original and partly containing previously scattered material, on nutrition and vitamins, cardiovascular system, and non-systemic disease (trauma, malignancy). Disease of skeletal muscle has been included in the chapter on the nervous system. With advances in laboratory use of DNA technology, inborn errors of metabolism now has a chapter to itself. There are separate chapters on therapeutic drug monitoring and on toxicology to take account of the importance of the work in chemical pathology today. Problems particular to the extremes of life are considered separately.

Tests that are no longer used in the United Kingdom may be employed in many parts of the world, because they are still reliable, and cheaper, and do not need elaborate laboratory facilities. For example, the World Health Organization recommends Benedict's test for glucose for health centre laboratories in developing countries. Such tests have been included therefore in a book that is used world-wide. At the other extreme, the reliability in unskilled hands of the increasing number of tests promoted to be available 'at the bedside' (or even by the public as over-the-counter purchases) has been examined critically. These take in the previous appendix on simple biochemical test procedures. There is an appendix on SI units (which should not be necessary in the next edition!) and reference ranges. There is considerable use of cross-referencing between sections and chapters, and an extensive index. Lists of further reading, mainly to reviews rather than to original articles, have been provided.

Acknowledgements: Dr Dimitri Mikhailidis, Dr Jolanta Sabbat, Dr Michael Thomas and Dr Elizabeth MacNamara have provided much assistance; Mrs Pamela Dale, Mrs Pat Windsor, Mrs Diane Reeves, Miss Tracey Turner, Mrs Maureen Baltazar and Miss Mandy Jones have been responsible for the typing and additional clerical help.

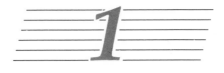

Introduction

Objectives

In this chapter the reader is able to

- follow the development of chemical pathology to its present-day position
- consider the principles of the biochemical investigation of disease: in patients by discretionary or profiling tests, in populations by screening.

At the conclusion of this chapter the reader is able to

- apply critical reasoning to the selection of tests for diagnosis and management
- apply critical reasoning to the interpretation of results in relation to reference ranges and previous results
- understand the concepts of sensitivity, specificity, and predictive values
- describe the main causes of non-pathological variation in measured biochemical values.

Definitions

Chemical pathology is the study of changes that occur in disease in the chemical constitution and biochemical mechanisms of the body – these changes may be either cause or effect. As a fundamental science, it applies physiology and biochemistry to the elucidation of the nature and cause of disease. As an applied science, it seeks by skilled analysis and interpretation to aid the clinician in diagnosis and treatment, and in the prevention of ill-health. Chemical pathology, the most popular term in Britain, will be employed throughout this book, though the widely used 'clinical biochemistry' and 'clinical chemistry' are almost synonymous. It is a relatively new discipline, though closely linked to other branches of medicine and science.

Historical development

The advance of chemical pathology has followed the development of clinical medicine, of biochemical knowledge, and of chemical analytical techniques.

By the middle of the nineteenth century it was possible to measure the concentration of hydrochloric acid in gastric juice; and to analyse urine for sugar by copper reduction, for protein by boiling with acidification, and for bile by nitric acid. The classical *Lectures on Chemical Pathology* of 1847 by Bence Jones, and many similar books of the time, were based mainly on quantitative analyses of urine. Increased sugar, uric acid, and urea had been demonstrated in blood using large volumes in diabetes mellitus, in gout, and in chronic renal disease, respectively, and decreased serum 'albumin' had been shown in 'dropsy', but there were no methods for their easy estimation, especially in small volumes of blood. In Germany, especially, laboratories for the chemical analysis of material from patients were set up. There were no important developments during the second half of the nineteenth century in the general application of chemical knowledge to medicine by the performance of biochemical analyses on patients, although many pioneers were laying the foundation for future advances.

The *first phase* of modern chemical pathology was from about 1910 to 1920, when important advances in methodology were made, notable pioneers being Bang in Sweden, and Folin and Van Slyke in the USA. By the early 1920s venepuncture had become routine practice, visual colorimeters were widely available, and analytical methods requiring only 1 ml of blood were generally adopted.

This led to the *second phase*. Because of this general acceptance of analyses of blood from patients, over the period 1920 to 1945 hospital laboratories that performed such biochemical analyses had a progressive increase in the number of investigations. These tests had been transferred from being performed by physicians in ward siderooms to being done and interpreted by trained staff, medical, scientific and technical, in special laboratories. The increase in the investigative work of biochemical laboratories played a part in the increase in knowledge of biochemical changes in disease. The next major methodological developments, in the 1940s, were flame photometers which permitted easy analysis of sodium and potassium; photoelectric colorimeters which afforded greater speed and precision than did visual colorimeters; and 'micro' techniques for 0.1 ml samples, developed in Britain particularly by King, which allowed more analyses to be done on single venous samples and permitted the use of capillary blood.

These brought in the *third phase*. Round about 1950 specialist societies, journals, and international congresses were established. Because of methodological advances, the greater knowledge of biochemistry applied by more scientifically minded clinicians, and the need for much greater biochemical control of potent therapy, a new steep increase in biochemical analytical work on patients began. A typical British laboratory in a large general hospital might have analysed 10 000 samples (20 000 individual tests) in 1950, and 150 000 samples (1 000 000 tests) in 1985. As appreciation of the meaning of the results has led to more knowledge, and this to more tests, the rate of increase has been continuous. Gradually more complex analytical procedures moved into the laboratories from the basic sciences – electrophoresis, chromatography, enzyme rate reactions, and isotopic and immunological procedures. Analytical procedures became possible on ultramicro samples (0.01 ml), thus allowing a more intensive biochemical study of paediatric and neonatal disease.

The *fourth phase* has been the introduction of automatic analytical equipment by continuous flow or discrete systems, of which the pioneer was the Technicon AutoAnalyzer, to cope with the demand for tests. Many manufacturers have developed further multichannel analysers, by which more than 20 simultaneous analyses may be done on a single plasma sample, and 200 or more of these samples processed per hour.

With this type of equipment we progressed to the *fifth phase*, when in large laboratories computers have become necessary to maintain the identification of the sample, to control the analytical machinery, and to calculate, store, and deliver the results.

When pathology, in any of its disciplines, is concerned with patient care (and may then be called *clinical pathology*, as opposed to *experimental pathology*), finance, efficacy, and priorities, as well as medical science, become involved. Health care resources can be spent once only; costs of this increase of laboratory services have been rapidly escalating, and are forcing control of hitherto unrestricted demands for analyses. One patient over-investigated at too great a cost may have to mean another patient under-investigated.

The *sixth phase*, which is now beginning, will have to involve much improved selectivity in the choice and frequency of biochemical investigations. Computer-based expert systems may help in the selection and grouping of tests and in the interpretation of results. On the one hand simple-to-operate machines for use at the bedside have been developed (p. 261), and these should reduce the load on the laboratory. However new (and expensive) procedures, derived from more basic sciences such as DNA technology (p. 248) or studies of receptor status (p. 217), will have to be added within the laboratory.

The investigation of possible abnormalities

Reasons for investigations

The clinician will decide, after the history and examination, whether instrumental or laboratory investigations are needed. In this book we are concerned only with decisions concerning investigations in chemical pathology. Laboratory tests are justified only when the clinician determines *beforehand* how the results will assist in diagnosis or management – or, do not ask a question unless you know what to do with the answer.

Discretionary tests

There are two main types.

Discriminating

The usual biochemical investigation of a patient can be put into a logical sequence, and better diagnostic information, with a gain in specificity, is obtained by testing in series than in parallel – testing in parallel has a higher sensitivity, but produces more false positives.

1 Decide what information is needed: you cannot get an answer unless you ask a question.
2 Choose the test(s) most likely to provide the information.
3 Use the analytical procedure(s) that best combines speed and quality.
4 Correlate the result(s) – which strictly is relevant only at the time of testing – with the existing information.

5 Decide, in the light of these results, whether further, different tests are needed.
6 Decide if and when to repeat the test(s).

A test that asks a specific question of an individual patient can be considered as one of six types.

(a) *Is anything wrong?* implies that a biochemical investigation is being used as the extension of a clinical examination to determine the presence or absence of an abnormality, under circumstances when the biochemical test is more sensitive than the clinical approach.

(b) *What is wrong?* implies that a general clinical abnormality has been identified, but the specific diagnosis is not known. A discriminating biochemical test (or preferably and more usually a particular combination of tests) can then be chosen which will give a different pattern of results in each of the several diseases of possible diagnosis.

(c) *How badly is it wrong?* implies that the specific diagnosis has been established, but it is necessary to use a biochemical test to assess progression or regression (perhaps after treatment) more sensitively than can clinical observation. On the whole, biochemical tests are probably more important for monitoring progress and treatment than for diagnosis.

(d) *What else is wrong?* implies that a biochemical test is being used to detect a complication of the disease, or an expected or unexpected side-effect of treatment, before it becomes evident clinically.

(e) *How can the wrong be corrected?* implies that in almost identical clinical disorders the choice of treatment depends on subtle biochemical differences.

(f) *Why is it wrong?* implies that the investigation is for research, to learn more about the chemical pathology of the disease. The patient being tested is not expected to benefit, and informed consent, and the approval of the local Ethics Committee, should be necessary. Investigations whose results are required only for teaching come into this category.

Base-line

It is usual to measure the initial values for biochemical components before a patient undergoes a procedure that may alter them significantly, e.g. plasma urea and electrolyte concentrations before major surgery or before diuretic drug therapy. However, it is unlikely that the 'routine' presurgery investigations on non-elderly and otherwise healthy subjects are of any value unless the patient has a reason, such as vomiting, for a possible abnormal baseline.

Screening tests

This is used in two different senses.

Population screening

It is feasible to examine a whole apparently healthy population for a particular disease or toxic effect which is present at low frequency, and which can be detected at a sub-clinical phase by a specific biochemical (or other) test. The population may be selected geographically as in a town, or by occupation, or by age or sex, or by choosing only members of affected families. There must be an advantage in treatment, or prevention of further toxic effects, by early detection of the disease being sought: if not, instead of giving patients, say, an extra year forward of life, they are merely being given an extra year in the knowledge of their disease.

The most widely used biochemical population screening test of generally accepted value is that of blood phenylalanine, done on week-old infants for diagnosis of phenylketonuria (p. 89). Neonatal biochemical screening for congenital hypothyroidism (p. 202), and antenatal screening for open neural tube defects (p. 225), are also now widely used. An example of a screening test of negligible value, because there is no sharp boundary between normal and abnormal, and be-

cause of doubts about the advantage of treating asymptomatic patients, is random blood glucose analysis for detection of sub-clinical diabetes mellitus in the general population.

A major consideration with screening is the efficiency of the test (p. 6).

Admission screening

This implies testing all hospital inpatient admissions, or perhaps outpatient referrals, or even 'check-ups' in a clinic just to see if there is 'anything wrong', for a large number (10–20) of biochemical variables on plasma at the same time. This screening is done irrespective of whether all these investigations are warranted by the patient's presenting condition. Such screening is made possible, and encouraged, by the above-mentioned availability of multichannel automatic equipment, and of computers. It had been hoped that such screening would be economical and provide a 'database' as many of the tests might eventually be requested anyway, and the patient's stay in hospital be shortened. It was also hoped that unexpected biochemical abnormalities would provide important diagnostic information. These hopes have generally not been fulfilled. Also the clinician may find it troublesome because the result wanted, or an unexpected and significantly abnormal result, may be swamped by 'noise' from unwanted results. Much effort is often spent in working up biochemical 'abnormalities' (p. 6) of no clinical importance: a healthy person is one who has not been sufficiently 'investigated'. Such multiphasic screening is not cost-effective.

Profiles, namely performance of an initial set small group of tests related to a specific organ or system, such as four or five tests in the investigation of all cases of jaundice (p. 151) or of metabolic bone disease (p. 183) are generally worthwhile and saving of time.

Types of test

In general, biochemical investigations of

function are first performed in the resting state as the patient presents clinically – *static tests*. This applies whether the function is of an excretory organ such as the renal glomerulus, of a secretory organ such as the pancreatic acinar cells or the adrenal cortex, or of a system such as the blood buffers. Gross changes are detected by such investigations, but a minor abnormality may well be covered by compensatory mechanisms. So, for the investigation of minimal changes it is often necessary to test the function when stressed – *dynamic tests*, and this may sometimes be helpful in determining the anatomical site and physiological level of an abnormality. One type of stress is an extreme load of a normal metabolite, such as using a large dose of ammonium chloride to test the ability of the renal tubules to acidify the urine: a small loss of function may be insufficient to destroy the ability to compensate for the acidity of a normal diet. Another type of stress test is to measure the reserve ability of a normal target organ to respond to an appropriate stimulus, such as the duodenal juice bicarbonate response to secretin to assess pancreatic acinar cell function. The response itself may be hormonal, such as the increase in plasma cortisol concentration after injection of adrenocorticotrophic hormone to measure adrenal function

(p. 213). The converse stress is a suppressant usually via a negative feedback mechanism. This is also usually hormonal, and tests both the integrity of feedback and the response of the target organ: as an example, the changes in plasma cortisol after dexamethasone test the suppression of adrenocorticotrophic hormone by the drug, and also assume the capability of the adrenal cortex to alter production of corticosteroids. (p. 213).

The meaning of diagnostic test results

Some of the reasons why clinicians over-emphasize the value of a test and have too much faith in laboratory diagnosis are lack of understanding of the possibility of laboratory variation and error (p. 9), and of important concepts related to the efficacy of a test which should influence their decisions (Table 1.1).

1 *True positives* (TP) are those ill patients who have that illness correctly diagnosed by the test relevant to the disease.
2 *True negatives* (TN) are those without the disease, who are correctly identified by the test as unaffected.
3 *False positives* (FP) are those unaffected subjects who are wrongly diagnosed by the test as having the disease.
4 *False negatives* (FN) are those affected

Table 1.1 Calculating true positive (TP), true negative (TN), false positive (FP), and false negative (FN) values

	Test positive	Test negative	Total
Disease present	TP	FN	TP + FN
Disease absent	FP	TN	FP + TN
Total	TP + FP	FN + TN	TP + FN + FP + TN

Table 1.2 Calculating the meaning of diagnostic test results

$$\text{Sensitivity} = \frac{TP}{TP + FN}$$

$$\text{Specificity} = \frac{TN}{TN + FP}$$

$$\text{Efficiency} = \frac{TP + TN}{TP + FP + TN + FN}$$

$$\text{Positive predictive value} = \frac{TP}{TP + FP}$$

$$\text{Negative predictive value} = \frac{TN}{TN + FN}$$

All terms are usually expressed as percentages (i.e. ×100%)

patients who are wrongly identified by the test as free from the disease.

Sensitivity, specificity, and predictive values (Table 1.2)

Sensitivity of a test
This is the percentage of diseased patients classified as positive for that disease by the test. The higher the sensitivity of a test, the less likely it is to fail to diagnose a patient as having the disease for which that test is relevant.

Specificity of a test
This is the percentage of negative results in subjects without the disease. The higher the specificity of a test, the less likely it is to misclassify an unaffected subject as having the relevant disease. Sensitivity and specificity do not depend on the prevalence of the disease for which the test is being made.

Efficiency of a test
This is the percentage correctly classified.

Predictive values
These take into account the prevalence of the disease in the population. Predictive value of a positive test is the percentage, in any given mixed population, with and without the disease, of positive results that are true positives. Predictive value of a negative test is the percentage, in a mixed population, of negatives that are true negatives.

The higher the predictive value of a test, the higher the likelihood, in any population, that a positive test means disease, or that a negative test means absence of disease. Most tests were developed in hospitals where a high proportion of patients had the relevant disease, so the tests would then have a high predictive value. If a disease has a low prevalence in the population being tested, such as an ambulatory population of non-disease subjects, then because of the higher proportion of non-diseased subjects there will a higher likelihood of false positives. A positive result then has a lower predictive value, that is a lower chance of being a true positive.

As an example, the parameters of Fig. 1.2 can be taken for a single test. Assuming a prevalence of the disease in the population tested of 1/3, then the predictive value of a positive test is 97 per cent, i.e. only 3 per cent of positive results will not be from patients with the disease. However if the prevalence was 1/100, then the predictive value would be only 30 per cent, i.e. 70 per cent of positive results would not be from diseased patients. Sensitivity, specificity, and predictive values should be reported whenever a new test is proposed.

Receiver operating characteristic (ROC) curve
This is another method of assessing the performance of a test. Sensitivity (or true positive rate) is plotted against one-minus-specificity (or false positive rate) at all possible reference limits or decision criteria.

Likelihood ratio

This further important index of the value of a diagnostic test is independent of prevalence, and ignores reference ranges. It expresses the odds, for any given level or range of test results, or positive/negative finding, that a patient with this result has the expected disease as opposed to being free from it.

Reference ranges, normality, and abnormal results

That there is a 'normal range' for any analysed body constituent is a convenient but artificial concept. A statement such as 'normal plasma sodium 135–145 mmol/l' implies that there is a strict boundary between normal and abnormal. This means that all normal subjects ('normal' is indefinable but implies the general population) have plasma sodium values within that range, and that it is abnormal to have a plasma sodium less than 135 mmol/l or more than 145 mmol/l. Because these

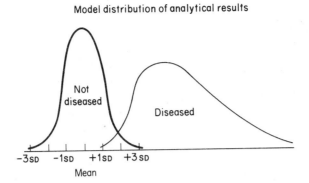

Model distribution of analytical results

Fig. 1.1   Theoretical Gaussian curve for the distribution of a component (e.g. measurements of plasma concentration) in a non-diseased population, showing the range at different multiples of 1 standard deviation (SD) from the mean. This is compared with a positively skewed curve for the same component in a theoretical diseased population, showing overlap between the values found with and without disease

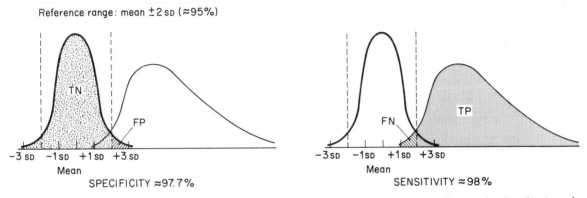

Reference range: mean ±2 SD (≈95%)

Fig. 1.2   The use of ±2 SD (≈95 per cent of population) as a reference range, and its effect on the distribution of true and false positives (TP and FP) and of true and false negatives (TN and FN), and on specificity and sensitivity. The distributions are the same as in Fig. 1.1

assumptions are not true, the term has been replaced by reference range (or reference interval), meaning a range of results to which the result in question can be compared, without making any assumptions about the meaning of 'normal'. It is fair to say that if a value falls within the reference range, then with regard to that component the subject is much more likely not to be diseased than to be diseased, whilst the converse applies to a value outside the reference range – though 'disease', like 'healthy' and 'unhealthy', is also undefinable (Fig. 1.1). In practice most analysed variables have either a roughly Gaussian or a log-normal distribution, and by convention the reference range is taken to include the central 95 per cent of the population under study (Fig. 1.2), thus

excluding 2.5 per cent at either extreme. This can usually be calculated as the mean ±2 standard deviations; if the distribution is non-parametric, then percentiles must be used.

However, for different circumstances different conventions may be used, and medical judgement is important. If a reference range of mean ±3 SD (99.7 per cent of the population) is used, then this will virtually eliminate the risk of a healthy subject being counted as unhealthy should this be considered necessary, as in measuring α-fetoprotein as an indication for therapeutic abortion (p. 220); but a greater number of unhealthy subjects will be missed (Fig. 1.3). Such a procedure will reduce the number of false positives, and operates the tests at high specificity. If the

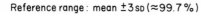

Reference range: mean ±3 SD (≈99.7%)

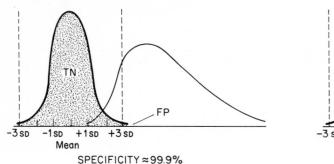

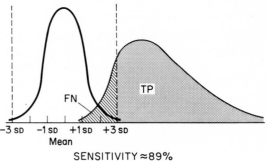

Fig. 1.3   The use of mean ±3 SD (≈99.7 per cent of population) as a reference range

Reference range: mean ±1 SD (≈67%)

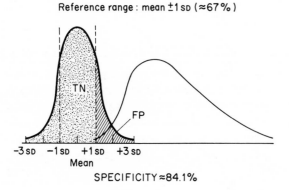

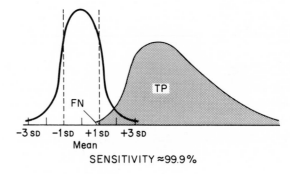

Fig. 1.4   The use of mean ±1 SD (≈67 per cent of population) as a reference range

risk may be the other way, and diseased patients must not be missed whilst occasional (perhaps temporary) misattribution of the unaffected is acceptable, as in screening for phenylketonuria (p. 89), then a narrower set of reference values than '95 per cent' could be chosen, such as mean ±1 SD, or 67 per cent of the population (Fig. 1.4). This procedure operates the test at high sensitivity, and reduces the number of false negatives.

It is possible to improve selection in screening by using a two-stage procedure, and this is done at present, for example, in testing for AIDS. A simple test of high sensitivity is first used. The positives from this test, now having a high prevalence of disease, are given a second (and possibly expensive) test of high specificity.

Relative risk of a test is the ratio of

percentage of positives that are true to percentage of negatives that are false, i.e. TP(TP + FP):FN(FN + TN).

Normality of a group of results
The accepted convention leads to the apparent paradox that if a population group of 'normal' subjects each has 15 independent tests performed by, say, a screening multichannel analyser, then more than half of the subjects will have at least one 'abnormal' result. It has been proposed, so as to reduce the incidence of such 'statistically abnormal' results, that mean ±3 SD would provide a better reference range for each item in such multiple analyses. More complex statistics employing multivariate analysis, and requiring a laboratory computer, can be used to consider the 'normality' of the pattern of all results together.

Other diagnostic indices

Another important value in investigating disease, independent of reference range, is the *action level* (or decision level) at which urgent measures need to be taken by laboratory or clinician. For example, if the upper reference limit for plasma potassium is 5.0 mmol/l, a value of 6.0 mmol/l (and *not* 5.1) could be an action level. In many cases this may be well outside the conventional reference range. Another value not dependent on reference range is the change between successive results that is meaningful, sometimes called the *delta check*, which depends both on precision and on biological variation. A value for plasma potassium of 4.9 mmol/l would be important if yesterday's result were 4.2 mmol/l.

Problems of methods

Reference values are dependent on methodology, for this affects the absolute value of the results. A method is *accurate* if the results are close to the true concentration (or activity) of the substance being measured – which may be difficult to establish in a biological system, and often results in an arbitrarily agreed definition of the amount of a substance present. A method is *precise* if repeated analyses give very similar results – even though not necessarily accurate. Methods for all substances analysed in biological materials have varying precision and are never absolutely accurate. A measurement of plasma concentration requires dividing the amount of substance (or analyte) present as the numerator, by the volume of solution (or analysand) as the denominator. Choice of plasma, or serum, or plasma water as the analysand often makes a difference; as may the use of arterial, capillary, or venous blood. Today, analytical performance in the chemical pathology laboratory is generally adequate for clinical needs.

In the interpretation of possible clinical significance of changes in results, consideration of variability due to the method is important, and the local laboratory can provide information. For example, flame photometry for plasma sodium is precise (coefficient of variation 2 per cent), so a 5 per cent change, say from 140 to 147 mmol/l, is unlikely to be due to laboratory variation and represents a true change in the patient. Extraction and titration for faecal fat is an imprecise method (coefficient of variation 10 per cent), so the same 5 per cent change, say from 14.0 g/24 h to 14.7 g/24 h, may well be due to laboratory or collection variation.

Imprecision of a method leads to loss both of specificity and of sensitivity. Inaccuracy may be less important if the reference range takes account of any consistent bias from the 'true' value.

Limitations of measuring concentration

Most analyses in chemical pathology measure the concentration of the substance being studied, which means the total amount of that substance, or of similar substances detected by the analytical procedure, per unit volume of material analysed. However, it is not only concentration that is important.

Concentration is customarily expressed *arithmetically*, e.g. as mmol/l, but this is not necessarily most appropriate in biologically relevant terms to express the degree of anormality. For example, *logarithmic* transformation is often used for calculating reference ranges when the distribution is positively skewed. Hydrogen ion activities are almost always expressed not arithmetically but as a negative logarithm, to make more comprehensible the enormous changes which occur. It has been proposed that the best way of expressing plasma creatinine concentration, to show its true relation to failure of glomerular filtration, is as the *reciprocal* of the arithmetical concentration. Haematologists may use the *square root* of the leucocyte count as a better guide to the activity of leukaemia than is the total (arithmetic) count.

Concentration and activity

The effect of a substance on a biological process depends on its activity, which is not necessarily the same as its concentration. This applies in blood plasma, and even more in cells. Concentration in plasma water, though rarely determined, is a better reflection of activity than is concentration in whole plasma. An increase in the plasma concentration of other substances (p. 28) will lower the concentration in whole plasma of the substance studied without altering its true concentration in plasma water.

For electrolytes, the presence of free (active) and bound (inactive) forms has to be taken into account (p. 175); ion-sensitive electrodes can measure activity directly (p. 28). Many non-peptide hormones are present in plasma in free and bound forms; measurement of the free/active component may be possible (p. 190). For polypeptide hormones, it is possible that some current immunoassay methods also detect inactive derivatives; bioassay procedures (p. 190) have the advantage of measuring hormone activity. For enzymes, current methods generally measure activity, which is influenced by inhibitors and activators; sometimes immunological measurement of the concentrations of total enzyme protein is useful and feasible (p. 106).

Concentration and content

When intake or output of a substance is studied, the importance of making the conversion from concentration to content, for example in a 24 h urinary excretion, is rarely forgotten. Total blood loss does not alter concentrations in the blood until secondary fluid shifts develop, though the total content of all substances in the intravascular compartment is reduced. Loss or gain of water in blood plasma will affect the measured concentrations of substances in plasma, and such changes will mask any changes due to loss or gain of a substance in the plasma compartment (p. 13).

Measured changes in body constituents due to factors other than disease and drugs

Because of physiological variations, the concentration or excretion of a body component is affected by accountable factors such as time of day (p. 15) and of menstrual cycle (and pregnancy, p. 219), exercise and recumbency, mental state, general diet, fluid balance, and specific meals. Body build will affect the amount of some substances that are excreted (e.g. creatinine, p. 88) but influences few plasma concentrations. The existence of seasonal variations is controlled by environmental temperature, sunlight, and probably an endogenous rhythm. The causes of racial variation are partly nutritional, partly environmental (including endemic disease), and possibly genetic (including blood groups). The main causes of variation in the reference ranges of a healthy population are age and sex: these are being established for all analytes, and the changes with ageing are not always the same for men and women. Plasma concentrations usually (except for albumin and iron) tend to rise with age, probably because of diminution of renal clearance. In general, except for chloride and phosphate, and excluding the female sex hormones, plasma values in men are higher than those in women: this difference is hormone-mediated, as it tends to disappear after the menopause. If a substance, such as aspirin, ascorbic acid, alcohol, cigarettes, or hormonal contraceptive, is taken regularly by a high proportion of healthy subjects, should these be counted as normal?

Differences in reference ranges from those found in the ambulant healthy population may be seen in 'hospital normals', which implies that measurements are made on inpatients who do not have any disease that is known to affect the measured constituent. The differences may then be due to hospital diet, recumbency, and the 'stress' non-specific effects of hospitalization and of any illness. A severe illness may affect biochemical values for weeks after clinical cure.

The ideal diagnostic test

Can be done at the bedside
Painless for the patient
Free of risk

Quick and easy
Does not need great skill
Inexpensive equipment
Low cost for reagents
Accurate and precise

Sensitive and specific
No false positives
No false negatives

High predictive values
Easy to interpret

It does not exist!

Further reading

Baron DN. Ideas towards a general theory of clinical biochemistry. *Ann Clin Biochem* 1986; **23**: 615–623.

Benson ES, Rubin M, eds. *Logic and Economics of Clinical Laboratory Use*. New York: Elsevier, 1978.

Buttner J, ed. *History of Clinical Chemistry*. New York: de Gruyter, 1983.

Noe BA. *The Logic of Laboratory Medicine*. Baltimore: Urban and Schwarzenberg, 1985.

General Metabolism and the Steady-State

Objectives

In this chapter the reader is able to

- revise the physiology of maintenance of the steady-state
- study how changes in measured analytes are caused by disturbances of their steady state, due to physiological and pathological factors.

At the conclusion of this chapter the reader is able to

- differentiate between changes in effective concentration in a compartment due to alteration in the rate of entry into the compartment, in the rate of disposal, in intracompartmental binding, and in compartmental volume.

Compartmental exchanges

The body can be considered in some respects as a set of open steady-state systems whose composition varies regularly and irregularly with such factors as meals, exercise, and circadian (and other) rhythms. The body has many compartments, principally plasma, interstitial fluid, the differing intracellular fluids, lymph, and the transcellular fluids such as peritoneal fluid or intestinal contents. Each compartment has a different and slightly variable composition, and movement between the compartments is not necessarily free and will be different for different components.

The gut is the main site of intake; it is also a site of excretion, and this includes excretion via the bile, which is derived from the plasma after modification in the liver cells. The lungs are similarly sites of intake and of excretion. The kidneys are a site of excretion and to a certain extent of synthesis. Excretion takes place through the sweat glands, and to a limited extent from the skin. The plasma compartment exchanges its components directly with the blood cells, and through the interstitial fluids with body cells. Some material in the body is readily exchangeable and some may be in storage form. Within the cells metabolic processes of synthesis and degradation take place. The generally constant compositions of the various compartments are maintained by balances between inward and outward flows (Fig. 2.1)

Compartmental analysis

Measurement of only the plasma concentration of a body component in a disease (a *static* observation) therefore gives a very limited view of the *dynamic* changes of disturbed rates of flow of the component under study between the body compartments, and of any alterations in the size of the compartmental pool. All of these, as well as the altered concentrations or activities usually measured, are part of the chemical pathology of the disease. For example, a low plasma albumin concentra-

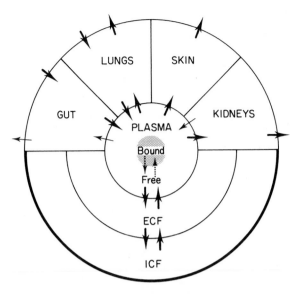

Fig. 2.1 A generalized representation of the exchanges between the exterior, the plasma, the extracellular fluid (ECF), and the intracellular fluid (ICF) that maintain the composition of the body compartments

tion may be due to diminished formation of albumin, or to increased loss or destruction, or to haemodilution. Only in occasional instances, by complex research procedures, is it possible to measure the actual exchanges between the compartments and their pool sizes. Measurement of actual secretion or production rate, usually of a hormone, is also usually difficult. An alternative approach which is sometimes useful is to measure input (food) and output (urinary and/or faecal) of the component under study by a balance technique (p. 83). Measurement of the urinary excretion of a substance is often a guide to the secretion or production rate of that substance or of its precursor, assuming unchanged renal function.

As long as inward and outward flow are equal, the plasma concentration of a component remains unchanged, unless there is also a change in plasma water volume, or (rarely) metabolism of that component within the plasma compartment. The plasma concentration of a component in a sample analysed is the ratio, at a given instant, between its total content in the plasma compartment, and the total volume of the plasma compartment, assuming even distribution. This concentration will rise when the rate of entry of the component exceeds the rate of disposal, provided that there is no diminution of plasma water: the rise goes on until, if possible, a new steady state is set up in which inward and outward flow are again equal. The reverse arguments apply to a fall in concentration in plasma. For example, in non-progressive renal failure the increased plasma creatinine concentration will stabilize when, with the reduced clearance, an excretion of creatinine develops once again equal to its production.

Cell assay

Analysis of particular cells, usually of skeletal muscle removed by biopsy, is done to obtain a view of the overall state of the intracellular compartment. This is a semi-research procedure but has been valuable particularly in elucidating disorders of water and electrolyte balance. The most obviously accessible cells, erythrocytes, are non-nucleated and atypical. Isolated leucocytes are used as model cells for the study of alterations of sodium and potassium transport.

The most practical use of cell analysis is to demonstrate particular enzyme defects in inborn errors of metabolism, when fetal cells from amniotic fluid, or chorionic villus biopsy, or leucocytes, are the most useful. A recent development, beyond the scope of this book, is the use of DNA analysis to identify prenatal cases or adult carriers of many genetic diseases, or to aid in their diagnosis.

Alterations of the steady-state

One of the main subjects of study of chemical pathology is to determine how derangements of steady-state mechanisms can cause disorders of a biochemical nature. For example, in diabetes mellitus the effective primary derangement is lack of insulin activity, causing (amongst other abnormalities) continuing release of glucose from liver cells and failure of glucose to enter muscle cells. Because glucose continues to enter the plasma at a faster rate than it leaves, this disturbs the steady-state primarily by increasing the concentration of plasma glucose. There results the secondary effect of increased filtration of glucose through the glomeruli, and so on. The steady-state is disturbed also within the peripheral cells because of the decreased rate of formation of glucose-6-phosphate from lack of available intracellular glucose.

A similar pattern can occur even when the primary disturbance is not biochemical but anatomical. For example, the urinary loss of albumin is maintained in health at a very low value by a balance between glomerular filtration and tubular reabsorption of albumin. Normal albuminuria thus does not significantly affect the plasma albumin concentration, which is maintained by a balance between the rates of synthesis and degradation of albumin. In the nephrotic syndrome the increased glomerular filtration of albumin becomes greater than the tubular reabsorptive capacity and there is massive albuminuria. This leads eventually to a fall in the plasma albumin because of the limited capacity to increase albumin synthesis. The plasma albumin would only remain unchanged, though with an increased turnover, if synthesis of albumin were increased in parallel with the increased loss.

In chronic disease a new steady-state will be set up, with altered concentrations of the affected components in the different compartments, and often altered volumes of the compartments and of rates of transfer of the components between them. This steady-state is not well maintained when there is the additional stress of an unphysiological load, and this may be useful in assessment. In chronic non-progressive disorders this is handled more slowly and less efficiently than in normal subjects.

The disturbance of the biochemical steady-state may be an effect of the disease, valuable for diagnosis or management but not part of the main metabolic disorder. For example, the normal level of concentration (and activity) of plasma aspartate transaminase, which is maintained by a balance between leakage of enzyme protein from cells and its disposal into the protein pool, is in chronic hepatitis set at a higher level because of increased leakage from the cells.

Disorders of transport

In many disturbances of the steady-state there are alterations of active or passive transport across the cell membrane, and in the example of diabetes mellitus given above this is secondary to deficient insulin activity. There are many disorders where the disturbance is primarily that of the cellular transport mechanisms, and many of these primarily affect the main transport organs, namely the mucosa of the small intestine and the renal tubules.

Disorders of binding

Within a given compartment, apart from any exchange with other compartments, there is an internal steady-state mechanism for many components because of the existence of free and bound forms. A proportion of many components of the body is held in an inactive or storage form. In the plasma this is due mainly to binding to proteins, often albumin, or to proteins that are relatively specific for some hormones and for metals. The mechanism in the cells is not known, but is probably also of a protein nature. In plasma, where these factors are better understood, what is biologically significant is not the total concentration of a component but its free (unbound) or active concentration. The concentration or capacity of binding proteins can be increased or decreased genetically, or by disease or hormonal changes, thus altering the amount of bound component. When this happens the total concentration of a component in the plasma changes in the same way, but the active fraction may remain unchanged. Free and bound forms for electrolytes are respectively also in the ionized and non-ionized states. Some substances, especially drugs, may displace components from protein-binding, thus increasing the free fraction without change in the total concentration.

Feedback

One way in which the steady-state is maintained is by negative feedback. A simple mechanism is when the concentration in the plasma or tissue compartment of a specific product (released from a body target cell) may be mainly controlled by a hormone through its influence on a metabolic process; and the secretion of that hormone be mainly controlled by the plasma concentration of the product (Fig. 2.2). Alternatively, the concentration of this hormone, or its activity, will often itself be controlled by another hormone from the anterior pituitary gland. The secretion of this pituitary hormone will be controlled directly, or through a hypothalamic mechanism, by the concentration in plasma of the hormone, or other substance, which is the end-product of the various stimulant activities (p. 192). The steady-state mechanisms attempt to maintain the final product approximately constant, because any alteration in its concentration will react back on the hypothalamus, anterior pituitary or other hormonal stimulant. This in its turn regulates directly or indirectly the concentration of the final needed product. An abnormality at any stage of the process will alter the steady state, and cause a biochemical abnormality – this is one of the fundamental disturbances of chemical pathology.

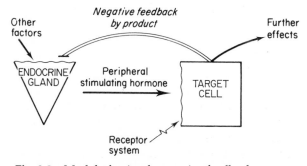

Fig. 2.2 Model of a simple negative feedback system

The opposite to the stabilizing negative feedback is the pathological *vicious circle*. A biochemical example may be found in gout. Hyperuricaemia can result in formation of uric acid calculi: these can damage renal function, which will further raise the plasma urate concentration.

Disorders of receptors

Both the control of secretion of hormones by negative feedback, and their direct actions on tissues, are dependent on the sensitivity of the appropriate receptors in the target organs. If receptor status (concentration or affinity) is altered, then a normal circulating concentration or activity of hormone, or other mediating substance, will elicit an abnormal cellular response – as in Cushing's syndrome (p. 209) or nephrogenic diabetes insipidus (p. 195). Little is known about pathological effects of such alterations, and measurement of receptor status is a research procedure.

Circadian rhythms

These are natural biological rhythms whose mean time is between 20 and 28 h. They have very complex control mechanisms, and amongst the known factors causing circadian rhythms are light and dark, and social influences, including meals, sleep, rest and work; the causes have not been completely elucidated, and there is an innate biological rhythm over about 25 h. Many of the circadian changes are mediated through a demonstrable fundamental rhythm of adrenocorticotrophic hormone, which affects plasma cortisol, which itself affects many metabolic activities: this is largely driven by a central nervous system 'clock', though the pituitary and the adrenal cortex have endogenous rhythms.

Various circadian rhythms will be mentioned where relevant: the marked circadian variation of plasma hormones (especially cortisol), iron, and phosphate must be taken into account when collecting blood for their analysis. Responses to many function tests, such as the glucose tolerance test or creatinine clearance, will also vary with time of day.

There are other natural rhythms. There may be a slight 28–30 day rhythm of hormone secretion in males, corresponding to the monthly changes in women (p. 218), of unknown primary cause. Seasonal rhythmical changes are mainly caused by changes in exposure to sunlight.

Failure of circadian rhythms can be an effect of a fundamental biochemical disturbance. As far as it is known such alterations do not in themselves cause disease.

Further reading

Baron DN. Ideas towards a general theory of clinical biochemistry. *Ann Clin Biochem* 1986; **23**: 615–623.

Noe BA. *The Logic of Laboratory Medicine.* Baltimore: Urban and Schwarzenberg, 1985.

Riggs DS. *The Mathematical Approach to Physiological Problems.* Baltimore: Williams and Wilkins, 1963.

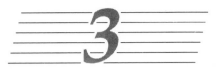

Water and Electrolytes

Objectives

In this chapter the reader is able to

- revise the physiology of osmotic pressure, of the distribution of water, sodium and potassium, and of their metabolic control.

At the conclusion of this chapter the reader is able to

- understand the causes and presentation of the primary syndromes of water and sodium depletion/excess and of their combinations
- investigate a patient with suspected disorder of water and/or sodium balance, and use the results as a guide to treatment
- understand the causes and presentation of potassium depletion/excess
- investigate a patient with suspected disorder of potassium balance, and use the results as a guide to treatment.

Normal distribution

Water

Water makes up 50 to 60 per cent of the body of a healthy adult, to a total of about 45 l in the average 70 kg man. Of this, 25 to 30 l (30–40 per cent) is intracellular fluid (ICF) and 13 to 16 l (15–20 per cent) is extracellular (ECF) of which plasma takes up 3 to 3.5 l (Fig. 3.1). About 1.5 l is lymph, and another 1.5 l is transcellular fluid – a

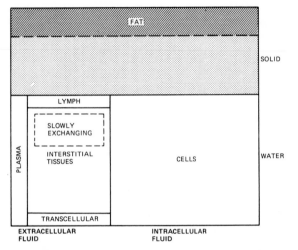

Fig. 3.1 Proportional distribution of solids and water in a healthy adult

term used to include alimentary secretions, cerebrospinal fluid, pleural and peritoneal fluid, aqueous humour, and synovial fluid. A sub-compartment of extracellular fluid, with a volume of about 4 l, is the slowly exchanging interstitial fluid of connective tissue and bone. Solids comprise 40 to 50 per cent of the body. About a third of the solid is fat, but this is very variable; adipose tissue contains less than 10 per cent of water which is poorly exchanged.

In infants a smaller proportion of the body is intracellular water. About 25 per cent of the mass of an infant is solid, 30 per cent ICF and 45 per cent ECF.

The boundary between the ICF and the ECF is normally permeable to water and small organic molecules, selectively permeable to ions (active cell metabolism maintains the sodium pump), and to a very limited degree permeable to protein. The boundary between interstitial fluid and plasma is freely permeable to water and ions, but only to a small extent to protein or lipid. The protein content of interstitial fluid, a plasma ultrafiltrate, is low (less than 200 mg/l) despite the high protein content of plasma and of cells. The water content of plasma is about 92 per cent and of most cells is about 70 per cent.

The movement of water is controlled by osmotic pressure which is dependent upon the total solute content of the fluid; it is normally about equal in all the body spaces. Water moves freely from one compartment to another to adjust any temporary imbalance of osmotic pressure. For example, if hypertonic saline were ingested or infused, the ECF would become temporarily hypertonic; water then moves from the ICF to the ECF to lower the osmotic pressure in the plasma and tissue fluid. There is a dynamic not a static equilibrium; movement of water and of ions is continuous, and this maintains osmotic and electrolyte equilibrium.

Electrolytes

In the intracellular fluid the dominant cation is potassium and there is little sodium or chloride: the dominant anions are protein, organic acids and organic phosphate. Inside cells there is about a tenth as much sodium and 30 times as much potassium as in the ECF. These gradients of concentrations are maintained by energy-dependent membrane pumps.

In the extracellular fluid the dominant cation is sodium and the predominant anion is chloride. Interstitial fluid has a very low protein concentration (less than 1 g/l) while intravascular fluid (plasma) has a high protein content of about 70 g/l. Protein acts as an anion, so diffusible anions are at a lower concentration in plasma than in interstitial fluid, whilst the opposite is true for diffusable cations: this is known as the Gibbs–Donnan equilibrium. However the effect is small, and the measurement of

plasma electrolyte concentrations may be used to assess those of the ECF as a whole.

Osmotic pressure, osmolarity, osmolality

The total solute content of body fluid determines its osmotic pressure. The movement of water between compartments depends on the difference in concentrations of the dissolved particles (solutes) on either side of the separating membrane which is impermeable to them. Osmotic effect is expressed in osmoles which is a measure of the number of osmotically active particles released by a molecule in solution. Thus for a non-dissociated molecule, such as glucose, 1 milliosmole is equivalent to 1 millimole, but for a completely dissociated molecule, such as sodium chloride, 1 millimole provides 2 milliosmoles. Osmotic activity therefore depends upon the dissociation constant of ions and may be expressed per volume of solution (osmolarity) or per weight of solvent (osmolality). In clinical practice the use of osmolality is favoured and values are reported as 'mmol/kg' and less often as 'mosmol/kg'. The normal plasma osmolality of 275–295 mmol/kg water is made up as shown in Table 3.1.

Table 3.1   Plasma osmolality

Ions or molecules in plasma	mmol/kg
Sodium and associated anions	270
Potassium and associated anions	7
Calcium and associated anions	2.5
Magnesium and associated anions	1
Glucose	4
Urea	4
Protein	1
Total approximately	290

Osmolality may be measured by depression of freezing point or elevation of boiling point, but in the case of plasma may be calculated with reasonable accuracy from the measured concentrations of the predominant solutes. As sodium and its associated anions, glucose and urea, comprise 95 per cent of the osmotically active particles normally present in plasma, the following calculation may be used:

Plasma osmolality =
$(2 \times Na) + (glucose) + (urea)$

e.g. $(2 \times 135) + (5) + (7) = 282$ mmol/l.

In urine such a calculation is not possible as there are more ions present contributing significantly to the osmolality but a reasonable estimate of solute content may be made by measurement of specific gravity (p. 254).

Under normal circumstances sodium and its associated anions provide 90 per cent of plasma and ECF osmolality and thus rapid changes in concentration (before equilibrium across cell membranes can occur) will cause water to enter or leave cells. The contribution of glucose and urea to osmolality is normally constant but in diabetes and renal failure levels may rise rapidly enough to cause the ECF osmolality to exceed that of the ICF with consequent cellular dehydration. Exogenous solutes that may contribute to the ECF osmolality are mannitol, ethanol, methanol and ethylene glycol. For example, a plasma ethanol level of 100 mg/dl contributes about 20 mmol/kg.

The high protein content of plasma as opposed to interstitial fluid results in an osmolality difference of 1–2 mmol/kg between these two compartments. This is known as the oncotic pressure and is balanced by a difference in hydrostatic pressure between the vascular and extravascular compartments.

Control of water and electrolyte metabolism

Water

The water content of the body is regulated by a combination of thirst and antidiuretic hormone (ADH) secretion. Both are controlled by hypothalamic centres which respond to the osmotic gradient across specialized neurones. ADH is produced in the hypothalamus, stored in the pituitary

gland, and released in response to increases in ECF osmolality of about 1 mmol/kg (p. 193). It increases the reabsorption of water by the renal collecting ducts. In addition to control by changes in osmolality, ADH is secreted in response to moderate falls in plasma volume (10 per cent or more).

Sodium

The sodium content of the body is regulated by renal tubular reabsorption (p. 114). This is determined by renal blood flow, aldosterone, and natriuretic hormones. The main stimulus to sodium reabsorption is volume depletion which stimulates renin production from the kidney and thence aldosterone production from the zona glomerulosa of the adrenals (p. 206). This results in enhanced sodium reabsorption in the proximal tubule of the kidney.

Loss of sodium from the ECF will result in a fall in osmolality. This will inhibit ADH secretion and water will be excreted until the osmolality is corrected. There will thus be a fall in ECF volume which will override the osmotic control of ADH secretion, switching it on when the plasma volume

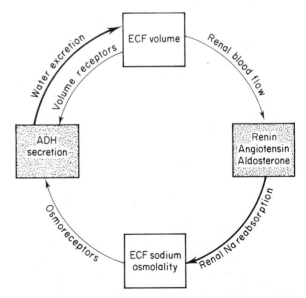

Fig. 3.2 Summary of factors regulating sodium and water balance showing their interdependence

has fallen by about 10 per cent. It is clear that osmolality and thus sodium concentration (the major contributor to ECF osmolality) controls the water content of the body under normal circumstances. The relationship of sodium to water regulation is shown in Fig. 3.2

Balance of water and electrolytes

Water balance

In a healthy subject, water output is equal to water intake and any minor short-term discrepancies result in an alteration in the volume of the total body water. Water is utilized for temperature regulation (sweating) and excretion of waste products in urine and faeces.

Table 3.2 shows the typical daily water balance of a healthy 70 kg adult. The normal daily solute load of waste products is approximately 600 mmol and as the urine can be concentrated to some 1 200 mmol/kg this can be excreted in 500 ml of urine. If to this minimal urine output is added the insensible fluid loss through the lungs and the skin, the daily obligatory water loss of a normal active adult in a temperate climate is seen to be 1 500 ml – which is about 2 per cent of the body weight; the insensible loss is less from a patient at rest in bed. An adult patient who is completely deprived of fluid may lose, therefore, up to 2 per cent of his body weight per day. If there is no additional loss of fluid, the daily fluid intake, to prevent any risk of water depletion, should be 2 000 to 2 500 ml.

If the concentrating power of the kidneys is diminished through disease, or if the renal load of metabolic waste products is increased, then the minimum volume of urine which is required for excretion of the waste products will be higher. For example, if the urine cannot be concentrated to an osmolality greater than 600 mmol/kg, then the obligatory minimal urinary output becomes about 1 000 ml.

In hot climates, or when there is severe fever, considerable water loss can occur as sweat; even minimal obvious sweating may lose 100 ml per day. In health the endogenous gastrointestinal tract water turnover is about 8 000 ml/24 h – 1 500 ml saliva, 2 500 ml gastric juice, 500 ml bile, 500 ml pancreatic juice, 3 000 ml intestinal secretions. In any disorder of the gut in which fluid is lost to the exterior, enormous water losses can also occur.

Paediatric problems

Infants develop water deprivation more easily than do adults. An infant utilizes about three times as much water per unit weight, has a relatively greater energy production, and a relatively large surface area. This leads to relatively greater losses of fluid through the skin and lungs, and to a relatively greater load of metabolic waste products for the kidneys. The kidney of an infant has less concentrating power than that of an adult; the adult kidney needs less than a litre of water to excrete 1 000 mmol of solute, whereas the infant kidney needs at least two litres for this purpose. The daily turnover of fluid in an infant is about one-half of its ECF volume, compared to one-fifth in an adult. As a result of these factors an infant deprived of fluid may lose 4 per cent of its body weight per day.

Table 3.2   Water balance

Intake	(ml)	Water pool	(ml)	Output	(ml)
Moist food and drink	2000	Plasma	3 000	Lungs	500
Water from oxidation and dry food	500	Tissue fluid	12 000	Insensible skin	400
		Cell fluid	30 000	Urine	1300
				Faeces	200
				Sweat	100
Total	2500		45 000		2500

Table 3.3 Sodium balance

Intake	(mmol)	Sodium pool	(mmol)	Output	(mmol)
Food, drink, and seasoning (10 g as sodium chloride)	170	*Exchangeable*		Insensible loss	Nil
		Plasma	450	Urine	155
		Tissue fluid	1600	Faeces	5
		Rest of body		Sweat and skin	10
		soft tissue	350		
		bone	500		
		Non-exchangeable			
		Bone	1000		
Total	≈170		≈4000		≈170

Sodium (and chloride) balance

In a healthy subject, sodium and chloride intake equals output (Table 3.3), and any minor discrepancies are balanced by an alteration of the sodium and chloride concentrations in the ECF. The reference range for plasma sodium concentration is 135–145 mmol/l, and for plasma chloride concentration is 98–107 mmol/l. The normal muscle cell sodium is about 10 mmol/kg wet weight (15 mmol/l cell water), and muscle chloride is about 3 mmol/kg wet weight (5 mmol/l cell water).

Table 3.3 shows an approximate typical daily sodium balance of a healthy adult in a temperate climate. Ample sodium is normally present in the diet: if there are no extra losses, then an adequate intake of sodium to prevent depletion is probably about 20 mmol (i.e. about 1 g of sodium chloride). In health the endogenous gastrointestinal tract sodium turnover is about 1500 mmol. However, considerable losses can occur in disease; 200 mmol may be lost in the sweat of tropical fever, and more than 500 mmol in severe diarrhoea and vomiting.

When assessing sodium balance in patients, drugs given as salts must not be forgotten: for example, 20 g of carbenicillin contains 94 mmol of sodium.

Although it is customary to speak of salt deficiency and salt replacement, it is the sodium that is osmotically important. The body fluids do not, however, contain equal proportions of sodium and chloride; for example gastric juice contains much less sodium than chloride. Average anion and cation concentrations (compared to plasma) in those body fluids which may be lost in disease are shown in Table 3.4. The salt content of sweat may vary considerably, and falls on adaptation to a hot climate.

Because of their variable sodium/chloride content, losses of body fluids may result in disturbances of acid–base balance as well as causing water- or salt-depletion. The healthy kidney, by its power to excrete sodium and chloride differentially, can usually redress the imbalance when adequate saline treatment is given. The deficient ion is retained, the unwanted ion is excreted.

Table 3.4 Composition of body fluids

	Na^+	K^+	Cl^-	HCO_3^- (mmol/l)
Intracellular	10	110	10	10
Extracellular				
Plasma	135	4	100	25
Saliva	30	20	30	Variable
Gastric juice	70	10	140	0
Bile	130	4	110	25
Pancreatic juice	130	4	60	60
Sweat	60	12	40	Variable

Disorders of water and sodium balance

Clinical syndromes due to loss of water or sodium are common. The word 'dehydration' is commonly applied to all forms of water and sodium loss, but the word means loss of water and should not be used to describe conditions in which redistribution and loss of body water is secondary to loss of sodium. It is advisable to consider water depletion and sodium depletion separately as their causes, metabolic effects, and clinical courses are different, and appropriate replacement therapy depends on correct appreciation of the initial deficiencies and on experienced judgement of the patient's responses. Pure water depletion or pure sodium depletion are rare, but combined depletion usually favours one or other component. It must be remembered that changes in the general body store of water or ions do not necessarily take place in the same direction as do changes in the plasma concentrations.

The osmotic gradient across cell walls is the most important determinant of the clinical effect of disturbances of sodium and water metabolism. Thus changes of sodium concentration without a change in other extracellular solutes will alter the osmotic gradient. Large changes in glucose will have similar effects. Gradual changes by allowing redistribution of water, and movement of diffusible solutes, such as urea, may produce little effect.

Water and sodium depletion

Causes and metabolic aspects

Water and sodium may be lost in roughly equal amounts in plasma, secretions from the small intestine, bile, pancreatic juice and the urine passed when tubular function has failed. Water and sodium depletion is also seen when ECF is removed from the general circulation in pools of fluid without being lost from the body, for example in ascites, gross oedema or paralytic ileus. Under these circumstances aldosterone is secreted in response to volume depletion and sodium is retained by the kidney (only if tubular function is normal). The resulting increase in osmolality causes increased ADH secretion, maximal water reabsorption in the renal collecting ducts, and oliguria together with thirst. If fluid is unavailable and losses continue hypovolaemia, decreased cardiac output and a falling glomerular filtration rate will occur with a rising plasma urea.

Therapy

This is iso-osmolar volume depletion and must be treated by replacement with sodium and water. If water alone is taken then the hypovolaemia cannot be corrected (p. 25). Treatment must be based on the presenting disturbances and previous losses of the patient, and (as in all these disorders) a well-kept fluid balance chart is essential, and is the easiest method of assessing the patient's needs. If, for a few days after an operation, an adult patient requires fluid intravenously because he cannot take fluid by mouth, and if there is no renal functional impairment or additional loss of secretions, then combining 500 ml of isotonic saline solution and 2000 ml of isotonic glucose solution provides a suitable daily infusion. Unless oral feeding can begin within a few days, potassium should also be given intravenously as 50 mmol of potassium chloride included in the above infusion. In the first 24 h following operation no potassium, and not more than 2000 ml of total fluid per day, should generally be given because of the oliguria, resulting from stress-induced ADH secretion (appropriate ADH secretion). If intestinal secretions have been lost they should if possible be collected, analysed, filtered, and replaced: valuable enzymes and bile contents will not then be wasted. Two or three days (but no more) without energy from food or intravenous nutriment can be easily tolerated. Daily weighing of the patient helps assessment.

Oral glucose (or perhaps sucrose) and electrolytes may often be used together in water for the treatment of severe fluid loss in diarrhoea. This simpler procedure – about 8 g glucose, 1 g sodium chloride in 1 litre water – is important for infants in the tropics.

Water depletion

Causes

The syndrome of predominant water depletion develops when fluid intake is insufficient and there is continuing loss of fluid of low sodium concentration. It is important to appreciate that most body fluids contain less sodium than plasma and ECF. Water depletion due primarily to deficient fluid intake may be seen postoperatively when oral fluid intake has ceased because of surgical necessity, or because the patient is unconscious, or has severe dysphagia or is old and feeble. When intake of water ceases, the insensible fluid loss from lungs and skin, and obligatory secretion of urine, continues. Postoperatively, after the immediate oliguria and sodium retention of the first few days, there is a water and sodium diuresis and any tendency to water depletion is increased.

Water depletion due to excessive fluid loss may result from sweating, hyperventilation, aspiration of gastric juice, vomiting and diarrhoea. Typical examples of gastrointestinal loss would be in cholera and infantile gastroenteritis. Water depletion of renal origin may develop in primary or nephrogenic diabetes insipidus (p. 195), in chronic nephritis and pyelonephritis, or in the diuretic phase of acute renal failure (p. 119), and in osmotic diuresis such as may occur with heavy glycosuria (p. 61). In all these cases water depletion may be avoided by increasing intake to match output. If this is done without any sodium intake predominant sodium depletion will however result (p. 24). After brain injury, there may be a combination of hyperthermic sweating and diabetes insipidus.

Metabolic aspects

In predominant water depletion the concentrations of sodium and chloride in the ECF and the osmotic pressure of the ECF gradually rise. If pituitary and renal function are normal this promotes the release of antidiuretic hormone which results in a small volume of concentrated urine. A fall in circulating blood volume stimulates aldosterone secretion causing maximal sodium retention and a low urinary sodium concentration. The volume depletion results in a falling glomerular filtration rate, but retention of nitrogenous waste products and a rise in the plasma urea occurs late, usually only when the urine flow falls below about 30 ml/h. Water depletion is accompanied by polyuria and a dilute urine if the loss is of renal origin. Effects tend to be more severe in infants and in old people because of poor renal compensating capacity, and in infants also because of relatively smaller fluid reserves.

The primary loss of water from the ECF is replaced from the ICF to maintain, as far as possible, the osmotic pressure of the plasma and tissue fluid. The concentrations of the ions in the plasma rise because there is a lag in water adjustment. The osmotic pressure of the ICF rises. As replacement of the ECF is not complete, there is a sustained fall in the plasma volume, and slowly progressive haemoconcentration and circulatory changes.

Clinical aspects

Symptoms begin to appear when about 2 l of water have been lost. The main symptoms, which reflect hyper-osmolality of the ECF and consequent cerebral dehydration, are apathy, thirst, and dryness of the mouth and tongue; there is a slight loss of skin turgor. The patient complains of general weakness and there is an oliguria with urine of high osmolality (and specific gravity). If renal function is unimpaired a daily urine volume of less than 750 ml means that a patient has water depletion; a severely dehydrated patient may excrete in a day only 500 ml of urine at an osmolality of more than 1200 mmol/kg (specific gravity 1.040). Measurement of the fall in body weight is an important method of detecting the extent of loss of water. The plasma sodium level is increased sometimes to as high as 170 mmol/l, but the level depends on the degree of equilibration between the ECF and ICF. Death after coma, possibly due to a rise in intracellular osmotic pressure, occurs when about 15 per cent of the body weight has been lost: in adults this happens after about 10 days without water, and in infants after less than 7 days.

Therapy

The treatment of choice is water orally until the daily urine volume exceeds 1500 ml. The amount of water required can be calculated from the plasma sodium concentrations according to the formula

$$\frac{(\text{plasma [Na]} - 135)}{135} \times \frac{\text{total body water (l)}}{(60\% \text{ of body weight in kg})}$$

Thirst is not necessarily a reliable index of water depletion. If the oral route is not possible or insufficient, water must be given intravenously, and 5.0 per cent w/v glucose (50 g/l, 280 mmol/l) is acceptably isotonic. Most pharmaceutical companies still label glucose for intravenous use as 'dextrose': this can be confusing. The rectal route is a last choice because of its relatively limited absorptive capacity. Oral salt or intravenous saline must not be given unless there is also sodium depletion; any addition to the extracellular sodium will withdraw more water from the cells.

Sodium depletion

Causes

The syndrome of predominant sodium depletion develops most commonly when there is general loss of both water and sodium which is replaced only by water or solutions of low sodium content. It occurs more rarely when there is a greatly diminished intake of sodium with normal water intake.

Loss of sodium-containing fluid results from burns, from severe exudative skin lesions, or through massive sweating ('heat exhaustion'). Large amounts of sodium and water can be lost in alimentary secretions, through fistulae, vomiting and diarrhoea (especially in cholera), steatorrhoea, and intestinal aspiration or high intestinal obstruction. In these conditions predominant sodium depletion usually results from inappropriate replacement by intravenous infusion of fluids containing too little sodium. Thus the commonly used 'dextrose saline' contains only 30 mmol/l of sodium, less than any body fluid.

Many diuretics lead to excessive urinary sodium loss, as does Addison's disease (p. 212), chronic renal failure, and diabetic ketoacidosis (p. 55). In these chronic conditions urinary sodium loss exceeds dietary intake, often leading to sodium depletion only over long periods of time.

A mild sodium depletion may develop when sodium intake is greatly diminished, and this can happen without excessive sodium loss in prolonged starvation, e.g. due to anorexia nervosa or in chronic alcoholism. Before an operation, many patients are sodium deficient from a combination of these causes.

Considerable amounts of sodium may be lost from the general ECF into the gut in paralytic ileus, into oedema, into interstitial fluid in an injured limb, or into pleural or ascitic fluid; these pools take only a limited part in the general ionic exchanges of the ECF, and thus can be considered as 'lost'.

The sick-cell syndrome is part of many severe chronic illnesses, and is due to failure of the sodium pump. Sodium passes into the cells (which lose potassium and other intracellular ions) and the plasma sodium concentration falls, but the total body sodium is unaltered.

Metabolic aspects

When sodium-containing fluids are lost from the body (Table 3.4) there will be hypernatraemia unless water is taken orally when there will be a net loss of sodium

Table 3.5   Changes in body fluids in disorders of water and electrolyte balance

Predominant disorder	ECF volume	ECF osmolality	Plasma sodium concentration	Urine sodium concentration	Urine volume
Water depletion	↓	↑	↑	↓	↓
Sodium excess	Normal	↑	↑	↑	↓
Sodium depletion					
Renal, e.g. in Addison's disease	↓	↓	↓	↑	↓
Other	↓	↓	↓	↓	↓
Water excess	↑	↓	↓	↑	↑

from the body. The ECF becomes hypotonic and some water passes into the more hypertonic ICF. The fall in tissue fluid osmotic pressure switches off ADH secretion and water is lost in the urine until the osmotic pressure of the ECF is restored. Water and sodium are thus 'lost' in parallel and the ECF and plasma volumes fall, stimulating aldosterone secretion. In the presence of normal renal function, sodium is reabsorbed from the urine which contains less than 10 mmol/l. Typically, plasma sodium and chloride levels do not fall until 10 per cent of the ECF volume has been lost and ADH is secreted in response to volume depletion (p. 19). The decrease in circulating blood volume and decrease in glomerular filtration rate (GFR) usually result in a slightly raised plasma urea at this point. The decreased GFR and secretion of ADH can result in a fall in urine volume. The changes in plasma volume, urea and sodium concentration in predominant sodium depletion are shown in Fig. 3.3.

Clinical aspects

Symptoms begin to appear when the patient has lost the sodium equivalent of 4 l of isotonic (physiological) saline. Initial symptoms are of tiredness and muscle weakness followed by those of circulatory failure, hypotension, coma and death. It is important to realize that when hyponatraemia is due to sodium loss the patient will be depleted of ECF by at least 10 per cent and that this is usually accompanied by a raised plasma urea concentration. Thirst is often absent as the ECF is hypo-osmolar.

Therapy

The treatment of choice is saline in-travenously. Isotonic saline (155 mmol/l: 9 g/l, 0.9 per cent w/v) is suitable and the amount of sodium required may be calculated from the formula

$$(135 - \text{plasma [Na]}) \times \text{total body water}$$

This is usually far more than would be given by 'clinical judgement'. Thus a 70 kg patient with Addison's disease and a plasma sodium concentration of 110 mmol/l will require 1050 mmol of sodium or 6.8 l of isotonic saline to correct the defect. It is safer to give a slight excess as this can easily be lost in the urine. Labelling as 'per cent' instead of g/l is still done on infusion fluids by many pharmaceutical companies. It is incorrect and may be dangerous to call this concentration of saline 'normal'. The term 'normal' is used chemically for solutions of 1 equivalent per litre, i.e. for NaCl of 5.85 per cent w/v.

If large volumes of saline have to be given it may be advisable to add potassium chloride and sodium bicarbonate to the infusion to counteract the saline-engendered hyperchloraemic metabolic acidosis and hypokalaemia, because isotonic saline, when compared to plasma, contains excess chloride and is acid.

Water and sodium excess

There are a number of conditions in which adrenocortical hormone secretion is chronically increased. This results in sodium reabsorption and consequently water retention as a result of the increasing ECF osmolality stimulating ADH secretion; the ECF volume is expanded.

Continuing sodium retention does not occur, probably due to sodium excretion

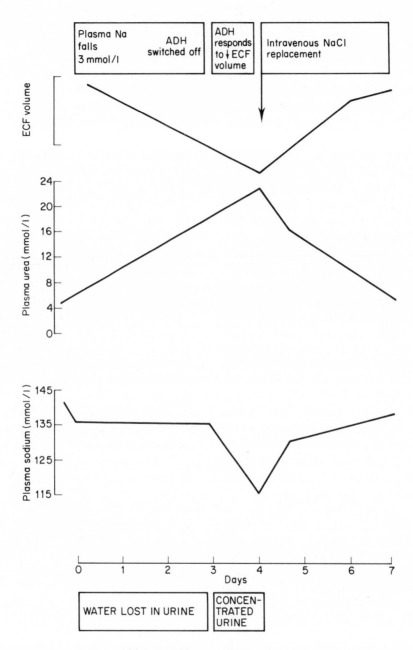

Fig. 3.3   Predominant sodium depletion induced by sweating. The water is replaced but excreted in urine. The fall in ECF osmolality (plasma sodium 137 mmol/l) switches ADH secretion off, and a negative water balance ensues. This results in a maintenance of ECF osmolality with a contraction of ECF volume and an increase in plasma urea. ADH secretion is stimulated by a significantly decreased (>10 per cent) ECF volume and this overrides the inhibitory effects of hypo-osmolality. ADH causes water retention and excretion of a concentrated urine. The ECF volume is increased at the expense of severe hyponatraemia (plasma sodium 115 mmol/l); plasma sodium only returns to normal after intravenous NaCl. Modified with permission from Walters G. Disorders of fluid and electrolyte balance. In Williams DL, Marks, V, eds. *The Scientific Foundations of Clinical Biochemistry.* Vol 1: Biochemistry in Clinical Practice. London: Heinemann, 1983: 1–23

caused by natriuretic hormones and the plasma sodium level is therefore usually on the upper limit of normal. Volume expansion causes hypertension but rarely oedema, and hypokalaemic alkalosis (p. 31) results from the action of mineralocorticoid on the distal renal tubule.

Decreased renal perfusion may result in stimulation of renin and aldosterone secretion causing the condition often referred to as secondary aldosteronism (p. 212). Renal vascular damage causes decreased perfusion in renal artery stenosis, malignant hypertension and essential hypertension. Decreased renal perfusion may occur as a result of cardiac failure where the cardiac output is low.

The plasma volume may be reduced if the interstitial fluid is expanded in oedema or ascites when the oncotic pressure is decreased due to hypoalbuminaemia. This occurs in kwashiorkor (p. 80), nephrotic syndrome (p. 123), and advanced liver disease (p. 159). The exact mechanism of this syndrome is complex and ill-understood. Despite the fact that the ECF volume is expanded and the total body water and sodium are increased, it is common to observe a low plasma sodium in these cases, especially if oedema is present.

More rarely, excessive mineralocorticoid secretion results from neoplasms of the adrenal in Conn's syndrome (p. 211) and Cushing's syndrome (p. 209).

Water excess

Water excess can only occur if normal homeostatic mechanisms have failed or, occasionally, if they are overridden.

In acute and end-stage chronic renal failure the urine volume and concentration are fixed and the administration of excessive amounts of salt-poor fluid will result in water overload.

ADH secretion is increased following major trauma or surgery and water retention is likely to occur if excessive amounts of low sodium-containing fluids are given to the patient. The secretion of ADH under these circumstances is often referred to as 'inappropriate' in that it continues even in the presence of ECF hypo-osmolality. It is however a relatively short-lived and normal response to conserve water following injury when 'in the wild' water to drink may not be available. Inappropriate ADH secretion is best used to describe those conditions where secretion of the hormone continues for days or weeks. Such a situation may occur following head injury, intracranial haemorrhage and encephalitis where the hypothalamic centres are damaged or with malignant tumours (especially carcinoma of the bronchus) which synthesize ADH or related peptides (p. 195).

Water intoxication due to 'psychogenic polydipsia' (p. 195) is rare and readily corrected when drinking stops.

Metabolic and clinical aspects

Water overload is an important cause of hyponatraemia and must be distinguished from predominant sodium loss. ECF volume expansion may result in cardiac failure if the heart is already compromised and occasionally oedema is seen. If hypo-osmolality has developed rapidly, cerebral oedema may lead to anorexia, lethargy, confusion, fits and coma. In the presence of normal renal function the increase in plasma volume and renal perfusion results in decreased aldosterone secretion with increased urinary sodium loss.

Therapy

The treatment of excess water intake is to restrict water intake to a negative balance of

$$\frac{(135 - \text{plasma [Na]})}{135} \times \text{total body water}$$

If the patient has clinical evidence of water intoxication (hypo-osmolality) then an infusion of hypertonic saline, e.g. 850 mmol/l, (1.5 per cent weight/volume) may be given over six to eight hours to replace the sodium deficit as calculated by the formula above. Water excess due to ADH secretion must not be treated with isotonic saline (as the sodium will be excreted) but if possible by treating the primary cause together with water deprivation. Drugs that inhibit ADH activity such as demeclocycline may be helpful.

Sodium excess

Causes

Excess sodium intake is relatively rare but may occur by drinking sea water (1200 mmol/kg) although it is often vomited due to its high salt content. Near-drowning in sea water is often associated with the absorption of sodium through the lung, and hypernatraemia may be seen due to this and also to the osmotic withdrawal of water through the pulmonary capillaries into fluid within the lung. In the past, high-sodium artificial milk has resulted in hypernatraemia and death in infants. The iatrogenic sodium excess may result from the administration of excess hypertonic bicarbonate following cardiac arrest and this is an important and avoidable cause of fatal hypernatraemia; 8.4 per cent sodium bicarbonate contains 1000 mmol/l of sodium.

Metabolic and clinical aspects

Predominant sodium excess is only important if water is unavailable. It invariably gives rise to hyperosmolality of the ECF with thirst and mental confusion, coma and death due to cerebral dehydration. This is because the increasing ECF osmolality results in water leaving the cells increasing the volume of the ECF. This results in plasma volume expansion, aldosterone is switched off and sodium is lost in the urine. At the same time the high osmolality results in maximum ADH secretion, the urine is therefore concentrated and of high sodium content. Treatment is by replacement of water according to the formula

$$\frac{(\text{plasma [Na]} - 135)}{135} \times \text{total body water}$$

Babies should not have their sodium content reduced at a rate greater than 2 mmol/kg·h as rapid changes in the water content of cerebral cells may give rise to fits.

Measurement of electrolytes in plasma and urine

Plasma

Plasma sodium and chloride estimations provide the most important information about disturbances of water and electrolyte metabolism. Urea measurement provides the all-important information about the renal function and also allows, together with glucose (which may be measured, or 'assumed' if there is no reason for it to be abnormal), calculation of the plasma osmolality (p. 19).

Hyponatraemia may result in ECF hypo-osmolality and is more commonly due to water excess than to sodium depletion. The plasma urea often helps in distinguishing these two conditions, being raised due to decreased renal perfusion in sodium deficiency and low due to dilution in water excess. It is important to appreciate that hyponatraemia may be appropriate to the osmolal state; thus with hyperglycaemia, uraemia, mannitol infusion, and high blood alcohol there will be an increase in osmolality. This results in withdrawal of water from cells and dilution of ECF sodium together with ADH switch on, water retention and volume expansion which switches off aldosterone and sodium is lost. Osmolality is restored at the cost of hyponatraemia. Treatment of this condition with sodium is thus dangerous. Occasionally, hyponatraemia may be due to the presence of lipids or proteins occupying a greater proportion of the volume of plasma than they usually do and thus diluting the measured sodium content. The sodium concentration in the plasma water will however be normal as will its osmotic activity on cell walls. This *pseudohyponatraemia* is only seen when measurements are made by flame photometry. The new ion-sensitive electrode measurements which measure ionic activity (p. 9) in plasma water do not suffer from this problem.

Hypernatraemia always reflects hyperosmolality and consequent cellular dehydration. It may result from water depletion or from predominant sodium overload. In either case it is dangerous and must be treated with water replacement.

Urine

The estimation of urinary sodium content may occasionally be helpful to the expert but is often misleading. In addition it is not a useful method of calculating loss in urine or other body fluids. The treatment of disturbances of sodium and electrolyte metabolism must be based on an assessment of fluid balance from fluid balance charts, an understanding of the underlying disease, and plasma electrolyte measurements. In general, urinary sodium output reflects intake unless there is increased aldosterone secretion when the concentration falls to 10–20 mmol/l.

Potassium

Potassium is the principal cation in the cells, and it is present in a relatively low concentration in the ECF. The reference range for plasma potassium concentration is 3.6–5.0 mmol/l: the plasma must be removed from the cells within three hours of venepuncture, and serum values are about 0.4 mmol/l higher due to the release of potassium from the clot. The potassium concentration in the erythrocyte is about 85 mmol/kg wet weight (160 mmol/l cell water). Potassium is freely filtered by the glomeruli and largely reabsorbed in the proximal tubules. Urinary potassium is derived from distal tubular secretion which is linked to sodium reabsorption and stimulated by aldosterone. Hydrogen ions compete with potassium for exchange with sodium. Potassium loss thus depends on the amount of sodium available for exchange, the relative amounts of H^+ and potassium in the tubular cells and the aldosterone level. Renal mechanisms are more competent in excreting excess potassium than in conserving diminished potassium.

Potassium moves from the ECF into the ICF either when protein is being deposited or glucose is being taken in and metabolized, or during extracellular alkalosis. Potassium moves from the ICF into the ECF and can then be lost from the body into the urine, when body protein is being catabolized in starvation or after stress or trauma (about 2.5 mmol potassium per gram protein), in severe illness (sick-cell syndrome), during exercise, in hypovolaemia when aldosterone is being secreted, or during acidosis.

The body contains about 3500 mmol (150 g) of exchangeable potassium and about another 1000 mmol of slowly exchangeable potassium. The average intake in an adult is about 100 mmol (4 g) per 24 h, of which at least 80 per cent is excreted in the urine and less than 20 per cent in the faeces. Up to 10 mmol may be lost in shed skin and sweat. If there are no additional losses of potassium the daily potassium intake, to prevent potassium depletion, should be about 30 mmol (1.2 g); about 20 mmol/24 h is lost in urine even if there is no intake. In disease potassium may be lost in any body secretions, most of which contain potassium in higher concentration than in the plasma (Table 3.4). Intake of salts in drugs must not be forgotten: for example, 20 g of penicillin G contains 52 mmol of potassium.

Assessment of abnormalities

It is important to realize that changes in the body store of potassium do not always take place in the same direction as changes in the plasma concentration of potassium. So by measuring the plasma potassium only a limited view is obtained of the changes in the total body potassium. In general, a change of 1 mmol/l in the plasma potassium implies a change of 200 mmol in body potassium. In practice the clinical degree of abnormality of potassium balance is usually reflected fairly adequately by the plasma potassium concentration, and measurement of cell potassium is not readily practicable: important exceptions such as diabetic coma are considered below. Neuromuscular conduction and the electrocardiographic changes which are characteristic of abnormal plasma potassium levels possibly depend on the ECF/ICF potassium gradient and not on the plasma concentration of potassium. These may be abnormal, with a normal plasma potassium level, when the cell potassium concentration is altered.

Hyperkalaemia and potassium retention

Causes

In clinical practice hyperkalaemia is not as common as hypokalaemia. A high plasma potassium level may occur when there is excessive intake, diminished excretion, or shift of potassium from the cells to the ECF. This may be caused by acidosis when hydrogen ions displace potassium ions from the cells. Conversely, loss of potassium from cells will promote an extracellular acidosis and intracellular alkalosis. Because of the high potassium content of cells, haemolysis or breakdown of leukaemic leucocytes after blood has been taken from the body will result in a falsely high plasma potassium. This effect may also be seen if samples are stored for 8 to 12 h in the refrigerator, when the sodium/potassium pump may not function adequately to prevent potassium leaking from the cells. It is also important to appreciate that sample tubes containing the anticoagulant EDTA may also contain potassium.

Hyperkalaemia due to excessive intake may develop during treatment of hypokalaemia, especially if large doses of potassium are given intravenously when renal function is impaired; also the potassium content of the plasma of stored blood which is used for transfusion may be much higher than that of normal plasma, increasing by 1 mmol/l per day of storage. In severe renal failure, due to disease of the glomeruli or to a diminished renal plasma flow, potassium is retained, and the rise in the plasma potassium concentration can be correlated with the fall in the glomerular filtration rate

– symptoms which are attributed to hyperkalaemia are part of the uraemia symptom complex (p. 120). In adrenocortical deficiency, particularly in Addisonian crisis (p. 210), and rarely in hypopituitarism, there may be hyperkalaemia due to decreased potassium excretion as a result of deficient mineralocorticoid activity. Potassium-retaining diuretics, such as spironolactone (an aldosterone antagonist) may have a similar effect. Potassium is released from cells when there is increased cellular catabolism such as after crush injury, burns, or in the early postoperative phase, or whenever much sodium is lost from the ECF (due to secondary aldosteronism). There may then be a raised plasma potassium level – but urinary excretion eliminates most of the cellular potassium and the body as a whole is potassium deficient.

Metabolic and clinical aspects

The chief toxic effect of hyperkalaemia is on neuromuscular conduction, especially in the heart, and signs develop at a plasma potassium level of about 7.5 mmol/l. Bradycardia develops with distinctive electrocardiographic changes of an absent P wave, broad QRS complex, and particularly high T waves. At high plasma levels (9 mmol/l), atrioventricular (AV) block and cardiac arrest can develop.

Therapy

Treatment is required in all severe cases. The cause of the hyperkalaemia can often be remedied by stopping the excessive intake, or by correcting the acidosis and any water and salt depletion. Reversal of toxic effects on the heart may require intravenous calcium. Hyperkalaemia of renal origin is difficult to treat. Insulin (with glucose) may be given to transfer potassium to the cells. Potassium may be withdrawn from the ECF into the gut and thence excreted by the use of a suitable ion-exchange resin that binds potassium. Peritoneal dialysis and haemodialysis will correct hyperkalaemia as well as the other abnormalities of uraemia.

Hypokalaemia and potassium deficiency

Causes

Hypokalaemia, which is commonly seen, is usually associated with general cellular deficiency of potassium.

All foods that contain cells contain potassium, and deprivation of food, with inadequate intravenous replacement, is an additional reason for the potassium deficiency that may develop in a severe illness or after an operation. Protein malnutrition such as kwashiorkor leads to severe potassium depletion though hypokalaemia may be masked by water depletion.

Hypokalaemia due to potassium loss is most commonly seen in patients with disease of the gastrointestinal tract, especially when this is associated with diarrhoea (or steatorrhoea) and vomiting, and may be marked in children; it often occurs after gastrointestinal surgery, especially with ileostomy, or after prolonged use of purgatives. In these conditions potassium intake is often also reduced. It is commoner in old people because of long-standing poor intake. There is increased catabolism of protein postoperatively, and potassium is lost from the cells to be eventually excreted in the urine; this process is exacerbated by water loss and aldosterone secretion. Patients with chronic gastrointestinal disease who require surgery are usually potassium-deficient even before the operation. The resultant body potassium deficiency and hypokalaemia are an important cause of postoperative 'weakness', morbidity, and mortality.

In diabetic coma (p. 55) there may be considerable loss of body potassium into the urine due to fluid loss stimulating aldosterone secretion. Because of dehydration, the initial plasma potassium may be normal or raised. Insulin treatment halts the loss of potassium because restoration of intracellular glucose metabolism with correction of acidosis fixes potassium in the cells, but the shift to the cells and fluid replacement lowers the plasma potassium level. Prolonged treatment with intravenous glucose likewise shifts the potassium from plasma to cells.

Many drugs can cause hypokalaemia including liquorice derivatives (with aldosterone-like effects), and diuretics, such as the thiazides and especially frusemide which inhibit sodium reabsorption making more available for direct tubular exchange with potassium. Because of increased activity of the sodium–potassium exchange mechanism there is urinary loss of potassium (causing hypokalaemia) in Cushing's syndrome, primary or secondary aldosteronism, or from overdosage with ACTH or adrenocortical hormones. Excessive potassium loss may occur in chronic pyelonephritis with mainly tubular disease, and in the Fanconi syndrome (p. 90) when proximal tubular damage prevents reabsorption. Decreased availability of H^+ for sodium exchange promotes potassium loss in renal tubular acidosis and treatment with carbonate dehydratase inhibitors. There may be excessive urinary loss of potassium due to prolonged diuresis from any cause, including the diuretic recovery phase of acute renal failure, and excessive potassium will be excreted in any prolonged acidosis. A urinary potassium of more than 20 mmol/24 h when there is hypokalaemia suggests that this is due to urinary loss.

In the rare disease familial periodic paralysis, attacks of paralysis are associated with temporary hypokalaemia due to passage of potassium from the ECF to the cells, although there is no change in the total body potassium.

Alkalosis accentuates hypokalaemia due to increased loss of potassium in exchange for sodium in the distal tubule. In addition, chronic potassium deficiency is a frequent cause of metabolic alkalosis (p. 41) as in this case H^+ is lost in exchange for sodium reabsorption.

Metabolic and clinical aspects

The ill-effects of potassium deficiency depend both on the plasma levels and on the total loss of potassium from the body:

symptoms appear after about 500 mmol have been lost. Potassium deficiency affects principally the neuromuscular system; the presenting symptoms are lethargy, muscular weakness, and ileus. If the diaphragm is affected there will be respiratory weakness and dyspnoea. The heart may be affected, and there are distinctive electrocardiographic changes with depression of the ST segment and a low or inverted T wave, and prominent U wave; arrhythmias, such as paroxysmal fibrillation, may develop, and hypotension is common. Prolonged hypokalaemia can lead to renal tubular damage, loss of concentrating power, and further loss of potassium (pathological vicious circle, p. 15). At first, losses of potassium from the ECF are replaced from the cells; thus mild potassium deficiency may exist with a normal plasma potassium level. The plasma levels fall when the rate of loss from the plasma exceeds the rate of potassium transfer from the cells to the plasma. If a patient has, as well as potassium deficiency, sodium depletion which has caused loss of extracellular water, this volume depletion may cause functional renal impairment and a secondary rise of the plasma potassium concentration. When the ECF volume is restored, the plasma potassium concentration falls to its appropriate low value. Hypokalaemia may develop during recovery from intracellular potassium deficiency.

It has been suggested that, in the absence of anaemia (which alters the electrolyte values), erythrocyte potassium changes are a guide to whole body changes.

A plasma potassium concentration below 1.5 mmol/l is often fatal. It is not fully known why potassium depletion causes death, but respiratory depression and cardiac arrhythmias play a part.

Therapy

Treatment is required if there is a history indicative of potassium loss from the body, electrocardiographic changes of potassium deficiency, or if the plasma potassium levels fall below 3.0 mmol/l. If the 24h urinary potassium is less than 10 mmol, then urinary loss is unlikely to be the cause of the hypokalaemia. Potassium should be given orally, if possible, as slow-release potassium chloride. The intravenous route is indicated if this is not possible or if the need is urgent, but must be used with great care if there is oliguria, renal damage, or heart failure. A daily input of 120 mmol of potassium chloride in divided doses is generally suitable for the treatment of the potassium deficiency of diabetic ketosis (after insulin therapy), or of moderate secretion loss.

A variety of intravenous potassium solutions have been recommended. Except in emergency, solutions stronger than 60 mmol/l of potassium should not be used. Potassium (as the chloride, generally 40 mmol/l) is nowadays usually given to adults by addition to isotonic glucose or saline.

Unless for emergency treatment of dangerous hypokalaemia, not more than 20 mmol of potassium may be infused in an hour, and not more than 120 mmol should be given in a day. Great care must be taken, by using serial plasma potassium estimations or electrocardiograms, to avoid hyperkalaemia.

Further reading

De Fronzo RA, Bia M, Smith D. Clinical disorders of hyperkalaemia. *Ann Rev Med* 1982; **33**: 521–54.

Jamieson MJ. Hyponatraemia. *Br Med J* 1985; **290**: 1723–8.

Morgan DB. Electrolyte disorders. *Clin Endocrinol Metab* 1984; **13:2**.

Penny MD, Walters G. Are osmolality measurements clinically useful? *Ann Clin Biochem* 1987; **24**: 566–71.

Walmsley RN, Guerin MD. *Disorders of Fluid and Electrolyte Balance*. Bristol: John Wright, 1984.

Walters G. Disorders of fluid and electrolyte balance. In: Williams DL, Marks V, eds. *The Scientific Foundations of Clinical Biochemistry. Vol 1: Biochemistry in Clinical Practice*. London: Heinemann, 1983: 1–23.

Acid–Base Regulation

Objectives

In this chapter the reader is able to

- revise the physiology of the control of acid–base balance and of the buffering and compensatory mechanisms.

At the conclusion of this chapter the reader is able to

- understand the relation between the measured variables and clinical acid–base status
- understand the causes and presentation of the primary syndromes of respiratory and metabolic acidosis and alkalosis, and of their combinations
- investigate a patient with suspected disorder of acid–base balance.

Basic concepts

pH is a measure of hydrogen-ion activity, a_{H^+}. The pH is defined as the logarithm of the reciprocal of the hydrogen-ion activity. Thus, for a pH of 7.0

$$pH\,(7.0) = \log\frac{1}{a_{H^+}} = -\log a_{H^+}$$
$$a_{H^+} = 10^{-7} \text{ or } 0.000\,000\,1 \text{ mol/l}$$

or 100 nmol/l. Thus, a change of 1 pH unit represents a tenfold change of hydrogen-ion activity (or approximately, concentration), and a change of 0.3 of a pH unit represents a doubling or halving of H^+ activity. The logarithmic scale is used for convenience to describe the enormously wide range of hydrogen-ion concentrations encountered in nature.

The pH of peripheral blood, measured as the pH of plasma in contact with erythrocytes, is normally within the range 7.35 to 7.45: in any individual healthy subject it varies only within narrow limits. Venous blood is slightly more acid than arterial blood and typical values are: arterial blood pH 7.40, venous blood pH 7.37. The average arterial plasma pH 7.40, corresponds to a hydrogen-ion activity of about 40 nmol/l.

An acid is defined as a potential donor of hydrogen ions (protons), when it dissociates. A strong acid such as HCl is highly dissociated producing more H^+ than a weak acid such as carbonic acid. This may be described thus

$$HCl \rightleftharpoons H^+ + Cl^-$$
$$H_2CO_3 \rightleftharpoons H^+ + HCO_3^-$$

A base is defined as a proton acceptor, e.g. (sodium) hydroxide, the bicarbonate ion, namely containing groups that bind hydrogen ions. The terms are restricted here to substances that act as proton donors or acceptors in the aqueous solutions of living systems. The term 'alkali' can be used for a potential donor of hydroxyl ions (OH^-) and is usually confined to compounds of alkali metals. An ion or molecule that is neither an acid nor a base is termed an aprote. In practice, in biological solutions, sodium (a cation) or chloride (an anion), may be considered as aprotes; however, in the presence of hydroxyl ions or hydrogen ions, they can form, respectively, the strongly ionized base, sodium hydroxide, and the strongly ionized acid, hydrochloric acid. The ammonium ion is an acid, and the bicarbonate ion is a base, because they can form respectively the readily metabolized ammonia with consequent release of hydrogen ions, and the weakly ionized acid carbonic acid by combining with hydrogen ions.

A buffer is the salt of a weak acid which, on exposure to the high H^+ concentration of a highly dissociated strong acid, forms a weak acid which is poorly dissociated thus 'mopping up' free H^+ and rendering it 'inactive'. The salt of the strong acid is also formed thus

$$H^+Cl^- + NaHCO_3 \rightleftharpoons H_2CO_3 + NaCl$$

| strong acid | buffer | weak acid | neutral salt |

The maintenance of the pH of the blood

On a mixed diet, metabolic processes cause an overall production of acid, 50–100 mmol H^+ per day. To meet this constant tendency to acidify the extracellar fluid (ECF), and to deal with changes in the acid–base balance of the body in disease, the blood contains buffering mechanisms. Final compensation for any change in the hydrogen-ion concentration of the ECF is performed by the lungs and the kidneys (see Fig. 4.2). The principal acid produced from the solution of the metabolic product carbon dioxide is carbonic acid, a valuable buffer which is excreted by the lungs as carbon dioxide, leaving H_2O behind in the ECF. Oxidation of sulphur-containing amino acids, and of organic phosphates (especially phospholipids), produces sulphate and phosphate together with equimolar amounts of H^+; sulphate and phosphate are excreted by the kidneys. Excess hydrogen ions are excreted by the kidneys as ammonium ions, and as organic acids – which are weak acids. A vegetarian diet, containing less protein, results in net production of base and a tendency to alkalosis, as oxidation of food then produces salts of organic acids such as sodium lactate, and not lactic acid, whose metabolism then utilizes hydrogen ions.

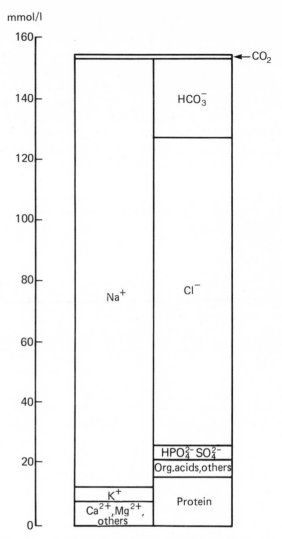

Fig. 4.1 Average electrolyte composition of normal plasma, expressed as millimoles of ion charges per litre of plasma

Aerobic metabolism of compounds containing carbon, hydrogen and oxygen produces H_2O and CO_2 with no net H^+ production. Anaerobic metabolism of carbohydrate and fats does however lead to net H^+ production. Many anabolic or synthetic processes utilize H^+.

Buffering

In plasma, the carbonic acid–bicarbonate mechanism is the most important buffering mechanism, although plasma proteins (and also phosphate) play a part. In interstitial fluid, protein buffering is absent. In the cells, buffering by proteins is more important. Haemoglobin, within the erythrocytes, plays a major part in the total buffering power of the blood. Buffer base is the sum of all these blood buffer ions.

The pH of erythrocytes is about 7.2 (60 nmol/l a_{H^+}) and of muscle cells is about 6.9 (120 nmol/l a_{H^+}). Figure 4.1 shows the normal distribution of anions and cations in plasma in terms of electrovalency. The buffering power of plasma may, for practical purposes, be considered solely dependent on the carbonic acid–bicarbonate mechanism

$$H_2CO_3 \rightleftharpoons H^+ + HCO_3^-$$

The Henderson–Hasselbalch equation

By the laws of mass action, at equilibrium

$$K \times [H_2CO_3] = [H^+] \times [HCO_3^-]$$

where K is the dissociation constant of carbonic acid.

Therefore, in the Henderson–Hasselbalch equations, as originally expressed without replacement of concentration by activity

$$[H^+] = K \times \left(\frac{[H_2CO_3]}{[HCO_3^-]} \right)$$

$$or \; pH = pK + \log \left(\frac{[HCO_3^-]}{[H_2CO_3]} \right) \text{ where } pK \text{ is } \log (1/K)$$

The plasma carbonic acid forms a small part (about 1/700) of, and is in equilibrium with, the dissolved carbon dioxide

$$[H_2CO_3] \rightleftharpoons K_2[CO_2] \times [H_2O]$$

The above equations can now be rewritten as

$$pH = pK' + \log \left(\frac{[HCO_3^-]}{[CO_2]} \right)$$

i.e. the hydrogen ion activity of the plasma depends on the ratio of dissolved carbon dioxide (the concentration of which is controlled by the lungs) to bicarbonate (the concentration of which is controlled by the kidneys). The combined constant of K and K_2 is K' and the pK' is about 6.1. The plasma

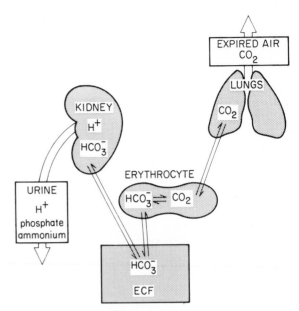

Fig. 4.2 Buffering mechanisms

carbon dioxide concentration is a function of its partial pressure (P_{CO_2}) and its solubility coefficient (α). If P_{CO_2} is expressed in kilopascals (kPa) this constant is 0.23, if in mmHg it is 0.03. Thus the equation can now be expressed as

$$pH = 6.1 + \log \left(\frac{[HCO_3^-]}{P_{CO_2} \times 0.23} \right)$$

The importance of this buffering system (Fig. 4.2) is that the amount of available HCO_3^- to buffer H^+ is controlled by HCO_3^- 'production' in the kidney (i.e. excretion of H^+ without HCO_3^- – see below) and the H_2CO_3 dissociates in aqueous solution to form H_2O and CO_2. The CO_2 can be lost in the lungs and thus H^+ has been effectively 'neutralized' by conversion to H_2O. However, buffering power (HCO_3^-) has been lost and this must be regenerated by the net excretion of H^+ and reabsorption of HCO_3^- in the kidney.

Methods of measurement

The pH of the plasma (in contact with erythrocytes) is measured with a special glass electrode, and requires anaerobic and iced handling of the blood (arterialized capillary, or arterial) between collection and analysis, to prevent metabolic products of red and white cells from altering the pH.

Plasma bicarbonate cannot be measured directly: plasma total carbon dioxide (T_{CO_2}) is mainly bicarbonate but includes dissolved carbon dioxide, carbonic acid and carbamino compounds for which an allowance (1–2 mmol/l) can be made in calculation. It is measured usually by acidifying plasma, and assaying the carbon dioxide liberated.

Plasma carbonic acid cannot be measured directly, and assessment is made by measuring P_{CO_2} on anaerobically collected blood by a special (Severinghaus) electrode (or indirectly by analysis of alveolar air).

Modern automatic blood-gas analysers simultaneously measure P_{O_2}, P_{CO_2}, and pH, and can calculate a value for bicarbonate from the second and third of these results, assuming a constant pK'. These have largely replaced the Astrup apparatus, which measured the pH of blood after equilibration with gas mixtures of different carbon dioxide tensions and, by application of the Siggaard–Andersen nomogram to the results, calculated the other values. Some workers find other measurements, that are less physiological, useful in patient care. Standard bicarbonate is the bicarbonate concentration of fully oxygenated blood equilibrated to a P_{CO_2} of 5.3 kPa (40 mmHg) at 37°C: this value is presumed to be independent of respiratory changes. Base excess is the amount of acid required to titrate (metabolically alkalaemic) whole blood to pH 7.40 at 37°C, P_{CO_2} 5.3 kPa: 'base deficit' is the reverse concept, for assessment of metabolically acidaemic changes. At a further remove from the *in vivo* situation are 'standard base excess' and 'corrected base excess'; these values 'corrected' for P_{CO_2} make the incomplete assumption that *in vitro* and *in vivo* correction are necessarily equal. Such 'artificial' derivatives are now rarely used.

Fundamental changes

Figure 4.3 shows the possible ways in which the plasma carbon dioxide and bicarbonate may be altered. Equally valid diagrams are available with pH and P_{CO_2} or with pH and [HCO_3^-], on the principal axes. The reference range for the partial pressure of blood carbon dioxide is 4.5–6.0 kPa (35–46 mmHg) corresponding to a concentration in solution of 1.1–1.4 mmol/l: the concentration of bicarbonate (derived from T_{CO_2}) is 24–30 mmol/l, and at pH 7.40 the bicarbonate/dissolved carbon dioxide ratio is approximately 20/1. A primary disturbance which causes (A) an increase in the plasma carbon dioxide or (B) a decrease in plasma bicarbonate leads to a fall in the pH of the plasma. Similarly, (C) a decrease in the plasma carbon dioxide or (D) an increase in the plasma bicarbonate leads to a rise in the plasma pH.

The terminology is confusing. Acidosis and alkalosis are used here for conditions which promote an increase of decrease in the hydrogen ion concentration, and hence respectively a fall or rise in the pH, of the blood. If terms are needed to describe the actual changes in blood pH, then 'acidaemia' and 'alkalaemia' have been suggested, though these terms have not become popular. Increase or decrease of plasma CO_2 is sometimes called hypercapnia or hypocapnia.

Compensatory mechanisms for acidosis and alkalosis

Immediate buffering of H^+ is carried out by the erythrocyte and ECF mechanisms, followed by equivalent changes in the general intracellular fluid (ICF). The cell membrane (and the cerebrospinal fluid) is readily permeable to H_2CO_3 and CO_2, but much less so to H^+ and HCO_3^-. Both H^+ and CO_2 are toxic metabolic products and need to be eliminated from the body by the kidneys and lungs respectively. Some CO_2 is converted to HCO_3^- which is then used to buffer H^+. The majority of the HCO_3^- is generated in the renal tubules but some is

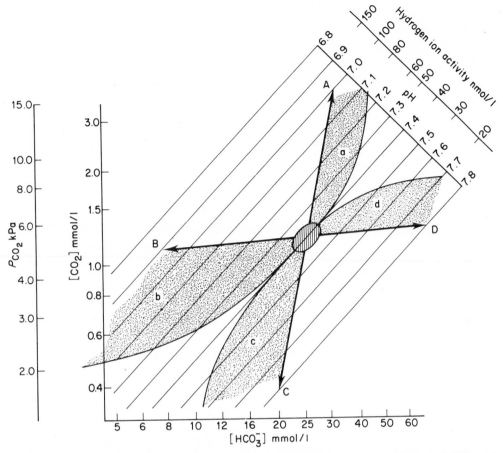

Fig. 4.3 Simplified chart showing the relation between bicarbonate concentration, P_{CO_2} and pH in normal and abnormal blood plasma. The central shaded area represents the reference range. Direction of changes in primary disturbances are shown by arrows. A, respiratory acidosis: B, metabolic acidosis: C, respiratory alkalosis: D, metabolic alkalosis. The shaded areas, a, b, c, d, adjacent to these arrows show the range of values found during compensation for the respective primary changes A, B, C, D.

produced by erythrocytes and the equimolar amounts of H^+ produced are buffered by haemoglobin. This process relies on the equation

$$CO_2 + H_2O \rightarrow H_2CO_3 \rightarrow H^+ + HCO_3^-$$

the first step of which is catalysed by the enzyme carbonate dehydratase which is present in both erythrocytes and renal tubular cells. Erythrocytes passing through capillaries in the tissues where CO_2 is being produced thus convert this to HCO_3^- while buffering the H^+. The reverse process releases CO_2 into the lungs. Excess H^+ are buffered by removal of the reactants with the generation of CO_2 and H_2O.

Respiratory mechanisms (Fig. 4.4)

This compensation for disturbances of the $[HCO_3^-] / [CO_2]$ ratio is rapid, and depends on the sensitivity of the respiratory centre to changes in both the P_{CO_2} and the pH of the blood, and to changes in cerebrospinal fluid pH. When there is an acidosis the respiratory centre responds by causing hyperventilation: this leads to an increased output of carbon dioxide by the lungs, and fall in plasma carbonic acid and correction of the pH at the cost of lost buffer (HCO_3^-). The erythrocyte carbonate dehydratase system is essential for the process to occur rapidly. When there is an alkalosis the

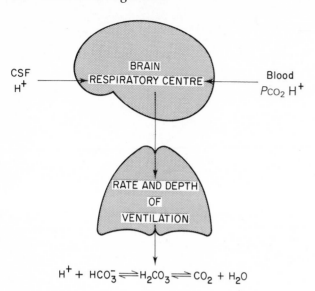

Fig. 4.4 Respiratory compensation for acid–base disturbances

reverse mechanism applies, and the depression of respiration leads to carbon dioxide retention and rise in plasma carbonic acid with production of HCO_3^- and H^+ by erythrocytes. However, the respiratory control of carbon dioxide excretion is ineffective when a respiratory disturbance has caused the acidosis or alkalosis and it is unable to compensate for an acidosis caused by gross additions of acid to the ECF. A normal adult excretes about 20 000 mmol of acid as carbon dioxide each 24 hours.

Renal mechanisms (Fig. 4.5)

This compensation for the normal tendency to acidification of the ECF, and for correction of pathological disturbances of the $[HCO_3^-]$ / $[CO_2]$ ratio, is less rapid, requires a normal glomerular filtration rate, and depends principally on the production of hydrogen ions by the distal tubular cells and requires carbonate dehydratase exactly as in the erythrocyte. The equimolar amounts of HCO_3^- produced enter the ECF thus replenishing the buffer system. Two basic mechanisms are thought to operate whereby the secreted H^+ is buffered by anions present in the glomerular filtrate.

(a) H^+, secreted by the tubular cell, combines with filtered HCO_3^- (which cannot itself be reabsorbed as tubular cells are impermeable to it) to form H_2CO_3 which dissociates to H_2O and CO_2 under the influence of carbonate dehydratase on the luminal surface of the proximal tubular cells. The CO_2 diffuses into the tubular cells where, again under the influence of carbonate dehydratase, it produces H_2CO_3 which then forms H^+ which is pumped back to the lumen and HCO_3^- which enters the ECF. The direction of these reactions is maintained by high levels of filtered HCO_3^- and H^+ in the tubular lumen and by low levels of H^+ in the tubular cell. The net effect of these processes is to reabsorb filtered HCO_3^-.

(b) In the distal tubule, where all HCO_3^- has been removed from the filtrate H^+ is produced as above (from cellular CO_2), and is buffered by other anions such as phosphate and sulphate ions forming the titratable acid (fixed acid) of the urine; they also combine with the ammonia secreted into the tubular lumen (produced mainly from glutamine by glutaminase activity) and are excreted as ammonium ions (NH_4^+) (acidosis stimulates glutaminase production by adaptive enzyme formation). Throughout the tubule Na^+ is reabsorbed in exchange for H^+ secreted. In addition, K^+ and H^+ appear to compete with each other for excretion.

A normal adult on a mixed diet excretes daily about 25 mmol of titratable acidity and 40 mmol of ammonium, and less than 5 mmol of bicarbonate. When there is acidosis, more hydrogen ions and ammonium are secreted, and the urine contains no bicarbonate and more ammonium and titratable acidity (ketoacids are also titratable acids); excess ammonium production requires a week to develop fully. When there is alkalosis, less hydrogen ions and often no ammonium are secreted; the urine contains increased bicarbonate, and titrat-

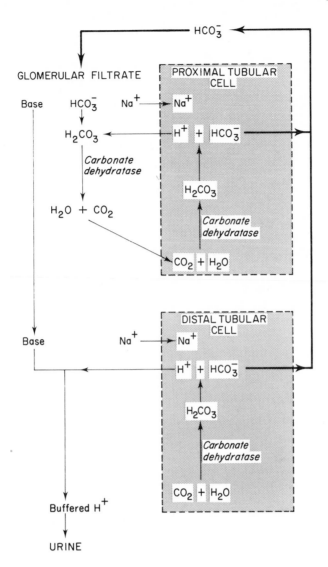

Fig. 4.5 Renal H^+ secretion and HCO_3^- reabsorption

able acidity may be replaced by titratable alkalinity ($H_2PO_4^-$ is replaced by HPO_4^{2-}). Even in mild acidosis bone salts release more Ca^{2+} and HPO_4^{2-}, the latter producing increased urinary buffering. It is important to note that urinary Cl^- cannot buffer H^+ as HCl is a strong acid almost wholly ionized.

During renal compensation for either acidosis or alkalosis there is usually a diuresis. When there is renal damage the resultant loss of compensatory power will diminish the body's capacity to maintain the constant pH of the ECF and acidosis may result.

When the disturbance in the acid–base balance of the body is greater than can be reversed by the compensatory mechanisms, a change in blood pH results. In Fig. 4.3 the shaded areas (a, b, c, d) show, in respect of each of the four primary disturbances (A, B, C, D), the range of values for the acid–base variables that are usually found during the normal processes of compensation.

Clinical acidosis and alkalosis

Mild acidosis causes few specific symptoms but when it is severe there will be increased ventilation and there may be vomiting and drowsiness. The symptoms of alkalosis are more specific. There may be confusion, nausea and anorexia, there is usually neuromuscular irritability with tetany due to decreased ionized calcium (p. 180); and, if it is chronic, there is often potassium depletion and there may be renal damage due to this (p. 32). In severe alkalosis respiration is depressed, and both oxygen uptake and the release of oxygen from haemoglobin to the tissues are diminished.

Acidosis and alkalosis may be respiratory or non-respiratory (metabolic) in origin (Fig. 4.3). Respiratory disturbances are associated primarily with an increase or decrease of the plasma carbonic acid concentration: in them excretion of carbon dioxide is no longer equal to production of carbon dioxide, and there is a change in pH due primarily to alteration in the ratio

$$\frac{[HCO_3^-]}{P_{CO_2} \times 0.23}$$

Metabolic disturbances are associated primarily with an increase or decrease in production or excretion of H^+: in them there is a secondary alteration of the ECF bicarbonate.

As with sodium and water, mixed disturbances are common; but the single disorders must be appreciated first.

Primary alteration in carbonic acid

Respiratory alkalosis

This results from hyperventilation, which leads to reduction of plasma carbonic acid. As P_{CO_2} falls, the equilibrium

$$H_2O + CO_2 \rightleftharpoons H_2CO_3 \rightleftharpoons H^+ + HCO_3^-$$

shifts to the left, so $[H^+]$ and $[HCO_3^-]$ also fall. The ratio

$$\frac{[HCO_3^-]}{P_{CO_2} \times 0.23}$$

however rises and the plasma pH may reach 7.8. The fall in P_{CO_2} decreases HCO_3^- generation in the erythrocytes and renal tubular cells and there is a compensatory fall in $[HCO_3^-]$. The features of respiratory alkalosis are thus a raised pH together with a low P_{CO_2} and low plasma bicarbonate. The urine is alkaline as less H^+ is secreted into the tubular lumen and filtered HCO_3^- is not reabsorbed.

Hyperventilation may occur in fever, at high altitudes (due to compensation for oxygen deficiency), or due to encephalitis, increased intracranial pressure, hepatic coma, anaesthesia and/or automatic ventilation, anxiety, or acute salicylate overdosage (which directly stimulates the respiratory centre (p. 242).

Respiratory acidosis

This results from depression of ventilation, which causes retention of carbonic acid. As P_{CO_2} rises, the equilibrium

$$H_2O + CO_2 \rightleftharpoons H_2CO_3 \rightleftharpoons H^+ + HCO_3^-$$

shifts to the right, so $[H^+]$ and $[HCO_3^-]$ also rise. The ratio

$$\frac{[HCO_3^-]}{P_{CO_2} \times 0.23}$$

falls and the plasma pH may reach 7.0. Compensation results in HCO_3^- generation in the erythrocyte and renal tubular cell with maximal HCO_3^- reabsorption and an acid urine. Typical findings are of low pH, high P_{CO_2} and raised bicarbonate.

Artificial respiration, by anaesthetist or machine, may produce an acidosis or an alkalosis. Diminished respiratory excretion of carbon dioxide results from obstruction, or may occur in chronic lung disease (either primary such as severe emphysema or secondary to heart failure), may be due to drugs which depress respiration, such as morphine and certain anaesthetics, and can be found in bulbar poliomyelitis and in hypothermia. It is important to appreciate that CO_2 is much more soluble than O_2 in body fluids and diffuses about 20 times as fast as O_2. For these reasons pulmonary oedema results in a low P_{O_2} but P_{CO_2} is usually normal as the hyperventilation removes the more soluble CO_2.

In chronic respiratory failure (due to chronic bronchitis and emphysema) where P_{O_2} is low and P_{CO_2} is raised, the respiratory centre becomes tolerant to the high P_{CO_2} and the predominant drive to respiration becomes the decreased P_{O_2} (in contrast to the normal situation). It is thus extremely dangerous to give such patients high concentrations of oxygen to breathe, despite severe hypoxaemia, as respiratory drive will be decreased and P_{CO_2} will rise to toxic levels. Carbon dioxide toxicity results in cerebral oedema, coma and muscular twitching. It is occasionally seen in industrial accidents when workers are exposed to accumulation of CO_2, which, being heavier than air, collects in low-lying enclosed areas.

In both respiratory acidosis and alkalosis the major changes in plasma HCO_3^- result from compensation. Figure 4.3 shows that the changes in P_{CO_2} have only a small effect on the HCO_3^- level.

Primary alteration in bicarbonate

Metabolic alkalosis

This is associated with an increase in the plasma bicarbonate concentration which is accompanied by either a decrease of the other anions of the plasma (principally chloride) or an increase of cationic sodium. The plasma pH may reach 7.8.

Gain of external base

Patients who treat their indigestion by taking unlimited quantities of sodium bicarbonate (or any other antacids that are alkaline) may become severely alkalotic, with a plasma bicarbonate concentration greater than 50 mmol/l. Alkalosis may be induced for therapeutic purposes by the use of sodium citrate or sodium lactate, as the catabolism of the anion consumes hydrogen ions.

Loss of hydrogen ions

This occurs with a rise in plasma bicarbonate following hydrochloric acid loss due to vomiting or gastric aspiration. The parietal cells of the stomach generate H^+ from the reaction

$$CO_2 + H_2O \rightarrow H_2CO_3 \rightarrow H^+ + HCO_3^-$$

The HCO_3^- is reabsorbed into the plasma together with Na^+ producing the 'post prandial alkaline tide' and the H^+ together with Cl^- is secreted into the lumen. The alkalosis is thus accompanied by hypochloraemia. It is commonly seen as a result of the vomiting of pyloric stenosis (including congenital pyloric stenosis of children). Patients with a juxtapyloric ulcer, who are vomiting and are also taking alkali therapeutically, develop a very severe alkalosis. However, if vomiting occurs in a patient who has achlorhydria then alkalosis does not result. If vomiting is prolonged the ketosis of starvation will complicate the clinical and biochemical picture. Alkalosis does not significantly depress the respiratory centre so compensation is by urinary bicarbonate loss. The increased ECF HCO_3^- inhibits the formation of H^+ and HCO_3^- by carbonate dehydratase in the renal tubular cells and decreased H^+ secretion results in loss of filtered HCO_3^- and decreased HCO_3^- generation. This process is also impaired if vomiting causes dehydration and a reduced GFR. In addition, hypochloraemia results in decreased Cl^- which must be reabsorbed with Na^+ to maintain electrochemical neutrality in the proximal tubules. Increased Na^+ is thus available for exchange with H^+ and K^+ giving rise to an inappropriate acid urine and aggravating the hypokalaemia which tends to develop when there is decreased H^+ secretion in the tubules. Though serious metabolic alkalosis due to gastric acid loss is rare, it demonstrates several important principles in acid-base metabolism.

Potassium deficiency (p. 31) is an important cause of alkalosis. This ECF alkalosis is partly due to hydrogen ions entering the cells to replace lost potassium ions (which compete in exchange for sodium ions), or to alterations of renal tubular function – tubular intracellular potassium deficiency results in increased loss of H^+ in exchange for Na^+. The reaction

$$H_2CO_3 \rightarrow H^+ + HCO_3^-$$

thus moves to the right (as H^+ is removed) and enhances bicarbonate generation and reabsorption, leading to an inappropriately acid urine with an alkalosis. It is commonly seen in patients taking diuretics such as frusemide and the thiazides.

Combined therapy (diuretics, low dietary NaCl, steroids) of chronic respiratory acidosis often leads to metabolic alkalosis.

Metabolic acidosis

This is due to either a retention of H^+ or loss of HCO_3^-. In the former HCO_3^- will be decreased due to consumption in buffering H^+ and loss in respiration as CO_2, or failure of its generation in 'kidney damage'. The ratio

$$\frac{[HCO_3^-]}{P_{CO_2} \times 0.23}$$

is thus decreased and the plasma pH may reach 6.9.

Gain of external acid
Acidosis can be induced by administration of substances whose metabolism yields hydrogen ions, such as ammonium chloride, hydrochlorides of organic bases, methanol producing formic acid, ethylene glycol producing oxalic acid, and para-ldehyde producing acetic acid. As the bicarbonate falls there will be a compensatory fall in cation, plasma Na^+, or retention of other anions such as chloride, phosphate, lactate, 3-hydroxybutyrate or acetoacetate. Increased ECF H^+ enters cells displacing K^+ which is lost in the urine if the GFR is normal. Respiratory compensation results from H^+ stimulating ventilation. P_{CO_2} decreases and both HCO_3^- and H^+ are effectively removed as H_2O and

CO_2. The ratio

$$\frac{[HCO_3^-]}{P_{CO_2} \times 0.23}$$

increases and the pH returns towards normal. Buffer HCO_3^- is however lost. H^+ is buffered in the erythrocyte by haemoglobin via the carbonate dehydratase mechanism again converting H^+ and HCO_3^- to H_2O and CO_2. Final compensation is effected by the renal tubule (in non-renal causes of acidosis) by H^+ and HCO_3^- generation from water with HCO_3^- being returned to the ECF. H^+ is thus buffered by HCO_3^- to form H_2O which acts as the 'carrier' to the kidney where it is finally excreted.

Increased internal production of acid
Excess production of keto acids (due to diabetes or starvation) or lactate (in anaerobic metabolism) results in the simultaneous production of H^+. HCO_3^- is consumed in buffering and respiratory compensation and may fall as low as 5 mmol/l. The chloride remains normal as electrochemical neutrality is maintained by 3-hydroxybutyrate, acetoacetate and lactate anions. Overdosage of salicylate results in uncoupling of oxidative phosphorylation and lactic acidosis (p. 61).

The organicacidurias are important in the neonate.

Failure to excrete acid
Chronic renal failure results in loss of nephrons and failure to adequately excrete H^+. In addition there is retention of anions such as phosphate and sulphate which maintain electrochemical neutrality.

Renal tubular failure (p. 121), especially proximal tubular damage (Fanconi syndrome), results in failure of HCO_3^- reabsorption and generation with loss of base and retention of H^+. Renal tubular acidosis comprises several, usually genetic, conditions in which failure to excrete H^+ and generate or reabsorb HCO_3^- occurs. Therapy with acetazolamide (a carbonate dehydratase inhibitor) has a similar effect while also decreasing erythrocyte buffering and CO_2 carriage. In all cases of tubular failure electrochemical neutrality is maintained by Cl^- retention which increases in parallel to the falling HCO_3^-.

Loss of bicarbonate (with sodium)

Pancreatic juice is alkaline (the pH of pancreatic juice is about 8 and its bicarbonate concentration may reach 100 mmol/l); bile and high small-intestinal secretions are also mildly alkaline. Such alkaline fluids can be lost through a fistula or ileostomy, or in severe diarrhoea (particularly from cholera) or steatorrhoea, or when there has been excess purgation: the plasma bicarbonate falls and acidosis is superimposed on the dominant biochemical picture of water and sodium depletion (p. 22). Electrochemical neutrality is maintained by parallel loss of Na^+ and K^+. The dehydration resulting from this causes a reduction in GFR thus impairing renal compensation.

Transplantation of the ureter (p. 121) into the intestine following total cystectomy for carcinoma of the bladder results in reabsorption of the urinary Cl^- by the mucosal cells in exchange for HCO_3^- from the ECF thus resulting in a net loss of HCO_3^- and acidosis. In this case chloride replaces HCO_3^- in the plasma in equimolar amounts. Large regular doses of oral bicarbonate are necessary to maintain a normal acid-base status in such patients.

Anion gap (Fig. 4.6)

In health

$$[Na^+] = [Cl^-] + [HCO_3^-] + [6 - 16]$$

the last value (in mmol/l) being called the anion gap. An increased anion gap usually indicates an acidosis where the H^+ is balanced electrochemically by an unmeasured anion such as phosphate, sulphate, lactate, or acetoacetate. In acidosis associated with increased Cl^- the anion gap is normal.

The diagnosis of disorders of acid–base balance

Acidosis or alkalosis are often associated with disorders of sodium or water balance. The body is less tolerant of osmotic pressure changes due to total electrolyte loss or gain, than it is of acidosis or alkalosis due to differential electrolyte loss or gain. In general, the osmotic pressure of the ECF is maintained as far as possible, even at the expense of a normal pH.

Acidosis and alkalosis, which cause their symptoms because of changes in the hydrogen ion activity of the blood, should be evaluated by measuring the pH, P_{CO_2}, and bicarbonate values in the blood; or less rigidly by measuring two and deriving the third. The pK' of carbonic acid in plasma,

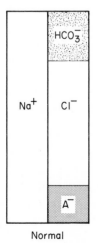

Normal

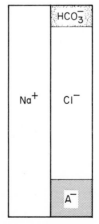

Hyperchloraemic acidosis:
Normal anion gap

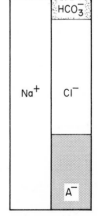

Metabolic acidosis:
Increased anion gap

Fig. 4.6   The anion gap. A^-: other anions, normally 6–16 mmol/l

and its solubility coefficient, are not constant in acute conditions of changing blood pH, and therefore all three components should be measured separately for the greatest accuracy. It is not possible in practice to measure changes in intracellular pH.

There is a need to distinguish between the primary cause of an acid–base disturbance, changes due to compensation, and changes due to complications. This is especially important in regard to treatment. Figure 4.3, with knowledge of the history, may be used as a guide. For example, blood values of pH 7.2, P_{CO_2} 4.0 kPa (30 mmHg), [HCO_3^-] 12 mmol/l fall within area b, and are therefore likely to represent partially compensated metabolic acidosis. The compensation is respiratory and reflected by the low P_{CO_2} due to hyperventilation. Blood values of pH 7.0, P_{CO_2} 8.0 kPa (60 mmHg), [HCO_3^-] 15 mmol/l fall between arrows A and B, and are therefore likely to represent combined respiratory and metabolic acidosis as in cardiac arrest (respiratory depression + lactic acidosis). The combination of respiratory alkalosis and metabolic acidosis occurs for example in salicylate poisoning.

The plasma bicarbonate concentration can be used as a measure of the degree of acidosis and alkalosis in all cases when the disturbance is solely metabolic in origin; this is the most commonly performed estimation as it has been automated. Some investigators prefer to use standard bicarbonate or the other P_{CO_2}-independent quantities. In respiratory acidosis or alkalosis the P_{CO_2} is the measure of the primary cause of the change in the plasma. In addition P_{O_2} measurement may be useful. Estimation of the plasma pH, sodium, potassium, and chloride levels is also valuable.

Some biochemical aspects of treatment

In cases of mild metabolic acidosis, or alkalosis, with water and sodium depletion, and in the presence of normal renal function, correction of the water and sodium depletion will eventually correct the acidosis or alkalosis as the kidney excretes the unwanted ions. Saline infusion corrects mild alkalosis efficiently by providing Na^+ for exchange with H^+ in the renal tubule, often the limiting factor if dehydration and a decreased GFR are present. Should intravenous therapy be required for the correction of severe acidosis that does not respond to saline replacement, then a suitable solution, which is approximately isotonic with plasma, is sodium bicarbonate (150 mmol/l; 1.26 per cent w/v), which has now generally replaced sodium lactate (165 mmol/l), for the treatment of acidosis. Hypertonic sodium bicarbonate is used for rapid correction, for example when metabolic acidosis is associated with cardiac arrest, and solutions up to 1000 mmol/l (8.4 per cent) are available. If potassium is required when there is acidosis it is usually given as the citrate. Ammonium chloride (165 mmol/l) for the treatment of alkalosis is rarely required and must be used with great care, as it is dangerous in liver disease; also it may accentuate sodium or potassium depletion, and in many circumstances potassium chloride, and occasionally dilute hydrochloric acid (150 mmol/l into a deep vein), is necessary. Arginine or lysine, being basic amino acids, may be used as their hydrochlorides.

Primary changes in P_{CO_2}, of respiratory origin, require therapy to that system.

The doses of such replacement fluids, and the duration of treatment and their combination with other therapy, must be judged by the biochemical and clinical degree of alteration of the normal electrolyte balance. It is essential to rely also on the history, on serial estimations of the changes, on a well-kept fluid balance chart, and on experience; and not just to use formulae (e.g. involving base deficit) for correction of disorders of acid–base balance and of sodium and water balance.

Unchecked over-correction of acidosis or alkalosis may lead to the opposite situation.

Oxygen

Oxygen tension

Measurement of arterial P_{O_2} is used in conjunction with that of P_{CO_2} in the assessment of respiratory disorders, as the analysis can be done on the same special blood sample with combined electrodes: the reference range of arterial blood is 11–15 kPa (85–105 mmHg) and this corresponds to 95 per cent saturation of haemoglobin with oxygen. A low P_{O_2} is a measure of anoxia, and is found frequently with a high P_{CO_2} whenever there is alveolar hypoventilation due to obstruction or depression of respiration. Less frequently a low P_{O_2} is seen with a low P_{CO_2} when ventilation and perfusion do not change in parallel, particularly when there is pulmonary oedema.

Oxygen availability

Oxygen release to the tissues, at a given P_{O_2}, is diminished by hypothermia, by alkalosis, and by a fall in erythrocyte 2,3-diphosphoglycerate (2,3DPG), as these affect the dissociation curve of haemoglobin. Acidosis causes depletion of 2,3DPG, accentuated in diabetic ketoacidosis by phosphate deficiency. Restoration of 2,3DPG is slow when correction of acidosis is rapid, so oxygen availability is then diminished.

Further reading

Bihari DJ. Metabolic acidosis. *Br J Hosp Med* 1986; **35**: 89–95.

Cohen JJ, Kassirer JP. *Acid–Base*. Boston: Little Brown, 1982.

Flenley DC. Arterial blood gas tensions and pH. *Br J Clin Pharmacol* 1980; **9**: 129–35.

Carbohydrate Metabolism

Objectives

In this chapter the reader is able to

- revise the biochemistry and physiology of carbohydrate, metabolism, especially the hormonal control of blood glucose
- study the biochemical bases of diabetes mellitus and its complications
- study the causes of and investigation of a patient with hypoglycaemia
- study the causes of and investigation of a patient with melituria/glycosuria
- study the main inborn errors of carbohydrate metabolism
- study the causes of lactic acidosis
- study the causes of ketonuria.

At the conclusion of this chapter the reader is able to

- perform and interpret the glucose tolerance test and related investigations
- use the laboratory in the investigation of diabetes mellitus and other causes of hyperglycaemia
- use the laboratory in the management of diabetes mellitus and its complications.

Dietary carbohydrate

A normal adult, living in a temperate climate, has a carbohydrate intake that averages about 400 g/day, and this supplies about half of the energy requirements – the energy value of carbohydrate is about 17 kilojoules (kJ) (4 kilocalories (kcal)) per gram. Dietary carbohydrate deficiency leads to a deficient energy intake and to starvation (p. 110); if the protein and fat intake remain normal when the carbohydrate intake is reduced, ketosis develops.

Digestion and absorption of carbohydrate

Most of the carbohydrate of food is the polysaccharide, starch; cellulose cannot be digested by man (both are polymers of glucose). Salivary amylase begins the digestion of carbohydrate by converting a little of the starch to α-limit dextrins, maltotriose, and to the disaccharide maltoses. No further chemical digestion of carbohydrate takes place in the stomach. Pancreatic amylase converts unchanged starch and dextrins to maltoses. In the brush border of the small intestine conversion of dextrins to maltose is completed, and the maltase is converted by the disaccharidase maltose into glucose which is absorbed into the portal circulation and passes to the liver. Similarly, lactase converts lactose to glucose and galactose, and sucrase converts sucrose to glucose and fructose. Glucose is the principal monosaccharide end-product of carbohydrate digestion; fructose and galactose are also produced when the subject is taking a normal diet. The amount of fructose is increased by a diet which contains excess fruit, or cane sugar (sucrose). The amount of galactose is increased when a high proportion of the carbohydrate intake is lactose, and this happens in infants and in patients on a milk diet.

Any of the disaccharidases may be deficient and this results in an osmotic diarrhoea due to intestinal accumulation of the appropriate disaccharide when it is present in food (p. 62).

Normally, more than 99 per cent of the carbohydrate in the diet is digested and absorbed and there is a negligible quantity of carbohydrate in the faeces. When there is an absorption defect of the intestinal mucosa (as in coeliac disease), or when there is intestinal hurry (as in severe diarrhoea), or in the disaccharidase deficiencies, absorption of glucose is reduced, and glucose may be detected in the faeces by the simple tests usually used for urinary glucose. Resection of the small intestine must be considerable to reduce the absorption of glucose significantly.

Absorption of glucose is more rapid in patients with hyperthyroidism, and is delayed in hypothyroidism.

Parenteral carbohydrate

The usual intravenous glucose solution is approximately isotonic with plasma (280 mmol/l:5 per cent w/v), but this provides only 800 kJ (200 kcal) per litre. For significant energy input higher concentrations must be used, e.g. 2800 mmol/l:50 per cent w/v (8000 kJ/l) but this is sclerosing and requires the use of central veins. The advantages of substances whose initial catabolism is not insulin-dependent, such as fructose, sorbitol or ethanol (29 kJ/g) are controversial – they may lead to lactic acidosis.

Normal glucose metabolism

Glucose cannot be further metabolized until it has been converted to glucose-6-phosphate by a reaction with ATP. This reaction is catalysed by the non-specific enzyme hexokinase, and also by the specific glucokinase in the liver. The reaction in the reverse direction, a simple hydrolysis of glucose-6-phosphate to glucose, is catalysed by glucose-6-phosphatase in the liver.

Once glucose has become phosphorylated it can be converted to glycogen for storage and cannot diffuse out of the cell. The liver also converts glucose to triglyceride which enters the systemic circulation whence it is stored in adipose tissue. The glucose which has not been so utilized passes from the liver via the systemic circulation to the tissues where it can be oxidized or stored as muscle glycogen. Glucokinase in the liver has a lower affinity for glucose than hexokinase in other tissues, the brain glucokinase has the highest affinity for glucose. This gives the energy-requiring tissues preference for glucose uptake. The glycogen in the liver acts as a reserve of carbohydrate, and releases glucose into the circulation whenever peripheral glucose utilization has lowered the concentration of glucose in the blood. In addition, the liver may produce glucose from glycerol, lactate, or the carbon chains resulting from deamination of amino acids. In the fasting state (see Fig. 5.3), when glucose is in short supply, the liver can convert fatty acids released from adipose tissue into ketones which can be used as an energy supply by all tissues. Muscle glycogen is converted to lactate by anaerobic glycolysis, thus releasing energy; it cannot produce glucose as muscle has no glucose-6-phosphatase.

For oxidation of glucose, or for conversion of carbohydrate to fat or protein, the glucose-6-phosphate can be converted in stages, via triose phosphates and phosphoenolpyruvate, to pyruvate – the Embden–Meyerhof glycolytic pathway of oxidative phosphorylation. There is an alternative metabolic pathway for the oxidation of glucose, the hexose monophosphate shunt, which leads to the formation of $NADPH_2$ and not of $NADH_2$. Fructose and galactose, after phosphorylation (mainly by fructokinase and galactokinase), enter the common metabolic pathways of carbohydrate. Pyruvate can enter the common metabolic pool or be converted to other

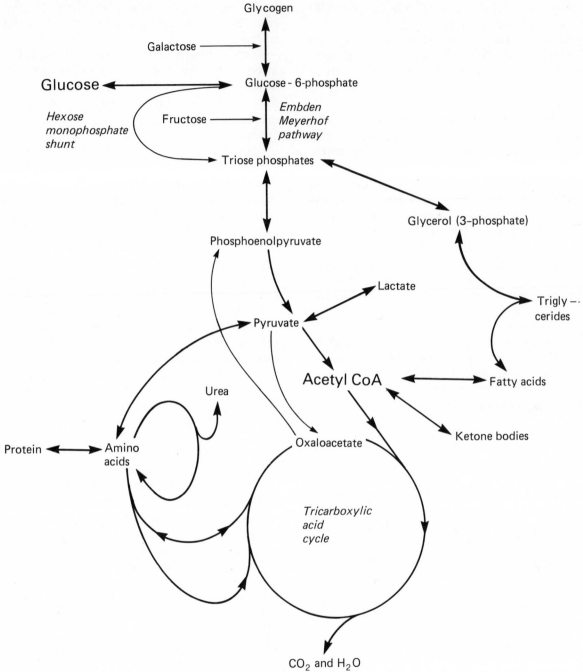

Fig. 5.1   Simplified scheme of the principal pathways of the general metabolism of carbohydrate, protein and fat (triglycerides). A double-headed arrow indicates that the metabolic process may go in both directions, but not necessarily by the same reaction or series of reactions

compounds. The common metabolic pool represents the series of reactions, based on acetyl coenzyme A and the tricarboxylic acid cycle (Krebs cycle), within which

carbon residues from protein, carbohydrate, or fat may be oxidized with release of energy, or converted one into another.

The basic biochemistry of the metabolism

of glucose, and its interrelationship with the metabolism of protein and lipids, is shown in Fig. 5.1.

The hormonal control of glucose metabolism

Insulin, a polypeptide secreted by the β-cells of the pancreatic islets of Langerhans, is synthesized as proinsulin, containing two chains connected by C-peptide. It is the principal hormone that controls the metabolism of carbohydrate and its interaction with the metabolism of proteins and lipids. Its structure has been completely elucidated: it binds to specific receptors on the membrane of cells such as adipose tissue and muscle although its modes of action are not fully understood. The secretion of insulin is primarily regulated by the arterial plasma glucose level with secondary influence by stimuli from the vagus nerve. Many other factors, including gastrointestinal hormones, and certain sugars, fatty acids and, amino acids, directly or indirectly may stimulate insulin secretion.

Insulin acts at the cell membrane to increase the rate of uptake of glucose into cells – particularly of muscle and adipose tissue, but not of brain, liver, or erythrocytes. Many of the other actions of insulin, such as promoting the phosphorylation of glucose, are secondary to this promotion of the passage of glucose into cells. The result is acceleration of the entry of glucose into further metabolic processes, either for storage as glycogen in liver and muscle, or for utilization by conversion or oxidation. Insulin is a storage hormone and the effect is to lower blood glucose. In the absence of insulin, glucose utilization is depressed and gluconeogenesis is enhanced. (The transport of fructose into cells is independent of insulin control.) Also, it is possible that insulin has a direct stimulant action on the oxidative phosphorylation of carbohydrate at a site further on in the metabolic path. Insulin promotes the conversion of acetyl CoA (derived from pyruvate) to fatty acids, thus promoting the synthesis of neutral fat:

it inhibits lipolysis and the release of free fatty acids while at the same time stimulating endothelial cell lipoprotein lipase (p. 68) in adipose tissue. This facilitates the breakdown and uptake of chylomicrons and VLDL for storage in fat. It inhibits gluconeogenesis from protein, and favours the synthesis of protein from amino acids. Insulin also promotes transfer of potassium, phosphate, and amino acids into cells. In the liver, the entry of glucose into the cells is only slightly dependent on insulin, and the major action is that glucose output is decreased by insulin.

The hypoglycaemic action of insulin is balanced by the action of hormones from the anterior pituitary and the adrenal cortex. Growth hormone, with the possible involvement of somatomedin, is responsible for the actions of what was formerly thought to be an independent diabetogenic hormone. It increases protein synthesis, induces lipolysis of adipose tissue, and opposes the glucose utilization actions of insulin – although the secretion of insulin is stimulated. Excess growth hormone causes hyperglycaemia, and the long-term effect of damage to the islet-cells may be due to the hyperglycaemia. Somatostatin (p. 194) inhibits the release of insulin. The glucocorticoids, and indirectly adrenocorticotrophic hormone, stimulate protein catabolism; this releases carbon residues and gluconeogenesis is increased. Glucose utilization is decreased; the increase of insulin secretion may be secondary to the increased blood glucose.

The pancreatic islets also secrete a hyperglycaemic glycogenolytic polypeptide hormone called glucagon from the α-cells. As well as having a glycogenolytic action and stimulating the release of insulin and of catecholamines, glucagon promotes protein catabolism, and is lipolytic and ketogenic.

Thyroxine stimulates the rate of intestinal absorption of carbohydrates, and increases the tissue needs for insulin, perhaps by its general promotion of tissue oxidation.

The adrenal medulla can be stimulated to release adrenaline by vagal impulses when the hypothalamus is stimulated by hypoglycaemia. Adrenaline (and to a lesser extent noradrenaline) raises the blood glucose level in two ways. It has a short-term effect of stimulating hepatic glycogenolysis, and a longer-term effect of promoting the secretion of adrenocortico-trophic hormone; it also inhibits insulin secretion.

Energy homeostasis – the relationship between fat and carbohydrate

The fed state (Fig. 5.2)

Under normal circumstances brain and muscle are able to utilize glucose preferentially as a result of the hexokinases in these tissues having a higher affinity for glucose.

Post-prandially, the rise in blood glucose level stimulates insulin secretion which promotes uptake of glucose into fat and

muscle, the remainder entering the liver by a non-insulin-dependent mechanism. Muscle stores a relatively small amount of glucose as glycogen. In the liver some glucose enters glycogen stores but the majority is converted to triglyceride for export as VLDL (very low density lipoprotein) particles. In fat, VLDL is hydrolysed by the insulin-dependent enzyme lipoprotein lipase, fatty acids entering the cells to be esterified with glycerol derived from glucose also entering the cell under the influence of insulin. Ultimately glucose is thus stored as fat. It is important to note that adipose tissue is unable to store glucose directly as triglyceride without the participation of the liver/VLDL mechanism.

The fasting state (Fig. 5.3)

In the fasting state the blood glucose level is

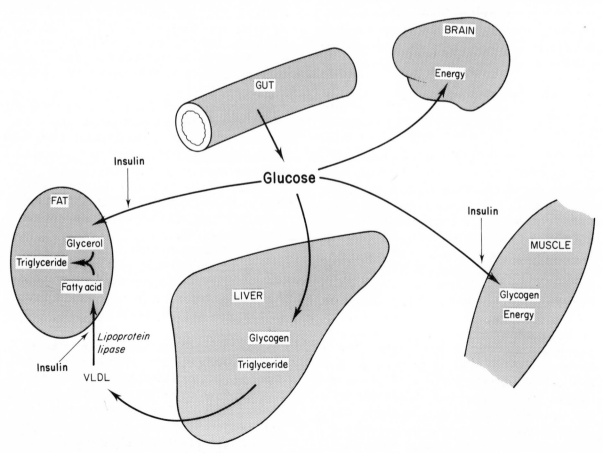

Fig. 5.2   Glucose metabolism in the fed state

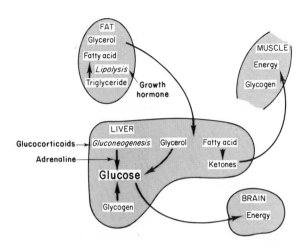

Fig. 5.3 Glucose metabolism in the fasting state

maintained from liver glycogen breakdown, and gluconeogenesis from amino acids and glycerol derived from adipose tissue lipolysis. Energy is also provided by the liver in the form of ketones derived from adipose tissue fatty acids. These may be used by all tissues. Lipolysis in adipose tissue is activated by growth hormone.

Blood sugar/blood glucose

The term 'blood sugar' is used loosely to include glucose and other sugars, and sometimes other reducing substances which may be present in the blood. Originally most methods for sugar analysis depended on glucose being a reducing substance. Blood for sugar determination is normally taken into fluoride, which inhibits glycolysis by erythrocytes.

Methods involving the specific enzyme glucose oxidase (or alternatively using hexokinase) measure only glucose: these are now universally employed, and all figures in this book are values for blood glucose. By using a commercial glucose oxidase stick preparation (p. 260) it is possible to perform a screening blood glucose estimation and to detect hypoglycaemia or hyperglycaemia. Precision is improved by using a reflectance meter to read the colour of the stick and some diabetic patients may thus monitor their own blood glucose levels.

The reference range for fasting venous whole blood glucose at rest is 3.0–5.5 mmol/l in adults, and is lower in infants (p. 57). In capillary blood (which represents arterial blood), the fasting value is about 0.2 mmol/l higher. Because of the widespread use of capillary samples, whole blood glucose is more commonly measured than is plasma glucose, the values for which are 10–15 per cent higher than whole blood.

Insulin can be measured in plasma or serum by radioimmunoassay and the assay is mainly used in the investigation of spontaneous hypoglycaemia. The reference range for fasting plasma insulin is 10–30 mu/l and in the presence of glucose levels below 2.2 mmol/l it should be less than 10 mu/l. There is also a variety of difficult biological assays which effectively measure 'insulin-like activity', and whose results may differ from those found by radioimmunoassay.

The excretion of glucose

Glucose is filtered by the glomeruli and the average normal tubule reabsorbs more than 99 per cent of the glucose that reaches it in the glomerular filtrate. The proximal renal tubules are responsible for returning glucose to the circulation. If the renal plasma flow is normal, and the kidney is healthy, then at a capillary blood glucose concentration of more than about 10 mmol/l sufficient glucose is filtered into the renal tubules to saturate a significant proportion of their variable reabsorptive capacity, and detectable glycosuria occurs. This concentration of 10 mmol/l is known as the renal threshold for glucose. A reduced renal plasma flow (as occurs in heart failure or volume depletion) or severe glomerular damage will reduce the rate of filtration of glucose through the glomeruli. In such cases a high blood glucose concentration will not result in as much glucose reaching the tubules as if the renal plasma flow were normal. If the reabsorptive power of the tubules is unaltered then there is a raised renal threshold for glucose and mild hyperglycaemia will not cause glycosuria. About 2 per cent of diabetic patients, mainly older people, have a high renal threshold for glucose.

Renal glycosuria

Diminution of tubular reabsorptive capacity for glucose, which may be due to specific or generalized abnormalities of tubular function or to gross tubular disease, can lead to glycosuria when the blood glucose level is normal. Renal glycosuria usually presents in the absence of other evidence of renal damage. The low threshold of pregnancy is attributed to an increase in glomerular filtration with an increased total amount of glucose being presented to the tubule.

The effect of carbohydrate on the blood glucose

When a fasting subject ingests glucose, or a meal containing carbohydrate, the blood glucose level rises as glucose is absorbed from the intestine. In a normal person, after a meal, the venous blood glucose level does not exceed 8.5 mmol/l and the capillary level (representing arterial blood glucose) should not rise above 10 mmol/l. The secretion of insulin greatly increases, and that of glucagon (after an initial rise), and of growth hormone, decreases. The mechanisms of tissue oxidation, storage of glucose as glycogen, and diminished gluconeogenesis (all 'antihyperglycaemic') are active and counteract the increased blood glucose which results from the absorption of glucose. At about an hour after the ingestion of carbohydrate the rate of removal of glucose from the blood becomes greater than the rate of addition of glucose to the blood, and the blood glucose level begins to fall – these antihyperglycaemic actions are not wholly insulin-controlled. The blood glucose may even fall below the fasting level at about 2 h – the slight hypoglycaemia then mobilizes the insulin antagonists and insulin and growth hormone return to normal, glycogenolysis

occurs, and the blood glucose level returns to normal at about 3 h after the meal.

The extent to which the body responds to a carbohydrate load is known as the glucose tolerance and primarily reflects the capacity of the tissues to take up glucose largely under the influence of insulin. Impaired glucose tolerance means that after taking carbohydrate (as glucose) the blood glucose level rises higher, and the rise is more prolonged, than in normal people. Enhanced glucose tolerance means that ingestion of carbohydrate causes a diminished rise in the blood glucose level. There is a normal circadian diminution of glucose tolerance in the afternoon.

The response to a carbohydrate load depends both on the previous carbohydrate diet and on the amount of glucose ingested. If a subject is fasting or on a low carbohydrate diet there can be impaired glucose tolerance: fasting increases gluconeogenesis. If a subject is on a very high carbohydrate diet (or has eaten just before the test) there can be enhanced glucose tolerance. The changes in glucose tolerance with alteration of the diet are related to changes in liver glycogen metabolism and also to changes in insulin and growth hormone secretion. The extent of the rise of the blood glucose level after glucose ingestion increases with the dose of glucose, up to a dose of about 1 g/kg body weight. Hence, if measurement of glucose tolerance is required for investigation of disease, standard conditions of diet and of glucose dose must be established.

The effect of insulin on the blood glucose

Insulin has no action orally, even when given in large doses, as it is inactivated by the gastric juice, and then digested. Insulin is given subcutaneously in the normal therapeutic control of diabetes, but for the treatment of diabetic coma or for studying the physiological response it may be injected intravenously. After the intravenous injection, to a fasting subject, of a small dose (0.1 units/kg) of soluble insulin, the blood glucose level falls for about half an hour to about 50 per cent of the resting level; the hypoglycaemia then mobilizes the insulin antagonists and the blood glucose returns to normal in about 2 h.

The response of insulin can be divided into two phases. The rate and degree of fall of the blood glucose concentration after the injection of insulin is known as the insulin-sensitivity – insulin-resistance means that the blood glucose does not fall as much as in a normal subject. The rate and degree of return to normal of the blood glucose concentration after the hypoglycaemia is known as the hypoglycaemia-response: hypoglycaemia-unresponsiveness means that the blood glucose fails to return to normal. Both insulin-resistance and hypoglycaemia-unresponsiveness may be present in pathological states.

Abnormal glucose metabolism

Hyperglycaemia and impaired glucose tolerance

The level of blood glucose depends on the balance between intake of carbohydrate and endogenous glucose synthesis and release by the liver on the one hand, and glucose storage utilization and excretion on the other. A carbohydrate meal in a normal person causes only a temporary rise in blood glucose level; the mechanisms for removal of glucose from the circulation, by storage or utilization, efficiently restore the normal level.

A temporary hyperglycaemia, due to increased glycogenolysis, may be due to excessive secretion of adrenaline: this occurs in patients who have phaeochromocytoma, and after emotional stress, asphyxia, and anaesthesia. The hyperglycaemia which follows cerebral injury, cerebrovascular accidents, and increased intracranial pressure may be due to increased glycogenolysis. Temporary hyperglycaemia follows over-rapid absorption of glucose from the gut and may occur after gastrectomy, gastroenterostomy, or pyloro-

plasty. It is also occasionally found, following a meal, in severe liver disease where there is delayed uptake of glucose by the liver. Peritoneal dialysis with hypertonic glucose solutions can cause severe hyperglycaemia.

An artefactual cause of hyperglycaemia is the blood sample being taken above, near, or even at the site of an intravenous glucose infusion.

Impairment of glucose tolerance, often with fasting hyperglycaemia may be seen in patients with cirrhosis, and as a result of stress, for example with severe staphylococcal infections. Glucose tolerance can also be impaired by the chronic action of various toxins, particularly alcohol and barbiturates, on the peripheral utilization of glucose; 'toxins' may be responsible for the impaired tolerance of chronic renal failure.

Diabetes mellitus

Sustained or episodic hyperglycaemia resulting from absolute or relative insulin deficiency is known as diabetes mellitus. It is defined as a fasting venous blood glucose level of 6.7 mmol/l or more, or if the fasting concentration is below this, a level of 10 mmol/l or more 2 h after an oral glucose load of 75 g (p. 59). Impaired glucose tolerance is considered to occur if the venous blood glucose 2 h following a 75 g load is between 6.7 and 10 mmol/l (Table 5.1). A small proportion of such people progress to diabetes mellitus, though the impaired glucose tolerance associated with obesity usually disappears on loss of weight.

Table 5.1 Classification of impaired glucose tolerance

	Venous blood glucose (mmol/l)	Condition
Fasting	>6.7	Diabetes mellitus
Two hours after 75 g glucose	>10	Diabetes mellitus
Two hours after 75 g glucose	6.7–10	Impaired glucose tolerance

Essential deficiency of effective insulin activity

The β-cell injury in insulin-dependent (juvenile) diabetes mellitus (IDDM or Type 1) is determined by genetic and immunological mechanisms, and possibly by viral and other factors. Endogenous secretion of insulin is diminished, and plasma insulin is always low at the time of diagnosis.

In non-insulin-dependent (maturity onset) diabetes mellitus (NIDDM or Type 2) the plasma insulin is higher than in juvenile diabetes, and may even be above normal; there is a delayed insulin response to hyperglycaemia. In this disease resistance to insulin is an important mechanism as well as genetic and possibly other factors. A high proportion of patients are obese, and insulin-resistance occurs in obesity.

Secondary destruction of insulin secretion

Insulin deficiency results when total pancreatectomy has been performed and may develop in severe chronic pancreatitis or haemochromatosis. After total pancreatectomy the patient's insulin requirement is only about 40 units per day, for in such patients there are no primary extrapancreatic metabolic changes, and glucagon secretion is also absent. When there is this type of deficient secretion of insulin, the patient's insulin sensitivity and hypoglycaemia responsiveness are normal, even though glucose tolerance is grossly impaired. Decreased glucose utilization is more important than increased glucose production.

Excess insulin antagonists

Excessive secretion of the 'anti-insulin' hormones may occur in acromegaly, Cushing's syndrome, phaeochromocytoma, or thyrotoxicosis, and the same effect can develop during treatment with adrenocorticotrophic hormone or corticosteroids; or in pregnancy (gestational diabetes). Impaired glucose tolerance occurs, because the balance of hormonal control of glucose metabolism is disturbed in the same direction as in deficient insulin activity. There may, however, be marked insulin resistance. Increased glucose production is more important than decreased glucose utilization.

Glucagonoma is rare, and presents with bullous dermatitis. There is hypoaminoacidaemia, and hyperglycaemia is inconstant.

Metabolic features of diabetes mellitus

Diabetes mellitus is a syndrome comprising many disturbances.

Permanent impairment of glucose tolerance is caused by similar deficiencies of insulin activity and alterations of normal glucose metabolism, whatever the initial cause of the disorder. There is impaired liver and tissue utilization of glucose, and hepatic glycogenolysis, and gluconeogenesis from protein and fatty acid carbon residues, are increased. The increased blood glucose level leads to increased glomerular filtration of glucose and if the renal threshold is exceeded glycosuria is present.

Protein metabolism is disturbed as excess protein is broken down in the process of gluconeogenesis. The disturbance of lipid metabolism may lead to ketosis. When there is relative or absolute insulin deficiency excess adipose tissue triglyceride is hydrolysed, which releases excess free fatty acids (FFAs): the latter if not oxidized, are converted to keto-acids if not reconverted to triglycerides. This reconversion is diminished because of deficient carbohydrate metabolism (p. 50) and the tissue oxidative power for keto-acids is overloaded. The result is retention of keto-acids in the plasma and their excretion in the urine. Excess glucose entering the liver is converted to triglyceride which is released into the circulation (along with that made from free fatty acids) as VLDL. Peripheral uptake of VLDL by lipoprotein lipase is deficient in the absence of insulin and hypertriglyceridaemia results.

Clinical features

The clinical features of a patient suffering from untreated diabetes mellitus are results of these metabolic disorders, which result from effective insulin deficiency.

The patient has impaired glucose tolerance combined with a high fasting blood glucose level. If the impairment of carbohydrate metabolism is more than minimal, protein and lipid metabolism are also affected. Tissue protein is destroyed during gluconeogenesis, with loss of potassium, nitrogen, and phosphate from the cells to the ECF, whence they are excreted. Fat is also drawn on to provide energy requirements as carbon residues for the common metabolic pool. The patient loses weight.

The levels of all the lipids in the plasma are raised. FFAs are released from adipose tissue lipolysis and the plasma may appear milky due to VLDL excess. Excess cholesterol is synthesized from acetyl CoA and there is an increase in the pre-β-lipoproteins. The increased plasma FFAs impair insulin sensitivity and further impair glucose tolerance.

The hyperglycaemia reduces the resistance to bacterial infection, causes itching, and leads to glycosuria. There is often a high level of salivary isoenzyme of amylase in plasma, coupled with a decreased pancreatic isoamylase and trypsin due to impaired exocrine function.

Long-standing diabetes mellitus often leads to intercapillary glomerulosclerosis (the Kimmelstiel–Wilson lesion in the kidney), which is accompanied by proteinuria and renal failure.

The relative parts played by the primary metabolic causes of diabetes mellitus, and by secondary effects such as hyperglycaemia and lipaemia, in the pathogenesis of the vascular and other complications of diabetes, are not decided.

The concentration of glycated haemoglobins, particularly HbA_{1c} (p. 139) is increased in diabetes mellitus: a value above 10 per cent indicates, and is a useful investigation for, poor long-term metabolic control.

Diabetic ketosis, acidosis, and coma

When treatment is inadequate, and in the presence of complicating factors such as infection and starvation or anorexia and vomiting, ketosis develops (p. 71); as this becomes severe (the total plasma ketones exceeding about 5 mmol/l), the patient slowly lapses into diabetic coma. The coma is due to the toxic effects of the acidosis and of the acetoacetate on the cerebral cortex. The ketoacids produce a severe metabolic acidosis with a plasma bicarbonate less than 10 mmol/l, and this leads to the characteristic deep respiration ('air hunger') due to stimulation of the respiratory centres by the low pH. Ketone bodies are excreted in the breath, which has the characteristic odour of acetone, and in the urine, where they can be easily detected (p. 258). The commercial strip or tablet tests for ketonuria can also be used for detection of excess ketone bodies in plasma: quantitation of plasma ketones is rarely needed. In a few patients there is also a contributory lactic acidosis (p. 61).

The blood glucose is generally above 20 mmol/l and the marked glycosuria (up to 1000 mmol/24 h) causes an osmotic diuresis. This diuresis, vomiting, the ketonuria, and the acidosis, cause severe dehydration with loss of intracellular and extracellular water and electrolytes (6–8 l of water and 500 mmol/l of potassium and sodium may be lost). The patient shows the symptoms of sodium and water depletion with a slight rise in plasma osmolality, and the loss of extracellular water eventually causes haemoconcentration, oliguria, and a rise in the plasma urea; vomiting causes chloride depletion. From inefficiency of the sodium pump due to inability to utilize glucose and because of the acidosis displacing it from the cells, the plasma potassium concentration may be increased, while the plasma sodium is usually slightly lowered. There is increased protein catabolism and a high plasma phosphate, and loss of liver and muscle glycogen. Potassium, nitrogen and phosphate released from the cells are excreted in the urine and a total body deficit of potassium is common.

Diagnosis is made both clinically, and on the demonstration of hyperglycaemia with glycosuria, ketosis with ketonuria, and acidosis – but impaired glomerular filtration may reduce the excretion of glucose and of ketones. Rarely, there is hyperglycaemia without ketoacidosis, or ketoacidosis without severe hyperglycaemia.

Treatment of ketoacidosis is directed to reversing the metabolic disturbances with insulin and by replacing the deficiencies of water and salt with intravenous saline and base (e.g. as sodium bicarbonate) as necessary. Potassium must be given, orally or intravenously, as soon as the plasma volume is restored and the potassium concentration falls below normal. Close biochemical control of glucose, electrolytes, and acid–base balance is necessary.

Hyperosmolar non-ketotic coma is an unusual complication, mainly in older patients, of unknown cause. The blood glucose usually exceeds 50 mmol/l, which yields a plasma osmolality above 350 mmol/kg and causes cell water deficiency. There is dehydration and often oliguria, and ketosis and acidosis are absent. Treatment is aimed at reducing osmolality by giving water intravenously into a central vein together with small doses of insulin to decrease blood glucose gradually. Patients are often sensitive to the action of insulin.

A milder diabetic syndrome occurs when glucose tolerance is impaired due to excess insulin antagonists. Ketosis and coma are rare in such conditions.

Hypoglycaemia

In normal adult subjects symptoms of hypoglycaemia occur at or below a capillary blood glucose level of about 2.2 mmol/l. If the brain is accustomed to a lower blood glucose level (as in hyperinsulinaemia or overtreated diabetes mellitus); symptoms occur only when the blood glucose is at a lower level, such as 1.7 mmol/l. If the brain is accustomed to a constantly higher blood glucose level (as in uncontrolled diabetes mellitus), then symptoms can occur at a higher blood glucose level, and the critical concentration may be above 3.3 mmol/l. Hypoglycaemic symptoms may also occur at a blood glucose of 2.8–4.0 mmol/l when the rate of fall is rapid. Early symptoms are faintness, dizziness or lethargy accompanied by sweating, tachycardia and feeling of anxiety due to adrenaline secretion. Progress to coma, permanent brain damage (seen where recovery occurs) and death occur rapidly.

Mechanisms of hypoglycaemia

Diminished absorption of glucose

A diet which has been low only in carbohydrate even for a prolonged period does not lead to clinical hypoglycaemia, as the blood glucose level is maintained at a slightly lower level from liver glycogen, which is itself synthesized from non-carbohydrate sources. In kwashiorkor, blood glucose is generally low, due largely to deficiency of glucogenic amino acids though clinical features of hypoglycaemia are absent.

If glucose absorption is diminished, a carbohydrate meal may make little difference to the blood glucose.

Urinary loss of glucose

A constant drain of glucose, due to a low renal threshold, may result in a persistently low blood glucose level, though this is rarely sufficient to cause symptoms. A patient suffering from renal glycosuria may develop diabetes mellitus as readily as may anyone else.

Inappropriately high level of insulin-like activity

This causes glucose entry into cells and hypoglycaemia. The main causes are

insulin-secreting tumours of the pancreas (insulinoma)
insulin or other hypoglycaemic drugs
excess insulin secretion in babies of diabetic mothers
excess insulin secretion induced by rapid absorption of glucose (reactive hypogly-

caemia) or by leucine (in children) or by alcohol

insulin activity derived from non-pancreatic tumours.

Failure to mobilize glycogen stores

This occurs in a number of conditions

severe liver disease
glucocorticoid deficiency
glycogenoses
galactosaemia
hereditary fructose intolerance
intrauterine malnutrition (absent glycogen stores).

Clinical presentation of hypoglycaemia

The individual causes of hypoglycaemia tend to present either in the fasting state or non-fasting. Such a clinical classification is useful in predicting the likely cause.

Fasting hypoglycaemia typically occurs at night or in the early morning and is caused by

insulinoma
production of insulin-like activity by non-pancreatic tumours
glucocorticoid deficiency
severe liver disease
intrauterine growth retardation
babies of diabetic mothers
glycogenoses.

Non-fasting hypoglycaemia typically occurs within 5–6 hours of a meal and may be related to an aggravating factor. Causes are

insulin (overdosage in a diabetic)
glucose (reactive hypoglycaemia)
alcohol
drugs
galactose (in galactosaemia)
fructose (in fructose intolerance)
leucine.

Childhood hypoglycaemia

This may occur at any age but different causes predominate in different age groups.

In the neonate plasma glucose levels of 2.2 mmol/l may be considered normal while levels as low as 1.1 mmol/l may occur in premature infants without ill effect. Clinical evidence of hypoglycaemia, such as convulsions, tremor and apnoea, require urgent treatment to avoid brain damage. In this age group babies suffering from intrauterine growth retardation have low glycogen stores and are particularly at risk, often tending towards hypoglycaemia for up to one week following birth. Babies of diabetic mothers suffer from islet cell hyperplasia and hyperinsulinism.

In early infancy the intake of milk or sucrose may reveal one of the rare inborn errors of carbohydrate metabolism leading to hypoglycaemia.

Glycogen storage diseases

In type 1 glycogen storage disease (von Gierke's disease), glucose-6-phosphate is absent and glycogen stores cannot be mobilized leading to fasting hypoglycaemia. There is enlargement of liver and kidneys. As well as the episodes of hypoglycaemia with ketosis and lactic acidosis, serum FFAs and lipids are increased, there is often hyperuricaemia, and the glycogen deposition in the kidneys may lead to a renal tubular syndrome (p. 121). As a diagnostic test the response of the blood glucose to glucagon is often valuable: normal subjects, after an intravenous injection of 1 mg of glucagon, have at least a 50 per cent rise in the fasting blood glucose within 20 min; this fails to occur in *von Gierke's disease*. The eight other rare types are each due to a deficiency of a different enzyme in the pathway of glycogen synthesis or degradation, and do not all show hypoglycaemia. Diagnosis may require enzyme assay on liver and other tissue biopsy.

Other causes

In galactosaemia and fructose intolerance the intake of galactose in milk and fructose in fruit results in the accumulation of the sugar monophosphate which inhibits glycogenolysis. Leucine present in the casein of milk stimulates insulin secretion in genetically susceptible individuals leading to hypoglycaemia following milk feeds.

In late infancy and childhood, hypoglycaemia is associated with fasting or febrile illnesses and may occur with or without ketosis. The mechanism of the ketotic and idiopathic hypoglycaemia of infancy and childhood are unknown.

Causes of hypoglycaemia

Treatment of diabetes mellitus

An overdose of insulin is probably the commonest cause of hypoglycaemia: chlorpropamide and other insulin-stimulating antidiabetic agents may rarely also produce hypoglycaemia.

Insulinoma

Benign or malignant tumours of the islet cells (which can be multiple), or rarely, hyperplasia of the islet cells, produce excess insulin. This results in a high fasting plasma insulin and a low fasting blood glucose level, and on occasion in attacks of severe hypoglycaemia, with mental or neurological symptoms. The blood glucose is lowest before breakfast, and three or four hours after meals.

As a diagnostic test it may be necessary to fast the patient for 24–48 hours in hospital under supervision. If hypoglycaemia develops, take blood to look for a diagnostically high insulin (assay of C-peptide may be more sensitive), and treat with intravenous glucose. Alternative tests are to give intravenous glucagon or leucine, and to look for the diagnostically high rise in the plasma insulin associated with the fall in blood glucose. The similar, and formerly popular, tolbutamide test is too dangerous. To detect autonomous insulin secretion during insulin-induced hypoglycaemia, either C-peptide can be assayed or immunologically-distinct fish insulin can be injected.

A variety of tumours of non-endocrine origin (particularly retroperitoneal fibrosa coma) may produce hypoglycaemia by secreting an insulin-like hormone or by stimulating or producing antibodies to insulin receptors.

Deficiency of insulin antagonists

In hypopituitarism, adrenal cortical deficiency and, rarely, in hypothyroidism, there may be fasting hypoglycaemia because of deficiency of hormones which normally act as insulin antagonists. Patients so affected have enhanced glucose tolerance and are hypoglycaemia-unresponsive.

Hepatic hypoglycaemia

In acute hepatic necrosis, and occasionally in viral hepatitis, there may be severe hypoglycaemia: renal gluconeogenesis continues on a small scale.

Alimentary hypoglycaemia

In patients who have had a gastrectomy or gastroenterostomy, a carbohydrate meal rapidly causes a high blood glucose level, often followed by hypoglycaemia after between 1 and 2 h. The high blood glucose level is due to rapid absorption of glucose, as the meal reaches the intestines more quickly than usual. There may be excessive vagal activity. Rapid absorption also occurs in hyperthyroidism. The hypoglycaemia results from rapid acceleration of glucose utilization due to reactive insulin secretion with a high plasma insulin at the same time as glucose absorption falls off. This postgastrectomy hypoglycaemia must be distinguished from the dumping syndrome (p. 165), which develops in these patients 20 to 60 min after a meal and which is due to plasma volume depletion as a result of fluid entering the gut due to the high osmotic load of carbohydrates rapidly entering the intestine.

Functional (reactive) hypoglycaemia

In some otherwise physically healthy subjects, hypoglycaemia often occurs about 2 h after a meal, possibly due to excessive insulin response to glucose. Alcohol may potentiate this effect. This response is also occasionally seen in early diabetes.

Investigation of abnormalities in carbohydrate metabolism

Investigation of glucose tolerance is of considerable importance in clinical and experimental practice. Conditions should be standardized so that consistent responses may be obtained.

Reliable and reproducible results are obtained only when the patient has been on a normal diet (containing at least 300 g of carbohydrate per day) for at least three days before the test, and is mentally and physically at rest before and during the test. The patient must fast 10 to 16 h overnight before all tests (water is allowed), and must not be allowed to smoke.

Consistent results are not found in children who are less than 2 years old. The present routine adult dose of glucose is 75 g, or 1.75 g/kg body weight in children to a maximum of 75 g. Diagnostic results can usually be obtained without extending the test beyond 120 min.

The test is not needed for diagnosis in cases of clinically overt diabetes mellitus, or if a fasting blood glucose exceeds 6.7 mmol/l, or a value exceeding 10 mmol/l 2 h after oral ingestion of 75 g of glucose or equivalent.

Standard (oral) glucose tolerance test

Method

Take a fasting blood sample for glucose estimation. Patient empties bladder; collect urine specimen.

Zero time: the patient drinks a solution of 75 g glucose in a glass of water (250 ml), preferably flavoured, e.g. with lemon.

At 30 min, 60 min, 90 min, 120 min take blood for glucose estimation.

At 60 min and 120 min patient empties bladder; collect specimens separately.

Send all blood and urine specimens to the laboratory, clearly labelled with the times of collection

Interpretation

The figures given here are for venous whole blood. If capillary blood is used, the fasting level is less than 0.3 mmol/l higher, the level at the peak is 1.1–1.7 mmol/l higher, and the 120 min level is 0.6–1.1 mmol/l higher; for venous plasma the levels are about 1 mmol/l higher. In diabetic patients there may be less difference between the venous and the capillary blood glucose levels.

The normal response (Fig. 5.4 a)

The fasting blood glucose level is 3.0–5.5 mmol/l. The blood glucose rises by 1.5–4.0 mmol/l to the 30–60 min level which is below 10 mmol/l, then falls to a 120 min level below 6.7 mmol/l. There is no glycosuria.

Impaired glucose tolerance (Fig. 5.4 b_1, b_2)

The curve is raised and prolonged. In diabetes mellitus the fasting blood glucose level is usually above 6.7 mmol/l; if it is not so raised then diabetes may be diagnosed when both an intermediate level and the 120 min level are above 10 mmol/l. Impairment of tolerance not amounting to diabetes is accepted when the fasting level is below 6.7 mmol/l, intermediate levels are below 10 mmol/l, and the 120 min level is between 6.7 and 10 mmol/l; though of course there can be no rigorous boundary between normal and abnormal (p. 6). Glycosuria is normally present, though not always, in the fasting specimen. It should be noted that special criteria apply in pregnancy.

For the diagnosis of diabetes mellitus, or other causes of impaired glucose tolerance, usually only the 120 min level is essential. A normal blood glucose found 120 min after the ingestion of 75 g of glucose under appropriate standardized conditions demonstrates normal glucose tolerance. In many cases of severe diabetes there is no 60 min peak as the blood glucose rises throughout the period of the test. The same type of diabetic curve is seen if there is

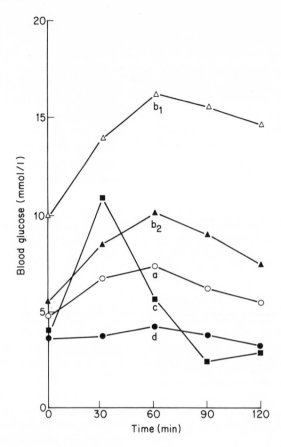

Fig. 5.4 Oral glucose tolerance test curves (75 g glucose: venous blood). (a) Normal, (b_1) diabetic, (b_2) mild impairment of tolerance, (c) lagstorage, (d) flat: enhanced tolerance

impairment of tolerance due, for example, to severe Cushing's disease.

Impairment of tolerance may be found in obesity, late pregnancy (or due to hormonal contraceptives), severe infections (especially staphylococcal), Cushing's syndrome, Conn's syndrome, acromegaly, thyrotoxicosis, gross liver damage, chronic renal disease, in old age, and in mild or incipient diabetes mellitus.

The urine results provide a guide to the renal threshold for glucose in that patient, and this is valuable in showing how much reliance can be placed on urine testing in patient management.

Steroid-augmented glucose tolerance tests are of some help in the detection of incipient diabetes. If, for example, 100 mg cortisone is given in the early morning before a glucose tolerance test, then the 120 min blood glucose may be raised above 7.7

mmol/l in potential diabetics.

The lag storage curve (Fig. 5.4 c)

The fasting blood glucose level is normal. There is a steep rise in blood glucose: the maximum level, found at 30 min, is above 10 mmol/l. The curve then falls sharply, and hypoglycaemic levels may be reached before 120 min. There is a lag in the initiation of the normal homeostatic processes, particularly storage of glucose as glycogen. Transient glycosuria is usually found. This curve was originally described in certain cases of severe liver disease, and sometimes occurs in thyrotoxicosis, but is more commonly seen due to rapid absorption following gastrectomy, gastroenterostomy, or vagotomy. The lag storage curve is occasionally found in apparently normal subjects.

The flat curve of apparently enhanced glucose tolerance (Fig. 5.4 d)

The fasting blood glucose is normal or low and throughout the test the level does not vary by more than about ±1.0 mmol/l. This curve may be seen in patients who are suffering from myxoedema (which reduces carbohydrate absorption), or who have deficiency of hormonal insulin antagonists, as in Addison's disease and hypopituitarism. There is no glycosuria.

A flat curve is often found in patients who have malabsorption of carbohydrate, as in coeliac disease. In lactase deficiency the blood glucose curve is normal after giving 25 g glucose + 25 g galactose (confirming normal absorption), but is flat (less than 1.0 mmol/l rise) after 50 g lactose because of diminished digestion of lactose to absorbable monosaccharide.

In renal glycosuria the glucose tolerance curve may be flat or normal depending on the rate of urinary loss of glucose.

The late hypoglycaemia of hyperinsulinism

In patients with hyperinsulinism, the fasting blood glucose is hypoglycaemic or normal, and late blood glucose estimated 4 h, 6 h, and if necessary 24 h after glucose has been taken may show hypoglycaemic levels.

Intravenous glucose tolerance test

Abnormal responses to the oral glucose tolerance test may be masked by defective intestinal absorption. For the investigation of glucose metabolism in such patients, the glucose may be given intravenously.

Method

Take a fasting blood sample for blood glucose.
Zero time: 50 ml of 50 per cent glucose is injected intravenously over 2 min.
At 10 min, 20 min and 30 min take samples for blood glucose.

Interpretation

The k value (percentage fall in blood glucose per minute) is calculated by plotting the results on semilogarithmic paper. In normal subjects k is about 1.5, in diabetic patients k is less than 1.0.

The test, though sometimes important, is little used because it is necessary to time the samples very accurately: injection of hypertonic glucose also carries a slight risk of thrombophlebitis. Cases for which it is an essential diagnostic measure, such as suspected diabetes in a patient with steatorrhoea, are rare. It is valuable for research on glucose tolerance, as variations in intestinal absorption are eliminated.

Lactate

The reference range for venous blood lactate is 0.4–1.4 mmol/l. Accumulation of lactic acid causes a metabolic acidosis, with an increased anion gap (p. 43).

Lactic acid is produced in excess by anaerobic glycolysis in anoxic tissues, e.g. occasionally during anaesthesia, in severe heart failure especially after cardiac arrest, in muscles after severe exercise, or generally after trauma. Alternatively, it may be normally metabolized, for example in liver failure and von Gierke's disease, diabetes mellitus, or due to phenformin therapy. Lactic acidosis is potentiated by alcohol.

Glycosuria

A 24 h specimen of urine from a normal subject contains a small amount of reducing substances, generally less than 1 g, of which 20–200 mg (0.1–1.1 mmol/l) is glucose. Glycosuria implies that sufficient glucose is present to be detectable by a simple clinical test – the 'correct' term glucosuria is rarely used. Tests for reducing substances depend on copper reduction, and these are semiquantitative. The traditional test employed is Benedict's solution, containing alkaline copper(III) citrate (cupric citrate) which is blue because of the presence of copper(III) ions. On reduction of Benedict's solution, by glucose or other substances, the blue colour disappears and an orange–red precipitate of copper(II) oxide (cuprous oxide) is formed. The colour of the reduced mixture varies from green to red, since the more glucose that reduces the reagent the more copper(III) ions are converted to copper(II) oxide. In general use Benedict's test has been replaced by Clinitest (p. 258), a commercial modification in which reagents in solid form are added to urine; no external source of heat is required as the heat of solution of the reagents boils the mixture. This is more useful for the ward side-room, for the general practitioner's surgery, and for issuing to diabetic patients to test their urine themselves.

Many substances that reduce copper can occur in urine: reduction due to any sugar is called melituria. Glucose is the commonest and most important, and reduction sufficient to form a precipitate must be considered to be due to glucose unless proved otherwise.

Many bacterial infections of urine (e.g. due to *E. coli*) lead to absence of urinary glucose. Detection of less than 0.3 mmol (5 mg) glucose per 24 h urine has been proposed as a screening test for bacteruria, but gives an unacceptably high proportion of false negative results.

Glucose

The causes of glycosuria may be summarized as

1 hyperglycaemia associated with impaired glucose tolerance
2 temporary hyperglycaemia
3 a low renal threshold for glucose.

The causes of these conditions have been discussed above. Hyperglycaemia without glycosuria may be found if there is a raised threshold due to diminished renal plasma flow: this is quite often seen in the elderly diabetic.

A reducing substance found in urine may be identified as glucose by

Use of the specific enzyme, glucose oxidase. Test strips incorporating glucose oxidase are commercially available for quantitatively testing urine (p. 258): they are simple, sensitive, specific for glucose, and do not react with other reducing substances.

Chemical tests. Identification of sugars other than glucose is performed in the biochemical laboratory by chromatography.

Other sugars

Lactose, galactose, fructose, and pentoses are other reducing sugars which may be found in urine. Sucrose is not a reducing sugar. Intestinal accumulation of any disaccharide can lead to some absorption and urinary excretion of that sugar as is seen in lactase deficiency (p. 47): a similar alimentary melituria may present when there is flattened intestinal mucosa (p. 168).

Lactose

This is often present in the urine of pregnancy after 20 weeks, and may be found either as the sole reducing sugar, or together with glucose. Lactosuria usually occurs in nursing mothers, and is occasionally found in patients on a milk diet. It is rare for the concentration of lactose in urine to exceed 14 mmol/l (0.5 g/100 ml). Lactosuria is benign.

Galactosaemia (with galactosuria)

This occurs as a congenital abnormality. It is due to deficiency of the hepatic enzyme galactose-1-phosphate uridyltransferase, which is concerned with the conversion of galactose through hexose phosphates to glucose: thus galactose cannot enter into further metabolic processes and there is hypoglycaemia. Accumulation of galactose-1-phosphate leads to renal tubular damage (p. 121) with aminoaciduria, proteinuria, and acidosis, and to liver damage with jaundice. The high blood galactose leads to cataracts. This disorder should always be considered as a possible cause of failure to thrive in an infant who is on a milk diet. It should be screened for by testing urine for reducing sugars, and confirming the presence of galactose by chromatography. The specific enzyme deficiency can be determined in erythrocytes or leucocytes before appropriate dietary therapy.

Fructose intolerance

This is a similar rare disease, due to deficiency of an isoenzyme of (fructose-bisphosphate) aldolase. Fructose-1-phosphate accumulates after ingestion of fructose or sucrose, and this causes hypoglycaemia and liver damage.

Benign congenital abnormalities

Fructosuria due to fructokinase deficiency, and galactosuria (which is associated with cataracts, due to galactokinase deficiency) are rare. Pentosuria (xylulosuria), due to L-xylulose reductase deficiency, is less rare. In addition various pentoses may occasionally be found in the urine after ingestion of large quantities of fruit.

Glucuronides

Glucuronides are conjugates of various compounds with glucuronic acid, and these are urinary reducing substances. Drugs in common use which are partially excreted as ester-glucuronides are the salicylates (including aspirin) and paracetamol.

The glucuronide of any salicylate drug, which is taken in therapeutic dosage, may be excreted in sufficient quantity in the urine to cause a greenish reduction. However, the reduction caused by the glucuronide of *p*-aminosalicylic acid, taken in the usual dosage, may mimic the reduction caused by (about 50 mmol/l) glucose.

Rare urine components

Amongst other reducing substances are homogentisic acid, phenylpyruvic acid, and melanogen. Homogentisic acid is found in the inborn error of metabolism alkaptonuria (p. 89). Phenylpyruvic acid, found in phenylketonuria (p. 89), can be further identified by the green colour it gives with iron(III) chloride (ferric chloride) or with the equivalent Phenystix. Melanogen is

produced by malignant melanoma: it blackens on oxidation to melanin, and is excreted in widespread disease (p. 234).

Normal constituents of urine

If urates are present in urine in sufficient quantity to form a sediment, the urine should be filtered before testing it for sugars. A high concentration of urates or of creatinine in urine will cause a slight reduction of copper.

Protein, or a high concentration of phosphates, may precipitate as greyish floccules on boiling the urine with Benedict's solution or Clinitest. This should not be mistaken for reduction.

Ketonuria

The ketone bodies which may be excreted in urine are acetone, acetoacetic acid, and 3-hydroxybutyric acid. There is a simple test available for ketone bodies in the urine. Rothera's test is sensitive to acetoacetic acid and acetone, and is a colour reaction with sodium nitroprusside in alkaline solution. This has now been developed into commercial tablet or stick preparations (p. 258).

Ketonuria occurs when there is ketonaemia. This may be found whenever, in a disorder of carbohydrate metabolism, insufficient carbohydrate is being catabolized to ensure proper oxidation of fat. This incomplete carbohydrate metabolism, combined with excessive fat breakdown, causes the ketosis of diabetes mellitus.

Ketonaemia and ketonuria also develop when the patient is suffering from carbohydrate deficiency. Thus ketonuria is found in starvation (or if the patient is on a badly balanced reducing diet) or after prolonged vomiting. Postoperative ketonuria is commonly seen. It is due to a combination of the starvation that precedes the operation, the vomiting that often follows it, and possibly to the effect of the anaesthetic which depletes liver glycogen.

Just as there may be hyperglycaemia without glycosuria, so ketonaemia without ketonuria may occur if there is a low renal plasma flow. This can be seen, e.g. in the ketosis due to prolonged vomiting associated with starvation and sodium depletion, or sometimes in severe diabetes.

Further reading

Cohen RD, Wood HF. *Lactic Acidosis*. Oxford: Blackwell Scientific Publications, 1976.

Gale E. Causes of hypoglycaemia. *Br J Hosp Med* 1985; **33**: 159–62.

Oakley WG, Pyke DA, Taylor KW. *Diabetes and its Management*. 3rd edn. Oxford: Blackwell Scientific Publications, 1978.

Watkins PJ. *ABC of Diabetes*. London: British Medical Journal, 1983.

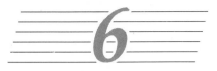

Lipid Metabolism

Objectives

In this chapter the reader is able to

- revise the chemistry, biochemistry and transport of triglycerides, phospholipids and cholesterol
- revise the physiology of fat metabolism and its inter-relationship with carbohydrate metabolism
- study the significance of alterations of plasma cholesterol and triglyceride.

At the conclusion of this chapter the reader is able to

- classify lipoproteins
- relate changes in plasma lipids to the problems of atheroma, coronary thrombosis, and hyperlipidaemias.

Chemistry and classification

The term 'lipid' is used to include all fats and substances of a fat-like nature. The principal lipids of clinical interest can be classified as below.

Triglycerides (neutral fat)

These are glycerol esters of medium- to long-chain fatty acids – i.e. triacylglycerols. The chief component of olive oil, triolein, is a typical neutral fat. However, most triglycerides are mixed, with more than one kind of fatty acid in the molecule.

Phospholipids

These are compounds that contain a nitrogenous base, a phosphoric acid residue, one or more fatty acids, and a complex alcohol, either glycerol or sphingosine. Lecithin (phosphatidyl choline) is a typical phosphoglyceride. Cerebrosides are similar compounds without phosphoric acid.

Cholesterol

This has a completely different chemical structure, and contains the cyclopentenophenanthrene ring system. Cholesterol is a member of the steroid family.

Carotenoids

The carotenoids and vitamin A are not

$$CH_2O.CO.C_{17}H_{33}$$
$$CHO.CO.C_{17}H_{33}$$
$$CH_2O.CO.C_{17}H_{33}$$

(a)

$$CH_2O. \text{Fatty acid}$$
$$CHO. \text{Fatty acid}$$
$$CH_2O. \overset{O}{\overset{\|}{P}}.OCH_2CH_2N^+(CH_3)_3$$
$$\underset{O^-}{|}$$

(b)

(c)

(d)

Fig. 6.1 Structures of (a) triolein, (b) α-lecithin, (c) cholesterol, (d) vitamin A

lipids. They are coloured fat-soluble compounds (lipochromes) and are absorbed with lipids from the small intestine.

The structures of triolein, α-lecithin, cholesterol, and vitamin A, are shown in Fig. 6.1. All these groups of substances are insoluble in water, and are held in solution in plasma by being in combination with specific carrier proteins – the apoproteins.

Lipid metabolism

Fat intake and output

Introduction

Members of the lipid family are more or less water insoluble and this property confers special requirements both for intestinal absorption and plasma transport. Fatty acids are a compact form of stored energy; different lipids are vital constituents of membrane structure not only because they form a water barrier but also by the nature of their structural interaction with other molecules associated with the membrane. Characteristically, membranes, plasma lipoprotein particles, and micelles have a hydrophobic core and a polar surface.

Dietary lipid

Triglycerides are the main lipid in the diet providing a concentrated source of energy: 37 kJ (9 kcal) per gram. The normal daily diet in the United Kingdom at present contains 40–80 g of triglycerides. Fat in the diet carries the fat-soluble vitamins A, D, E, and K.

The dietary triglyceride contains both unsaturated fatty acids (some of which, particularly linoleic acid, are essential, because they cannot be synthesized in the body) and saturated fatty acids. The proportion of saturated to unsaturated fatty acids is generally higher in animal fat than in vegetable fat. A high content of triglyceride in the diet containing saturated fatty acids increases blood cholesterol and is a factor in the aetiology of atheroma.

Fat absorption

Though there is a gastric lipase, negligible digestion of neutral fat takes place in the stomach. In the upper small intestine, under the influence of pancreatic lipase, about a quarter of the triglyceride is completely hydrolysed. There is both partial hydrolysis to monoglycerides, and also complete hydrolysis into glycerol and the constituent fatty acids. The glycerol, which is water soluble, is readily absorbed into the portal system. Most short-chain fatty acids can be absorbed directly into the blood; the long-chain fatty acids and monoglycerides (normally insoluble in water) combine with bile salts to form water-soluble micelles. Monoglycerides and fatty acids, with bile salts, promote the emulsification and dispersion of the remaining unhydrolysed fat which is then available for hydrolysis: a little finely dispersed fat can be absorbed directly. The water-soluble fatty acid-containing micelles are absorbed into the mucosal cells of the intestine, where the bile salts are released into the portal circulation; the fatty acids and monoglycerides are resynthesized in the intestinal wall to triglycerides. These triglycerides are absorbed into the lacteals as small particles known as chylomicrons, which have an average diameter of 1.0 μm and enter the general circulation via the thoracic duct. Chylomicrons contain about 1 per cent carrier apoprotein.

Cholesterol is absorbed directly from the bile salt-containing micelles into the intestinal mucosal cells.

Fat excretion

In a normal subject not more than 10 per cent of the fat that has been taken in the food can be recovered in the faeces. The daily faecal fat excretion of a person on an average diet, which contains about 70 g of fat, is under 5 g (18 mmol), and an increase to a high fat diet (150 g) will not raise this above 7 g (25 mmol); there may be considerable day-to-day variation. Much of the excreted fat is derived from non-dietary sources (bacteria, yeasts, intestinal secretions, and desquamated epithelium), for up to 2 g of lipid material is found in the faeces even in subjects on a fat-free diet. Fat excretion can be studied by a balance technique, which relates excretion to intake.

In clinical practice analysis for total fat of three to five days' excretion of faeces, from a patient on an average diet with a fat intake of 60–100 g, gives the same information. Examination of the proportion of fat by weight in dried faeces, or of the proportion of split fat present (as this depends on bacterial action as well as on pancreatic lipase), does not give information of value. Alternatively, the effect of an oral dose of vitamin A on its plasma concentration may be used as a measure of total fat absorption.

The investigation, effects, and differential diagnosis of an increase in faecal fat (steatorrhoea) are discussed in Chapter 15.

An insignificant quantity of fat is normally lost in the urine and the sebum. Fat is found in the urine in occasional cases of lipid nephrosis or the nephrotic syndrome (lipiduria), or when excess fat enters the blood, often as a fat embolus, after extensive injury to fat depots in bone marrow or subcutaneous tissue. *Chyluria*, the urine having the appearance of milk, is rarely seen. It is usually due to obstruction of the thoracic duct, when chylomicrons reflux through the lymph vessels of the urogenital tract. There can also be *chylothorax* and *chylous ascites* when chylomicrons from the intestinal lacteals leak into the pleural and abdominal cavities.

Intravenous lipid

Various commercial fat emulsions are available, prepared from soyabean oil with phospholipid emulsifiers. They are metabolized as chylomicrons. These preparations provide high energy in low volume for parenteral nutrition: 1 l of a 20 per cent preparation supplies about 8.4 MJ (2000 kcal).

Lipid transport

All lipids are relatively insoluble in water and are transported in the plasma as micelles, solubilized by proteins and the more polar lipids. These particles are known as *lipoproteins* and are comprised of an outer layer of relatively polar proteins, phospholipids and cholesterol with a core of insoluble triglyceride and cholesterol ester.

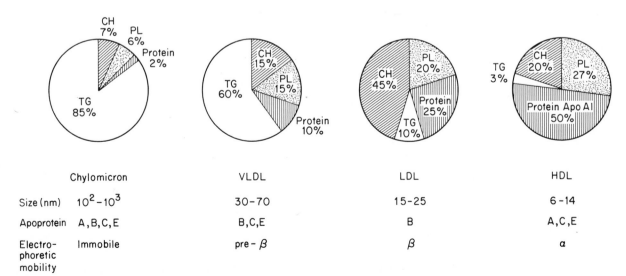

Fig. 6.2 Plasma lipoprotein particles. CH, cholesterol; TG, triglyceride; PL, phospholipid; A, B, C, E, apoproteins, A, B, C, and E

The proteins found in lipoproteins vary greatly in their molecular characteristics but all tend to form helical structures which have both a hydrophobic and hydrophilic surface. They function both to solubilize the lipids and also to interact with enzymes and cellular receptors which control the metabolism of the lipids. They are known as apoproteins and are divided into families, A, B, C, D, and E, on the basis of their structure and function.

Lipoproteins are classified according to their density, composition and electrophoretic mobility. Density is determined by ultracentrifugation and depends on the relative content of protein and lipid. Electrophoretic mobility depends primarily on the charge resulting from the apoprotein content. The composition and characteristics of the main lipoprotein classes is shown in Fig. 6.2. The larger particles (>50 nm) scatter light and cause plasma to appear turbid if they are present in high concentrations.

Lipoprotein metabolism

Chylomicrons (Fig. 6.3)

Triglycerides and cholesterol in the intestinal mucosal cell are packaged, together with the intestinal B apoprotein (known as B-48), A apoprotein, and phospholipid into chylomicrons which enter the lymphatics and pass through the thoracic duct into the systemic circulation. In the lymph and blood the particles acquire C and E apoprotein from HDL particles which have been produced by the liver. The chylomicrons then interact with the enzyme lipoprotein lipase on the surface of the capillary endothelial cells primarily in muscle and adipose tissue. The enzyme is activated by one of the C apoproteins and hydrolyses

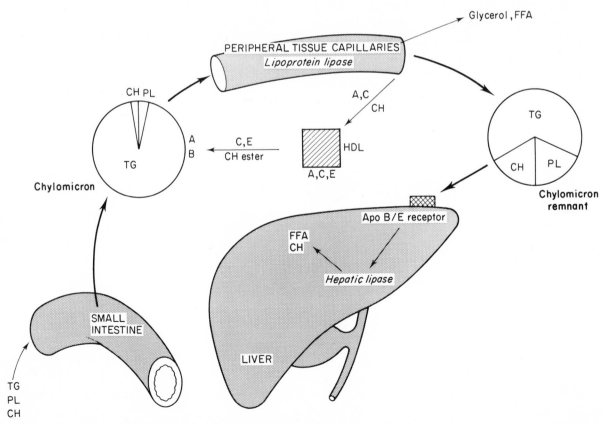

Fig. 6.3   The fate of dietary lipid. See Fig. 6.2 for an explanation of abbreviations

triglycerides from the surface of the chylomicrons releasing fatty acids and glycerol. The fatty acids are taken up by the fat cells where they are stored as triglyceride or by muscle cells where they are used for energy while glycerol passes in the blood to the liver where it enters the glycolytic pathways. Lipoprotein lipase of adipose tissue is activated by insulin (an energy storage hormone) resulting in storage of dietary fat.

As the triglycerides are removed from the chylomicron it shrinks and at the same time phospholipids and apoprotein C and A are transferred back to HDL. Apoprotein E which is present on the surface of the chylomicrons is altered by the loss of apoprotein C so that the chylomicron remnant is recognized by a specific receptor on the surface of the hepatocyte, bound and taken up into the cell by pinocytosis. Once inside the cell the proteins are catabolized in the lysosomes and the cholesterol is released into the cells where it enters the hepatic cholesterol pool. Cholesterol may then leave this pool to enter the circulation again in the VLDL particle, or undergo excretion in the bile either unaltered or in the form of bile salts.

Chylomicrons usually disappear from the circulation, with loss of plasma turbidity, within 12 to 14 h after a fatty meal.

Very low density lipoproteins (VLDL) (Fig. 6.4)

Triglycerides, cholesterol and apoprotein B, C and E are packaged into the VLDL particles within the hepatocyte and secreted into the blood.

Triglycerides are synthesized in the liver either from fatty acids derived from adipose tissue (free fatty acids) or from glucose. Cholesterol is synthesized in the liver or

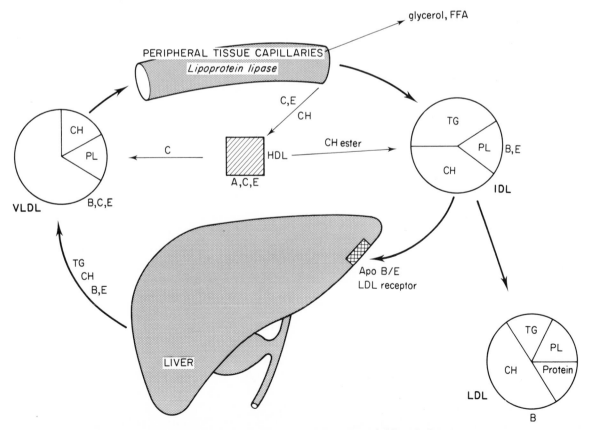

Fig. 6.4 The fate of liver-derived lipid. See Fig. 6.2 for an explanation of abbreviations

derived from chylomicron remnants (dietary cholesterol).

VLDL synthesis is increased in obese people and in diabetics when there is an excess of glucose available in the liver while it is inhibited by the uptake of chylomicron remnants. Interchange of apoprotein with HDL and hydrolysis of triglyceride by lipoprotein lipase occurs in exactly the same way as for chylomicrons. The VLDL remnant (sometimes known as intermediate density lipoprotein, IDL) may undergo pinocytosis by the liver but as a result of interaction with the B/E receptor on the hepatocyte. Some loss of the remaining triglyceride and apo-E occurs and the particles remaining enter the circulation as low density lipoprotein, LDL. It comprises the major source of plasma cholesterol.

Low-density lipoprotein (LDL)

Unlike the other particles LDL is metabolized slowly by uptake in most tissues of the body. This is mediated by specific B/E receptors (LDL receptors) and probably also by non-specific mechanisms known as the scavenger pathway. The LDL particle is internalized by endocytosis and the cholesterol released into the cells by lysosomal catabolism is used for cell membrane synthesis, and maintenance in all cells and for the production of steroid hormones. All cells are capable of *de novo* cholesterol synthesis which is inhibited by cholesterol entering through endocytosis. Increased intracellular cholesterol concentration also down-regulates the receptors. The scavenger pathway is most evident in macrophages whose cholesterol synthesis does not seem to be down-regulated by that entering from outside.

High-density lipoprotein (HDL)

HDL particles are secreted in precursor or nascent form from the hepatocyte and possibly from other tissues, such as the gut. They appear as discoidal particles comprised of a bilayer of phospholipids surounded by apoproteins A and C. In the presence of the liver-derived plasma enzyme lecithin acyl cholesterol transferase (LCAT) cholesterol derived from peripheral cell membranes or other lipoprotein particles is esterified and taken up by nascent HDL to form the spherical micelles of HDL. Both the apoproteins and cholesterol ester may be transferred to other lipoprotein particles before the HDL is taken up by the liver where the cholesterol enters the hepatic cholesterol pool whence it may be excreted in the bile or recycled in VLDL. HDL thus provides a mechanism for removing cholesterol from peripheral tissues to the liver and also for removing cholesterol from VLDL and LDL before it enters peripheral tissues. HDL enters the hepatocyte via the apoprotein B receptor for which the E interaction appears to be the major component. Uptake may be inhibited by high plasma concentrations of VLDL which compete for the B/E receptor.

General lipid metabolism

Triglyceride

Dietary triglyceride is stored in adipose tissue by the action of lipoprotein lipase breaking down chylomicrons preferentially in this tissue under the influence of insulin. Small amounts may be used for energy in muscle and any fatty acids not taken up by peripheral tissue passes in the blood to the liver, bound to albumin. This so-called free fatty acid either enters general carbohydrate metabolism, is converted to ketones or resynthesized to triglyceride and exported from the liver in VLDL.

Dietary carbohydrate can only be stored in very limited amounts as glycogen. The majority enters the liver where it is converted to triglyceride, packaged into VLDL and exported into the circulation where it is catabolized by lipoprotein lipase enabling the released fatty acids to be stored in adipose tissue as triglyceride. The glycerol released by hydrolysis of triglyceride from chylomicrons and VLDL by lipoprotein lipase passes in the blood to the liver while the fatty acids entering adipose tissue are esterified with glyceraldehyde-3-

phosphate derived from glucose entering the cells under the influence of insulin.

In fasting conditions the plasma contains no chylomicrons and only small amounts of VLDL. The fasting plasma triglyceride, which ranges between 0.3 and 1.8 mmol/l, comprises that present in VLDL, remnants of both chylomicrons and VLDL and a small amount present in the long-lived LDL particle.

Significant amounts of chylomicrons or VLDL result in opalescence or milkiness of the plasma known as lipaemia. The triglyceride level is about 5 mmol/l more under these circumstances. Chylomicrons may be distinguished from VLDL by their propensity to form a creamy layer on the top of the plasma when it is allowed to stand for 12 h or more. The relatively low content of cholesterol in these two types of particle means that even in severe lipaemia the cholesterol content of the blood is only slightly raised.

Free fatty acids (Fig. 6.5)

In starvation when glucose is in short supply (more than 3 h after a meal),

hydrolysis of triglyceride in adipose tissue occurs under the influence of adipocyte lipase, an intracellular enzyme, activated by growth hormone. Glycerol and fatty acids enter the circulation and pass to the liver and other tissues. The free fatty acids can be used by most tissues other than the brain as an energy source and in starvation about three-quarters of the energy requirement is provided in this way. The glycerol enters the liver taking part in gluconeogenesis and thus maintaining the blood glucose level while the free fatty acids may be converted to *ketones* which can be used as an energy source by the brain and other tissues when glucose is in short supply. The main ketone is acetoacetic acid which may be converted to the other 'ketone' bodies, 3-hydroxybutyrate (by reduction; not a ketone) and acetone (by decarboxylation). The state of ketosis exists when acetoacetate and other ketone bodies accumulate in the plasma. The principal causes of ketosis are starvation and diabetes mellitus. In starvation, because of lack of carbohydrates, energy requirements are met from depot fat via FFAs, and excess ketones are therefore produced in the liver and pass

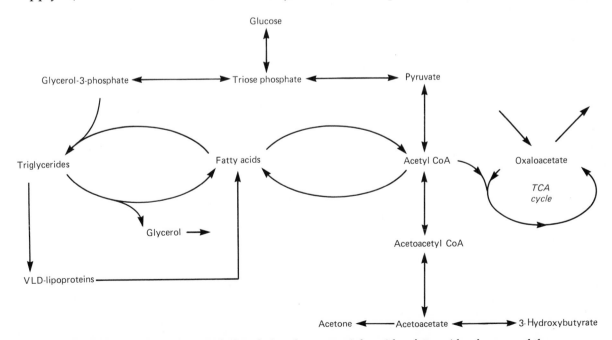

Fig. 6.5 Simplified scheme of the metabolic relations between triglycerides, fatty acids, glucose and the tricarboxylic acid cycle, and acetoacetate and the other ketone bodies

into the plasma – at a rate faster than they can be utilized in the muscles. In diabetes mellitus, glycerol-3-phosphate, derived from glucose entering the cell, is not available to take up the excess FFAs produced: it is possible that oxaloacetate (from amino acids etc.) has been excessively utilized for gluconeogenesis and is therefore less available to take up acetyl CoA. The excess acetyl CoA is converted to ketones.

Phospholipids

The most widely distributed phospholipids are the lecithins. They contain glycerol (as the base) and choline: sphingomyelins contain sphingosine as base, and no glycerol. A small quantity of phospholipid is present in food; this is probably hydrolysed before absorption. Phospholipid synthesis and degradation occur within each cell. Most of the lecithin in the plasma is derived from synthesis in the liver. The estimation of plasma phospholipid is technically difficult and rarely requested.

Cholesterol

Dietary cholesterol which is predominantly of animal origin is only absorbed to a limited extent though the amount entering the body in the chylomicrons is dependent on dietary intake. All cells are capable of cholesterol synthesis although the majority of endogenous cholesterol is produced in the liver from acetyl CoA via β-hydroxy-β-methyl glutaryl CoA. Liver synthesis is reduced by dietary cholesterol entering it and synthesis in peripheral tissues is reduced by cholesterol entering cells in LDL.

Cholesterol is removed from peripheral tissues by the HDL system and enters the hepatocyte cholesterol pool. Cholesterol cannot be degraded in any tissues of the body and excretion occurs from the hepatocyte into the bile as unchanged cholesterol or as cholic acid or chenodeoxycholic acid (bile salts). Cholesterol is held in solution in bile by bile salts and phospholipids. Bile salts are in part reabsorbed in the ileum and reused (enterohepatic circulation). Increased cholesterol excretion can be achieved by preventing this through chelation of bile salts in the gut when the liver increases the *de novo* synthesis thus reducing the hepatic cholesterol pool.

Hyperlipidaemia

Excessive circulating blood lipids may result from genetically determined disorders of lipoprotein metabolism: the primary hyperlipidaemias. More commonly, however, they result from excessive dietary intake of lipid or carbohydrate or

Table 6.1 Genetic classification of hyperlipidaemia

Disorders	Fredrickson type	Prevalence
Monogenic disorders		
Enzyme defects		
Familial lipoprotein lipase deficiency	I or V	<1:1 000 000
Transport protein defects		
Familial apoprotein CII deficiency	I or V	<1:1 000 000
Familial dysbetalipoproteinaemia	III	1:3000
Receptor defects		
Familial hypercholesterolaemia (heterozygous)	IIa	1:500
Possibly monogenic		
Familial combined hyperlipidaemia	IIa, IIb	1:300
Familial hypertriglyceridaemia	IV	1:500
Familial combined hyperlipidaemia	IIa, IIb	1:300
Polygenic		
Hypercholesterolaemia	IIa	

from the effects of another disease; these are the secondary hyperlipidaemias. In most cases it is impossible to distinguish primary from secondary hyperlipidaemia on the basis of the lipoprotein abnormality and indeed the disorders may share some of the same pathogenetic mechanisms. In addition systemic disorders may alter the expression of the primary hyperlipidaemias often greatly increasing their severity.

Hyperlipidaemia may be classified according to the lipoprotein abnormality observed in the plasma, as in the Fredrickson classification which is shown in Table 6.1, or by the pathogenetic mechanism resulting from either genetic changes or other diseases.

Primary hyperlipidaemias

A genetic classification of these disorders is shown (Table 6.1). The four monogenic disorders comprise defects in enzyme, transport proteins or receptors in which the molecular nature of the change and the mechanism of hyperlipidaemia is reasonably well understood. The other disorders are less well characterized but appear to be genetically determined.

Failure of peripheral tissue to catabolize chylomicrons and VLDL

The rare deficiencies of lipoprotein lipase and apoprotein C2 (this apoprotein activates lipoprotein lipase) both result in decreased peripheral tissue removal of chylomicrons and VLDL. The accumulation of chylomicrons after a fatty meal is most noticeable but there may be an associated increase in VLDL especially if dietary fat is restricted. Triglyceride levels are often markedly raised (as high as 20–30 mmol/l) with only slight to moderate increases in cholesterol (owing to the low cholesterol content of these particles) and the plasma appears lipaemic, the chylomicrons separating as a creamy layer on standing.

Accumulation of these large particles in the plasma does not give rise to atheroma but deposition of lipid in the skin results in eruptive xanthomata and in the liver, hepatomegaly. Abdominal pain is an important feature and acute pancreatitis may occur though the pathogenesis of this severe complication is unclear.

Failure of liver catabolism of chylomicrons and VLDL remnants

Familial dysbetalipoproteinaemia results from the inheritance of altered forms of apoprotein E which do not bind to the hepatic E receptor, or the B/E receptor. The result is decreased clearance from the blood of chylomicron and VLDL remnants. Although this form of dyslipidaemia in the homozygous form probably occurs in about 1 per cent of the population, overt hyperlipidaemia is much less prevalent and requires the additional presence of a primary or secondary hyperlipidemic tendency. The accumulation of VLDL remnants, so called β-VLDL, is a likely predisposing factor to atheroma and the development of characteristic tuberous xanthomas over the elbows and knees or cutaneous xanthomas in the palmar and digital creases. There is an increased plasma level of both cholesterol and triglyceride.

Increased plasma VLDL

Familial hypertriglyceridaemia is probably inherited as an autosomal dominant condition. The defect is unknown but may be due to increased liver VLDL synthesis or decreased clearance. It is uncertain whether this condition which increases over-production of VLDL triglyceride and also confers the risk of coronary artery disease. The plasma lipoprotein pattern is of an increased triglyceride causing lipaemia usually with a normal cholesterol but a low HDL, and this may be a factor in the increased atherogenic risk observed in some studies.

Familial combined hyperlipidaemia is thought to result from over-production of VLDL apoprotein B with or without an increase in triglyceride. Family studies show that about one-third of members have increases in plasma LDL levels, one-third have increases in VLDL and LDL levels, and the remaining one-third have increases in VLDL alone. There may be a single inherited metabolic defect though the triglyceride content of the VLDL particle is modified by other factors affecting VLDL turnover. Increased concentrations in the blood of LDL or cholesterol and apo-B rich VLDL increase the risk of atheroma.

Decreased peripheral tissue clearance of LDL

Familial hypercholesterolaemia (FH)
This is the best defined of the diseases causing hyperlipidaemia. It results from several defects in the cell surface receptor which is responsible for the uptake of LDL by peripheral tissue cells. Plasma levels rise in heterozygotes and much more so in rarer homozygotes. LDL is taken up by macrophages in the vessel wall (by the scavenger pathway), resulting in atheroma and in the skin causing xanthoma. Coronary artery disease develops prematurely with homozygotes rarely living beyond the age of 20 years and heterozygotes demonstrating an increased risk of death of between 10 and 50-fold. Heterozygote frequency is about 1/500 and homozygote frequency about 1/1 000 000. Plasma levels of cholesterol are raised often to levels between 10 and 20 mmol/l. Plasma triglyceride levels are normal or slightly raised.

Polygenic hypercholesterolaemia
It is common to find families with a tendency towards raised cholesterol levels. The members of such families have a spectrum of blood cholesterol concentrations from normal to moderately raised (10 mmol/l). This is probably due to more than one abnormality, and increased apoprotein B production in VLDL with decreased clearance of LDL by peripheral tissues have both been demonstrated. Environmental and dietary factors may influence the degree of hypercholesterolaemia which is the determining factor in the increased risk of arterial disease from which these people suffer.

Secondary hyperlipidaemia

A wide variety of diseases result in hyperlipidaemia though the mechanism is understood in only a few of these (Table 6.2).

Table 6.2 The causes of secondary hyperlipidaemia

Condition	Cholesterol	Triglyceride
Obesity		↑
Diabetes mellitus	↑	↑
Excessive alcohol intake		↑
Hypothyroidism	↑	↑
Nephrotic syndrome	↑	↑
Biliary obstruction	↑	
Renal failure		↑

Over-production of VLDL triglyceride with hypertriglyceridaemia is a feature of several conditions. Obesity results in a futile cycle of adipose tissue breakdown releasing free fatty acids which are converted by the liver to VLDL which enters the circulation and is hydrolysed by lipoprotein lipase in adipose tissue, allowing restorage of triglyceride. Diabetes mellitus due to decreased insulin results in increased entry of glucose into the liver (non-insulin dependent) and over-production of VLDL. Excess alcohol intake provides glucose for increased VLDL production.

Increased production of VLDL apo-B is a feature of hypothyroidism and the nephrotic syndrome. In the latter, hypoalbuminaemia results in increased synthesis of albumin and several other liver-derived transport proteins. Increased VLDL triglycerides may be seen in these conditions together with hypercholesterolaemia due to the accumulation of LDL resulting from over-production of apo-B.

Cholesterol rises in a unique form of hyperlipidaemia due to the regurgitation into the blood of cholesterol-rich biliary lipids which complex with albumin to form lipoprotein X in biliary obstruction.

Patients with renal failure, hypothyroidism or diabetes mellitus may have decreased lipoprotein lipase activity which results in an accumulation in the blood of both chylomicrons and VLDL. Over-production of VLDL triglyceride also occurs in these conditions and these factors combine to result in a raised VLDL level and triglyceride level.

Hypolipidaemia

Hypolipidaemia is much less common than hyperlipidaemia and it is often genetic in origin due to failure of lipoprotein produc-tion (Table 6.3). Absence of apoproteins results in inability to produce transport lipoproteins. Thus chylomicron deficiency results in accumulation of lipid in the gut and absence of VLDL and LDL causes accumulation of triglyceride in the liver and failure of delivery of cholesterol to peripheral cells. Failure of HDL production or of LCAT causes accumulation of cholesterol in peripheral tissues as it cannot be transferred to the liver.

Abetalipoproteinaemia is a recessively inherited condition causing failure of pro-duction of chylomicrons in the gut and absent VLDL production in the liver. As expected LDL is undetectable in the plasma. Malabsorption of fat results in growth retardation with steatorrhoea and accumulation of fat in the gut mucosa. Cell membranes throughout the body are abnor-mal due to a deficiency of dietary and liver-derived phospholipids. Progressive degeneration of the CNS is due to shortage of phospholipids.

Tangier disease is due to decreased production of apo-A and thus of HDL. It is characterized by accumulation of choles-terol esters in the reticuloendothelial sys-tem and other tissues.

Familial LCAT deficiency results in the accumulation of unesterified cholesterol in tissues which cannot be transferred to HDL for excretion. Premature atheroma, corneal opacity and renal damage are the predomi-nant features. Decreased LCAT production is seen in severe liver disease when plasma cholesterol levels may be low.

Table 6.3   Classification of hypolipidaemia according to plasma lipoprotein abnormality

Type	Prevalence	Lipoprotein abnormality
I	Rare	Chylomicrons
IIa	Common	LDL
IIb	Common	LDL + VLDL
III	Uncommon	Remnants
IV	Common	VLDL
V	Uncommon	VLDL + chylomicrons

Consequences of hyperlipidaemia

Atheroma

The mechanism of atherogenesis is incom-pletely understood but it is clear that high plasma levels of VLDL remnants containing apo-B (β-VLDL) and LDL are the prime culprits. The evidence suggests that these particles are taken up by macrophages in massive amounts at sites close to the blood such as vessel walls. Death of cholesterol-laden macrophages produces atheromatous

Table 6.4   Incidence of coronary heart disease after 10 and 20 years related to serum cholesterol concentration in men aged 33–49 years

Cholesterol concentration (mmol/l)	Rate/100	
	10-year incidence	20-year incidence
3.0–5.0	1.0	8.6
5.0–5.5	5.3	15.3
5.5–6.0	6.7	22.0
6.0–6.6	12.4	26.8
6.6–13.3	15.3	30.6

plaques. The removal of cholesterol from the macrophage by HDL is of great importance and the risk of atheroma is directly related to LDL cholesterol levels but inversely related to HDL cholesterol levels. In practice total plasma cholesterol is a major risk factor in atheroma, and prospective studies, as well as studies in different populations, have shown a clear relationship (Table 6.4). Even in the absence of a defined primary or secondary form of hyperlipidaemia this holds true. However, even if plasma cholesterol is at the lower end of the reference range this does not exclude the risk of atheroma or myocardial infarction. However it is now thought that dietary cholesterol intake itself is relatively unimportant as it has little effect on the levels of β-VLDL and LDL. Intake of saturated fat which induces LDL cholesterol synthesis by the liver appears to be much more important.

Xanthomatosis

Eruptive xanthomas which appear as clusters of itchy yellow nodules are associated with an increase in plasma concentrations of chylomicrons or VLDL. They rapidly reduce on correction of the plasma lipid abnormality.

Tuberous xanthomata are flat yellow plaques found over the elbows and knees together with deposition in palmar and digital creases that are typical of high levels of VLDL remnants such as occur in familial dysbetalipoproteinaemia.

Xanthelasma are flat pale lipid deposits in the periorbital area and together with the corneal arcus are usually unassociated with lipid abnormality but may, particularly in the young, be due to high levels of LDL.

Abdominal pain

Very high levels of triglyceride, present in VLDL or chylomicrons may result in abdominal pain and acute pancreatitis. The mechanism of this association is unclear.

Laboratory investigation of hyperlipidaemia

It is clear that an accurate diagnosis in both primary and secondary lipidaemia depends not only on clinical and family history but upon a knowledge of which particles are present in excess in the plasma. A simple approach is to measure the total level of cholesterol and triglyceride and to examine a fasting plasma that has stood overnight. In this way an increase in chylomicrons (creamy layer), VLDL (opalescence) and LDL (clear sample) will usually be identifiable. The presence of turbidity or opalescence in fresh plasma indicates a triglyceride level of greater than 4 mmol/l. Difficulty arises in distinguishing an increase in LDL together with VLDL from VLDL remnants. In both cases the cholesterol and triglyceride will be raised and the plasma will appear turbid. In addition moderately raised levels of cholesterol may be due to LDL (common) or HDL (rare).

Electrophoresis of plasma will separate HDL, LDL, VLDL remnants, VLDL and chylomicrons from each other and they may be recognized by staining the electrophoretic separation with fat-soluble dyes. VLDL remnants characteristically form a broad β-band. This is however a non-specific finding and should be confirmed by apo-E measurements or phenotyping of the apo-E protein by isoelectric focusing. A raised HDL as a cause of a moderately increased cholesterol may be suspected on electrophoresis by an increased α-band but should be confirmed by the measurement of HDL cholesterol. Final characterization of primary hyperlipidaemia may require separation of the lipoprotein classes by ultracentrifugation and the measurement of their lipid or apoprotein content.

Treatment of hyperlipidaemia

Hypercholesterolaemia if mild may be treated by dietary restriction of cholesterol (ineffective) and reduction of saturated fat intake. If this is insufficient cholesterol excretion may be enhanced by chelating bile salts in the gut with cholestyramine which induces bile salt synthesis and depletes the hepatic cholesterol pool. This results in decreased LDL cholesterol levels (due to a decrease in production of VLDL cholesterol).

Hypertriglyceridaemia is often remedied by decreased dietary fat intake, reduction of obesity and, in the case of increased VLDL production, decreased carbohydrate intake. Recalcitrant cases may be treated with clofibrate which both decreases VLDL production and increases clearance.

It is important to appreciate that cholesterol levels may be low for some weeks following severe illness such as myocardial infarction, probably due to alterations in the dietary saturated fat intake. Conversely the stress of illness may cause an acute increase in VLDL triglyceride levels, probably as a result of catecholamine secretion. Blood samples for analysis in patients with myocardial infarction should thus be taken either immediately before changes have occurred or on leaving hospital when the patient is on a normal diet.

Deposition disorders

Fatty liver

The liver is important in lipid metabolism, and in many diseases the fat content of the liver may be greatly increased. In starvation and diabetes mellitus, FFAs are produced in large amounts, and the excess which is not oxidized is deposited in the liver; liver function is not seriously impaired. Disturbance of liver metabolism by various poisons results in extensive fatty deposition in the liver without changes in plasma lipids: such toxins may be endogenous (as in toxaemia of pregnancy) or exogenous chemicals (e.g. carbon tetrachloride).

The lipotropic factors are substances responsible for the normal hepatic metabolism of lipids. Choline is an important dietary lipotropic factor, whose essential function may be the synthesis of lecithin.

Methionine, which can donate methyl groups for choline synthesis, is also lipotropic; consequently protein deficiency predisposes to the development of fatty liver.

Chronic alcoholism

Fatty liver is common. Alcohol has a direct hepatotoxic action (causing an early rise in plasma γ-glutamyl transferase), quite apart from the protein- and choline-deficient, and vitamins B-deficient, high-energy diet of alcoholic patients. There is diversion of fatty acids from oxidation to esterification as triglycerides. These both accumulate in the liver, and are released into the plasma as the characteristic Type IV hyperlipidaemia.

The lipidoses

Certain rare inborn errors of metabolism are associated with a disturbance of synthesis or disposal of intracellular lipid, whilst the levels of circulating lipids are within the reference range. They are generally due to specific enzyme defects within lysosomes which can be identified in affected organs. The same enzyme defects can often be found in leucocytes, which may be a simpler tissue to obtain for analysis; or in fetal cells to be cultured for prenatal diagnosis.

Hand-Schuller-Christian syndrome is a group of disorders in which cholesterol is deposited in the skin (where xanthomas appear), brain, spleen, lymph glands, and bones. *Niemann-Pick's disease* is a group of familial diseases in which the phospholipid sphingomyelin may be deposited throughout the body, particularly in liver and spleen. *Gaucher's disease* is a group of familial diseases in which a glycocerebroside called kerasin is deposited in the reticuloendothelial system: there is also a high plasma acid phosphatase, derived from the Gaucher's cells. *Tay-Sach's disease* (infantile amaurotic idiocy) is a familial disease in which an unusual cerebroside, called ganglioside, is deposited in the central nervous system. *Wolman's disease,*

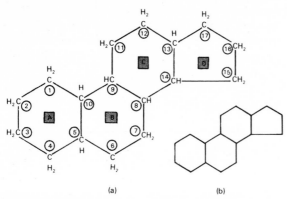

(a)   (b)

Fig. 6.6   (a) Structure of the saturated unsubstituted cyclopentenophenanthrene ring compound, with the carbon atoms numbered and the rings labelled. (b) Shorthand formula of this compound

with hepatosplenomegaly, has cholesterol esters and triglycerides as the abnormally stored components.

Other disorders

Hurler's syndrome (formerly called *gargoylism*) is a typical carbohydrate storage disorder. There is mucopolysaccharide deposition in brain, liver, reticulum cells and many tissues, and secondarily glycolipid deposition in the nervous system. Detection in the urine of excess sulphated mucopolysaccharides (dermatan sulphate and heparan sulphate), which have not been normally broken down, serves as a biochemical screening test.

The steroids

The steroids are a group of substances of great medical and pharmacological importance which contain the cyclopentenophenanthrene ring system (Fig. 6.6). Sterols are steroids which contain a hydroxyl(-OH) group. The steroids differ from one another in the spatial arrangement of their rings and side chains, as well as in the nature of the side chains attached to the rings.

The classes of steroids of interest in clinical biochemistry include cholesterol, precursors of vitamin D, bile acids, adrenocortical hormones, oestrogens, progestogens, and androgens.

Further reading

Lewis B. Plasma lipid concentrations: the concept of normality and its implications for detection of high risk. *J Clin Pathol* 1987; **40**: 1118–27.

Schaefer EJ, Levy RI. Pathogenesis and management of lipoprotein disorders. *New Engl J Med* 1985; **312**: 1300–10.

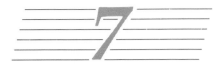

Protein and Nitrogenous Metabolism

Objectives

In this chapter the reader is able to

- revise the general biochemistry of protein anabolism and catabolism
- revise the biochemistry of the non-protein nitrogen components of plasma: urea, urate, creatine, creatinine, amino acids, ammonia
- study the factors controlling protein digestion and absorption
- study the causes and significance of an altered plasma urea concentration
- study the causes of an altered plasma urate concentration
- study the causes of an altered plasma and urine creatine/creatinine concentrations
- study the classification of aminoacidurias.

At the conclusion of this chapter the reader is able to

- understand the control of nitrogen balance, and investigate a patient with negative nitrogen balance
- investigate a patient with gout
- understand the presentation and investigation of patients with the main congenital aminoacidurias.

General metabolism of protein

Dietary protein

A reasonable protein intake for an adult is about 1 g/kg body weight per day, and the actual intake varies according to prosperity and local custom. Protein should provide 11 per cent of the energy requirements – the energy value being about 17 kJ (4 kcal) per gram. The protein allowance for children must be higher to allow for the protein needs of growth: 2–3 g/kg for infants and about 2 g/kg for children have been advocated. In late pregnancy and during lactation the mother requires at least 1 g of protein/kg body weight.

The diet must not only contain sufficient protein, but the protein intake must be qualitatively adequate. Proteins are sometimes classified as first-class and second-class proteins. First-class proteins are capable of supporting growth by themselves, since they contain all the essential amino acids in the right proportion and because these amino acids are readily released by digestion. An amino acid is called 'essential' if it must be provided in the diet because the metabolic requirements for it cannot be met by synthesis within the body. Second-class proteins do not satisfy these conditions. Most animal proteins are first-class proteins, a notable exception being gelatin, a hydrolysate of collagen. Most second-class proteins are vegetable proteins.

A normal good vegetarian diet, which includes the animal products milk and eggs, contains ample first-class protein. A vegan diet, which is a strictly vegetarian diet omitting all animal products, does not lead to protein deficiency in adults with no extra needs if the diet is otherwise satisfactory.

Effects of dietary protein deficiency

A diet which is moderately inadequate in protein may give rise to fatigue and irritability before symptoms of gross protein deficiency develop. In children protein deficiency retards growth. At all ages prolonged protein deficiency causes anorexia and apathy, muscle wasting, loss of weight (which may be masked by retention of water), poor wound healing, and slow convalescence after illness. There is often a hypochromic anaemia because synthesis of haemoglobin is impaired. Retention of water causes oedema, due, in part to hypoalbuminaemia. There is a progressive fall in the concentrations of the plasma albumin and transferrin. Alteration in the immunoglobulins is variable, depending on the presence of infections. The plasma concentrations of prealbumin and retinol-binding protein are reduced early, and these have also been suggested as markers of protein malnutrition (p. 108). Liver damage and pulmonary tuberculosis are diseases to which protein-deficient subjects are particularly vulnerable. Damage to the liver occurs because diets which are deficient in protein lack methionine which protects the integrity of liver cells. There are also usually associated deficiencies of the vitamin B complex (p. 110). In kwashiorkor, the protein-deficiency syndrome of children in the tropics who live mainly on carbohydrate, oedema and other symptoms are associated with skin and hair changes. Failure to produce proteolytic digestive enzymes reduces further the small amount of available amino acids. In marasmus, with protein and carbohydrate deficiency, there is less oedema or skin and hair change than in kwashiorkor.

In protein deficiency, 1 kg of body weight loss means about 30 g of nitrogen loss. For biochemical assessment of protein malnutrition, plasma albumin concentration is the most available measure. It is however affected by changes in plasma volume, distribution and the decreased liver synthesis accompanying inflammation (p. 95). In addition albumin does not respond to rapid changes in nutritional status, and for this the measurement of plasma prealbumin and retinol-binding protein (p. 97) is better.

Protein digestion, absorption, and metabolism

No digestion of protein takes place in the mouth. Gastric juice contains pepsinogen; hydrochloric acid activates pepsinogen to pepsin, and provides the optimum pH for pepsin to digest some protein to polypeptides. However, peptic activity is not essential for protein digestion which proceeds satisfactorily when pepsin is deficient, or is inactive due to achlorhydria. Pancreatic juice contains trypsinogen which is activated to trypsin by enterokinase, secreted by the small intestine; chymotrypsin(ogen) and carboxypolypeptidase are other pancreatic proteolytic enzymes. The alkaline pancreatic juice provides the optimum pH for their activity. Trypsin digests protein to short-chain peptides and to a limited extent to free amino acids. In chronic pancreatic disease (p. 167) protein digestion may be severely impaired due to trypsin deficiency. A group of intestinal peptidases completes the digestive process by converting peptides to amino acids, though some peptides are not fully digested.

Amino acids are readily absorbed by the small intestine. Peptides and possibly even traces of protein can be absorbed undigested. Intestinal disorders associated with malabsorption of fat, such as coeliac disease (p. 170), do not generally cause severe impairment of amino acid absorption.

Simple nitrogenous materials, such as ammonium ions, are readily absorbed.

The amino acids pass in the portal system to the liver and deamination of a proportion of these takes place there. The amino groups and carbon residues may be used for synthesis of other amino acids, or other nitrogenous compounds. Amino acids as such are not stored: the surplus amino groups are eventually converted to urea, whilst the carbon residues are metabolized in the common metabolic pool and converted to carbohydrate or lipid, or oxidised (p. 48). The remainder are used for protein synthesis in the cells.

Protein stores

Amino acids from tissue protein turnover are metabolized in the same way and form a common pool. A few hours after administration of labelled amino acids, isotopic nitrogen can be found in all the protein of the body – and an average adult turns over about 400 g of protein daily. The half-life of plasma albumin is about 19 days, of muscle protein is about 5 months, and of collagen is many years. When a cell dies, its protein is reconverted by lysosomes to amino acids. Although some proteins are more stable than others there is no specialized storage product or deposit protein. There is in the tissues a certain amount of labile protein, which can be utilized when protein intake is insufficient and which serves to delay the development of the protein-deficiency state.

Nitrogen excretion

A normal adult ingests 10–15 g (0.7–1.1 mol) of nitrogen per day in dietary protein – on average 1 g (70 mmol) nitrogen is derived from about 6 g protein. Faecal excretion of nitrogen is relatively constant, within the limits of 1–1.5 g (70–110 mmol)/24 h, despite changes in the protein intake. It consists partly of nitrogenous material of the diet which has not been digested or absorbed, partly of end-products of nitrogenous metabolism which have been actively excreted into the bowel from shed intestinal cells or digestive enzymes, and partly of intestinal bacterial nitrogen. In total protein starvation the faecal nitrogen excretion is about 0.5 g (35 mmol)/24 h. Most of the endogenous protein from intestinal secretion (principally enzymes) and des-

quamated cells, which amounts to about 50 g protein per 24 hours, is digested and reabsorbed. Some urea which diffuses into the gut is hydrolysed (by bacterial ureases) to ammonia which is reabsorbed.

Undigested muscle fibres are not seen in the faeces of healthy persons on a normal diet, but they may be found when faecal nitrogen is increased as a result of impaired protein digestion. Changes in nitrogen excretion in pancreatic disease and in coeliac disease are discussed in Chapter 15.

Losses of nitrogen in hair, desquamated skin and sweat, are about 1 g (70 mmol)/ 24 h. Nitrogen is also lost in the menstruum. The remainder of the end-products of nitrogen metabolism are excreted in the urine. Only traces of protein (p. 115) are found in the urine in health. Nitrogen is principally excreted in the urine as urea, and with a fall or rise in the protein intake the principal excretory change is in the urine urea; the normal urine urea nitrogen is 80 to 85 per cent of the total urinary nitrogen. Lesser quantities of nitrogen are lost in the urine as ammonia, as amino acids, as urate (the end-product of purine metabolism), as creatinine (the end-product of creatine metabolism in muscles), and as many other identified and unidentified nitrogenous compounds. There is probably no net gain or loss of nitrogen through the lungs as nitrogen or ammonia gas.

Nitrogen balance

A normal adult is in nitrogen equilibrium. A positive nitrogen balance is defined as a state in which the body is retaining nitrogen; and a negative nitrogen balance is a state in which nitrogen is being lost. When the nitrogen intake is reduced (but still remains above the minimum need for equilibrium) a negative nitrogen balance will occur for a few days, then equilibrium will be restored at the lower intake level. When the nitrogen intake is increased the opposite happens: after a short period of positive balance a new steady state is reached.

Effect of hormones

Anabolism and catabolism of protein are to a certain extent under hormonal control. Adrenocorticotrophic hormone and the glucocorticoids, and excess thyroxine, promote protein catabolism and a negative nitrogen balance. Growth hormone, the androgens, to a less extent the gonadotrophins and oestrogens, and thyroxine and insulin in physiological amounts, promote protein anabolism and a positive nitrogen balance.

Positive nitrogen balance

This develops during growth and pregnancy, and during recovery from periods of negative nitrogen balance, e.g. in the late postoperative period, if protein intake is adequate. A positive balance develops as a result of the action of excess of the nitrogen anabolic hormones, either due to excess secretion (e.g. of growth hormone in acromegaly) or when given as treatment (e.g. during androgen therapy). An increase of tissue protein is more likely if the diet is adequate in energy with sufficient carbohydrate, fat and vitamins of the B group.

Negative nitrogen balance

Deficient protein intake

When the protein intake falls below the appropriate minimum, a negative balance develops within 48 h. A negative balance also develops when protein uptake is just within the minimum needed for equilibrium and this protein is not qualitatively adequate or the total energy intake is deficient.

Table 7.1 Factors that affect nitrogen balance

Stimulate protein anabolism	*Stimulate protein catabolism*
GH	Glucocorticoids
'Normal' T_4	Excess T_4
Androgens	ACTH
'Normal' insulin	
Positive nitrogen balance	*Negative nitrogen balance*
Growth	Protein deficiency
Pregnancy	Trauma, burns etc
Late postoperative	Protein losing states

Diminished protein digestion

This results from deficiency of proteolytic enzymes due to chronic pancreatic disease (p. 167).

Diminished absorption of amino acids

This develops in severe intestinal disease, or after massive resection of the small intestine (p. 169), or as part of an inherited transport defect (p. 171).

Increased protein catabolism

When there is excess breakdown of body protein much of the released nitrogen is excreted and negative balance develops unless protein intake is increased. Certain types of endocrine disturbance directly increase protein catabolism – negative balance develops in thyrotoxicosis or Cushing's syndrome and sometimes at the menopause, and after prolonged treatment with adrenocorticotrophic hormone or glucocorticoids. In wasting processes, including diabetic coma, increased tissue protein breakdown is found. After severe trauma (due to wounds, fracture, or surgical operation), during the course of a severe acute or chronic infection, in malignant disease, or after rest in bed, negative nitrogen balance usually develops, which is partly due to excessive secretion of glucocorticoids and a proteolysis-inducing factor, interleukin-1, which causes skeletal muscle catabolism (p. 232). However, patients who have been on a protein-deficient diet show less negative nitrogen balance after injury. Equilibrium may be restored after easily mobilized tissue proteins are exhausted.

Increased protein loss

At each normal menstrual period up to 20 g of protein may be lost, but this is insufficient to cause protein depletion provided an adequate diet is taken. Considerable quantities of protein may be lost from severely burned areas (10–50 g/day), or into urine in the nephrotic syndrome or in myelomatosis. In exfoliative dermatitis, skin protein loss may be 20 g/day. Even larger quantities of protein may be lost as pus, for example from a lung abscess or through osteomyelitic sinuses. The *protein-losing enteropathies* are a group of disorders of the gastrointestinal tract, including malignant and inflammatory disease, in which there is excessive leakage of plasma proteins into the gut; although much of the protein is digested and absorbed, the liver cannot resynthesize sufficient extra protein (p. 148) and hypoproteinaemia occurs. Formation of ascites causes loss of protein from the circulation into the ascitic fluid (p. 159) where exchange is slow, though this loss is not strictly from the body until the ascites is tapped; peritoneal dialysis may remove 25 g of protein per day. In many diseases loss of protein happens at the same time as increased protein catabolism.

In haemorrhage (to the exterior or into the gut), albumin and globulins, as well as haemoglobin, are lost: 1 l of blood contains about 200 g of protein, so donation of a 'unit' of blood takes off about 80 g of protein.

Balance tests

Accurate measurement of the state of nitrogen metabolism may be done by means of a metabolic balance test. In this the patient's intake and output of nitrogen (or calcium, or other metabolite) are measured over an accurately timed period – usually between three and seven days. A balance test requires skilled ward staff, preferably in a special metabolic unit, to ensure that the dietary intake is controlled, and that all the patient's faeces and urine are collected at the correct times.

The result, in the case of a nitrogen balance, will be expressed as

Average 24 h intake A g (or A' mmol) nitrogen
Average 24 h output in urine B g (or B' mmol) nitrogen
Average 24 h output in faeces (or other source of loss) C g (or C' mmol) nitrogen
24 h balance = A−(B+C) g
(or A' − (B' + C') mmol)

The test has a reproducibility of about ±10 per cent, which is accounted for by slight short-term variations in the patient's nitrogen metabolism, and by errors in collection and analysis. A variation in nitrogen balance during the course of the test may be shown by a change in values for plasma nitrogenous components such as albumin, urea and creatinine.

Such tests are now rarely used but calculation of nitrogen balance in patients on parenteral nutrition (p. 112) may be important to ensure adequate intake. Losses of nitrogen may be calculated as shown in Table 7.2.

Table 7.2 Calculation of nitrogen loss

Nitrogen in urine (g) = 24 h urine urea (mmol) × 0.028

plus

24 h urine protein (g) ÷ 6.25
Nitrogen loss from skin/faeces (g) = 2.5 per 24 h

Change in body nitrogen (g) = Change in plasma urea (mmol/l) × total body water (body weight, kg × 0.6) × 0.028

Nitrogen in urine (mmol) = 24 h urine urea (mmol)

plus

$$24 \text{ h urine protein (g)} \times \left(\frac{71}{6.25} \right)$$

Nitrogen loss from skin/faeces (mmol) = 175 per 24 h

Change in body nitrogen (mmol) = change in plasma urea (mmol/l) × total body water (body weight, kg × 0.6)

Biochemical aspects of treatment

A state of prolonged negative nitrogen balance usually demands treatment, but it may prove impossible to correct the negative nitrogen balance fully by protein replacement, particularly when it is due to increased catabolism of protein or to renal loss. The balance will return to normal when the cause, for example protein loss, is removed, and the lost protein is replaced. In all circumstances the patient must be placed on as high a protein diet as possible, and the diet must also be adequate in its energy and vitamin content – 150 g of protein per day is generally suitable. If the patient is unable to digest ordinary protein food, suitably prepared milk protein or protein hydrolysate (an amino acid mixture) may be given by continuous intragastric drip.

Intravenous therapy

When protein loss cannot be replaced fully by oral feeding, protein substitutes (for general nutrition) or plasma (to replace plasma proteins) can be given intravenously. This method of administration may be used when there are disorders of amino acid absorption.

Commercial amino acid preparations are available for intravenous use that, given adequate carbohydrate and appropriate electrolytes, can maintain a positive nitrogen balance and may be used in connection with major surgery (p. 112). A 10 per cent solution (casein hydrolysate or a mixture of synthetic L-amino acids) provides about 12 g (340 mmol) of nitrogen per litre.

A number of 'indices' based on laboratory and clinical data have been derived to assess the response to nutritional replacement. Most of them compare the plasma albumin and transferrin concentrations, together with skinfold thickness and skin test reactivity to an antigen to which the patient has been previously sensitized. The serum prealbumin concentration is a sensitive and rapid indication of energy and protein intake (p. 110).

Non-protein nitrogen constituents of the blood and urine

The term blood non-protein nitrogen (NPN) comprises urea, urate, creatine and creatinine, amino acids, and minor components, and in health about 50 per cent of this consists of urea. Total NPN is no longer estimated, for changes in the plasma urea usually reflect adequately total protein catabolism, and the other NPN constituents are estimated individually when required.

Urea

Urea is formed, almost solely in the liver, from the catabolism of amino acids, and is the main excretion product of protein metabolism. The concentration of urea in the blood plasma represents mainly a balance between urea formation from protein catabolism and urea excretion by the kidneys: some urea is further metabolized and a small amount is lost in the sweat and faeces.

The reference range for plasma urea concentration throughout adult life is generally taken as 2.5–7.1 mmol/l. The plasma urea increases with age even in the absence of detectable renal disease, although the changes are certainly due to alteration of renal function; concentrations are also slightly higher in men. A single protein meal does not significantly increase the plasma urea. The fasting plasma urea is higher on a high protein diet than on a low protein diet. Urea diffuses freely, at the same concentration, through all the body water. The *whole blood* urea level is 5 to 10 per cent lower than the *plasma* urea level. In the USA results are still often expressed as blood urea nitrogen (BUN), the reference range being 7.5–22 mg/100 ml – about half of urea is nitrogen.

High plasma urea

This is one of the commonest abnormal findings in chemical pathology, and its causes are classified below.

Increased tissue protein catabolism associated with a negative nitrogen balance

This occurs for example, in fevers, wasting diseases, thyrotoxicosis (p. 201), diabetic coma (p. 55), or after trauma (p. 231), or a major operation. Unless the increase of protein catabolism is very large or there is concomitant renal damage, then urinary excretion will dispose of the excess urea and there will be no significant rise in the plasma urea.

Excess breakdown of blood protein

In leukaemia release of leucocyte protein contributes to the high plasma urea. Erythrocyte haemoglobin and plasma proteins can be released into the gut due to bleeding from gastrointestinal disease, and then digested: there is often an associated low blood volume with secondary impairment of renal function.

Diminished excretion of urea

This is the commonest and most important cause and may be prerenal, renal, or postrenal. In general the plasma urea (and creatinine) does not rise significantly until the glomerular filtration rate has fallen to about 50 per cent of normal, though it will happen sooner in the presence of tissue protein breakdown. A fall in the peripheral blood pressure (e.g. in shock), or in cardiac output (e.g. in congestive heart failure), or a low plasma volume (e.g. in sodium depletion from any cause, including Addison's disease (p. 212)), diminishes the renal plasma flow. Glomerular filtration of urea falls and there is a rise in the plasma urea. When there is no permanent renal structural damage, the plasma urea will return to normal when the renal perfusion is restored to normal (p. 119).

Renal disease of any kind that is associated with a fall in the glomerular filtration rate causes a high plasma urea. This is seen in acute and in chronic renal failure. In the complete absence of renal function the plasma urea will rise at a rate of between 7 and 20 mmol/l every 24 h depending on whether there is increased protein catabolism. The plasma urea is normal in the uncomplicated nephrotic syndrome.

Obstruction to the outflow of urine, for example by an enlarged prostate gland, leads to a high plasma urea by causing both increased reabsorption of urea through the tubules, and diminished filtration.

Azotaemia is the term sometimes used for a high blood/plasma urea concentration. *Uraemia* (as opposed to azotaemia) is the name given to the clinical syndrome that develops when there is marked nitrogen retention due to renal failure (p. 120).

Low plasma urea

This is sometimes seen in late pregnancy; it may be due to increased glomerular filtration, diversion of nitrogen to the fetus, or to water retention. In acute hepatic necrosis the plasma urea is often low, as amino acids are not further metabolized. In cirrhosis of the liver the low plasma urea is due partly to diminished synthesis, and partly to water retention (p. 158): the water retention of inappropriate antidiuretic hormone secretion lowers the plasma urea (p. 195). A low plasma urea caused by a high rate of protein anabolism may develop during intensive androgen treatment e.g. for carcinoma of the breast. The plasma urea falls in long-term protein malnutrition. Long-term replacement of blood loss with intravenous dextran, glucose, or saline may lower the plasma urea by dilution.

Uric acid/urate

Uric acid is the principal end-product of nucleic acid and purine metabolism in man via a final common pathway of conversion of xanthine, by means of xanthine oxidase, to uric acid. The reference range for plasma urate in men is 0.12–0.42 mmol/l, and in women is 0.09–0.36 mmol/l, increasing slightly with age. The plasma urate level is little affected by variation in the purine content of the diet and represents a steady state between endogenous production and urinary tubular secretion, for filtered urate

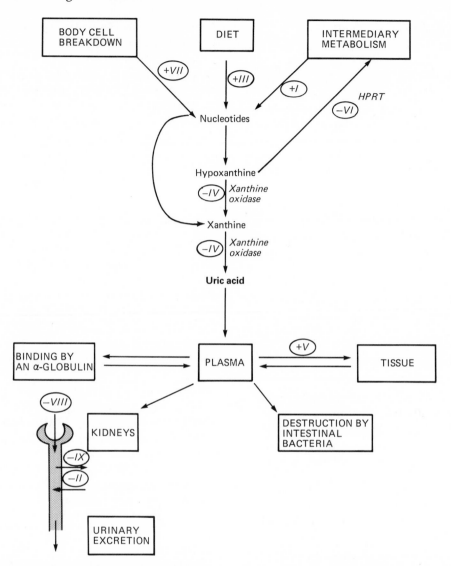

Fig. 7.1   The main pathways of uric acid metabolism and transport. The alterations in gout and other disorders, indicated by roman numerals, are described in the text

is normally almost wholly reabsorbed: there is also some intestinal destruction (Fig. 7.1).

Raised plasma urate

Gout
Uric acid is relatively insoluble in body fluids and urate crystals are easily deposited in various tissues if the plasma concentration rises above about 0.60 mmol/l (see Fig. 7.1(V)). Gout is a painful mono- or polyarthritis due to deposition of sodium/urate in the joints sometimes accompanied

by soft tissue deposits known as tophi. In gout the urate pool in the body may be over 10 times the normal 6 mmol. Shortly before, and during, an acute attack of gout the plasma urate rises, to a maximum level of about 0.9 mmol/l, this investigation being usually all that is necessary for diagnosis. In chronic gout, between acute episodes, the plasma urate is usually in the high normal range and moderately raised values may be found in male relatives of patients. The cause of the high plasma urate in gout is not known in all cases, but it is usually due to increased endogenous synthesis of uric acid as an inborn metabolic defect (Fig. 7.1(I)), though sometimes there is reduced renal tubular secretion (Fig. 7.1(II). Alcoholism, perhaps by producing lactic acidaemia (Fig. 7.1(II)), and an abnormal diet high in purines (Fig. 7.1(III)), may be predisposing factors: some patients have hypertriglyceridaemia, associated with obesity. Allopurinol is used in the treatment of gout because, as a xanthine oxidase inhibitor (Fig. 7.1(IV)), it blocks the synthesis of uric acid and allows excretion of purines as the more soluble xanthine. Secondary renal damage due to urate deposition, sometimes with calculi, may develop. Clinical gout occurs mainly when the raised urate is due to a metabolic defect and not usually when secondary to other conditions. Urate crystals may be found in synovial fluid of the affected joints, and their identification may be of diagnostic value.

In pseudogout, which is not a disorder of urate metabolism, the synovial fluid contains crystals of calcium pyrophosphate dihydrate.

Lesch-Nyhan syndrome

This rare inborn error of metabolism is due to deficient resynthesis of purines to nucleotides (Fig. 7.1(VI)), due to deficiency of hypoxanthinephosphoribosyl transferase and consequent excess production of uric acid. There is a high plasma and urine urate with urinary calculi, and sometimes gout, with mental retardation, self-mutilation, and other symptoms.

Breakdown of cell nuclei

A raised plasma urate is found in leukaemia (especially acute leukaemia during treatment), in myeloproliferative diseases including polycythaemia, in pernicious anaemia, and sometimes in psoriasis (Fig. 7.1(VII)). Treatment with adrenocorticotrophic hormone or corticosteroids, whose protein catabolic action accelerates nuclear breakdown, or with cytotoxic drugs, causes a rise in the plasma urate. Treatment with allopurinol may be necessary to avoid renal damage due to urate deposition.

Renal causes

In glomerular failure, or when there is obstruction to the outflow of urine, urate is retained with the other blood nitrogenous constituents (Fig. 7.1(VIII)). It may be difficult to distinguish between renal failure with hyperuricaemia or renal damage secondary to hyperuricaemia. The high plasma urate which can develop in eclampsia in the absence of azotaemia or uraemia may be due to a specific renal lesion or to altered uric acid metabolism. Both ketotic and lactic acidosis (p. 42) may increase the plasma urate by diminishing its renal tubular secretion, as do frusemide and thiazide diuretics (Fig. 7.1(II)). The high values (sometimes causing gout) which occur during acute starvation are due to a combination of cell breakdown and ketoacidosis.

Estimation of plasma urate is important principally for the diagnosis and monitoring of gout and toxaemia in pregnancy and in the management of leukaemia or cytotoxic therapy.

Low plasma urate

This results from urinary loss in renal tubular syndromes (p. 121), or from failure of synthesis.

Xanthinuria

This rare inborn error of metabolism is due to deficiency of xanthine oxidase (Fig. 7.1(IV)). The plasma and urine urate are therefore low, and excess xanthine and hypoxanthine may present as xanthine calculi.

Urine uric acid

This estimation is of little value; the quantity excreted depends to a large extent on the purine content of the diet and is normally 1.5–4.5 mmol/24 h. Uric acid is generally retained before an acute attack of gout, and the urine uric acid rises during the attack – though these changes are not diagnostic. Treatment of chronic gout with (e.g.) probenecid (which diminishes tubular reabsorption of many compounds, including uric acid) lowers the plasma urate, and improves the patient's condition, by increasing the urinary excretion of uric acid (Fig. 7.1(IX)). Adrenocorticotrophic hormone or glucocorticoid therapy increases uric acid excretion partly by diminishing tubular reabsorption, and partly by increasing endogenous synthesis of uric acid.

Creatine and creatinine

Creatine is principally synthesized in the liver and kidneys from amino acids. It is taken up from the bloodstream largely by the muscles, where it is phosphorylated and acts as the energy source of muscle – almost all the creatine of the body is in the muscles. The end-product of creatine metabolism in muscles is its anhydride, creatinine, which is metabolically inactive; creatinine diffuses into the plasma and is excreted in the urine. Abnormalities of plasma creatine and creatinine concentration and of their urinary excretion, reflect either changes in skeletal muscle metabolism (p. 229) or in renal function (p. 128).

Plasma values

In renal failure creatinine is retained with the other NPN constituents of the blood normally excreted by the kidneys. Plasma creatinine is widely used to measure failure of renal excretory function, especially in conditions where there is non-renal alteration of urea metabolism (e.g. a low protein diet). In general, if the plasma creatinine is less than about 90 μmol/l then glomerular filtration is normal. The reciprocal of plasma creatinine is a more reliable index than creatinine clearance (p. 129) in monitoring glomerular function in patients with chronic renal disease.

Urine values

The urinary excretion of creatinine in health in an individual varies little from day to day on a meat-free diet. A diet containing meat increases the 24 h urine excretion by up to 60 per cent. The magnitude of urinary creatinine excretion is considered to be representative of the total active muscle mass, and estimation of urinary creatinine is used as a very rough check of the accuracy of collection of successive 24 h urine specimens.

Amino acids

Estimations of all the individual amino acids can be done quantitatively, using expensive automatic apparatus for column chromatography, or semi-quantitatively by simple chromatography.

Plasma values

The plasma amino acid levels are raised in severe renal failure together with the other NPN constituents of the blood. The most marked rise in the plasma amino acid levels is a result of acute hepatic necrosis, because of impaired conversion of amino acids to urea. A slight rise is found in acute hepatitis and cirrhosis, or after severe shock. The plasma amino acid levels are lowered by the protein anabolic effects of growth hormone or androgens.

Aminoaciduria

Glutamine/glutamic acid, glycine, serine, and alanine are normally detected by simple chromatography of the urine of a healthy adult.

Excess urinary amino acids (Fig. 7.2) can be classified as below.

Overflow aminoaciduria without primary renal disease

The plasma amino acid levels may be high or normal, depending on their thresholds (p. 117). The overflow aminoacidurias comprise conditions detailed in (a) and (b) below.

(a) *Acquired secondarily to other diseases.* Generalized aminoaciduria is seen regularly, to a mild extent, in cirrhosis and other chronic liver diseases, and to a marked

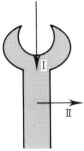

Fig. 7.2 Renal processing of amino acids. Plasma amino acids are filtered at the glomerulus (I); increased plasma amino acids results in 'overflow aminoaciduria'. Failure to reabsorb amino acids (II) can be due to defective transport mechanisms or damage to the renal proximal tubules

extent in acute hepatic necrosis. Slight aminoaciduria is seen in wasting diseases, eclampsia, and when there is tissue damage, and also after infusion of amino acids (p. 84).

Hydroxyproline is an amino acid specific to collagen, and is normally excreted in small amounts. Hydroxyprolinuria is a measure of increased collagen turnover, which includes bone growth, Paget's disease, hyperparathyroidism, and malignant disease of bone. The measurement is more sensitive as the hydroxyproline/creatinine ratio.

(b) *Caused by an inborn error of metabolism.* There are a considerable number of congenital disorders due to enzyme defects, in which one or more amino acids are incompletely degraded, and may present as themselves or metabolites in increased concentration in the plasma, and are excreted in excess in the urine. The examples given are disorders which have specific symptoms and involve different types of amino acid.

Phenylketonuria, a group of related disorders of aromatic amino acids, is in its main variety the commonest aminoaciduria and causes mental retardation; the high phenylalanine also inhibits tyrosinase and lessens melanin formation. Due to deficiency of phenylalanine hydroxylase (phenylalanine 4-monooxygenase), or other related enzymes, the normal conversion of phenylalanine to tyrosine is almost absent and phenylalanine and its derivatives, particularly phenylpyruvic acid and phenyllactic acid, are present in excess. Partial deficiency, due to delayed maturation with prematurity, gives the benign hyperphenylalaninaemia. Phenylketonuria should be screened for in all children by detecting a raised blood phenylalanine (from the normal <0.2 mmol/l to >12 mmol/l in homozygotes) at 6 to 14 days after birth, either using the Guthrie test which is a microbiological assay, or by chemical estimation. Screening by detection of the excess phenylketones in urine (p. 259), though much simpler, is not satisfactory as there are many false negatives and has been abandoned. Further brain damage may then be avoided in affected children by the use of phenylalanine-free diet. By the use of a modified Guthrie test, or by chromatography, it is possible to screen for many other inborn errors of amino acid metabolism.

Alkaptonuria involves the further metabolism of tyrosine and is relatively benign. Due to deficiency of homogentisate 1,2-dioxygenase, homogentisic acid cannot be further oxidized. It is deposited in cartilage causing arthritis, and excreted in the urine, which turns dark brown on becoming alkaline or oxidized.

Homocystinuria involves sulphur-containing amino acids. In one variety, due to deficiency of cystathionine β-synthase, methionine, homocysteine, and homocystine (excreted in the urine) are present in excess. Diverse clinical features include mental deficiency, skeletal abnormalities, and dislocation of the lens.

Maple syrup urine disease involves branched-chain amino acids. Due to deficiency of 'branched-chain ketoacid decarboxylases', there is a block in the metabolism of valine, leucine and isoleucine. These and their derivatives accumulate in blood and urine (which smells like maple syrup). Mental damage is severe: its special interest is that treatment by an artificial diet may be possible.

In other (sometimes transient) disorders of which tyrosinaemia and histidinaemia are examples, symptoms may be absent or not certainly attributable to the metabolic error.

Organicacidurias, which include isovaleric acidaemia, are important as a cause of metabolic acidosis in the neonate.

Renal aminoaciduria due to diminished tubular reabsorption

These comprise the renal tubular syndromes, with normal or low plasma amino acids and can be divided into groups as detailed in (a) and (b) below.

(a) *Aminoaciduria due to specific inborn disorders of the tubular reabsorptive mechanisms,* e.g. cystinuria (p. 121). In some syndromes the same transport defect is present in the small intestine.

Hartnup disease involves intestinal and renal transport of neutral amino acids, especially tryptophan. The patient has nicotinic acid deficiency (p. 111), with skin and mental effects of pellagra, and cerebellar symptoms. Urinary indoles also are increased, derived from intestinal tryptophan.

(b) *Non-specific aminoaciduria secondary to acquired proximal renal tubular damage.* The *Fanconi syndrome* describes generalized proximal tubular damage with aminoaciduria and other reabsorptive defects; it is commonly due to exogenous toxins (e.g. heavy metal poisoning, p. 113) or to abnormal metabolites (e.g. galactose-1-phosphate, p. 57).

In the rare *cystinosis* the primary defect is of cystine metabolism, with deposition of excess cystine intracellularly in various tissues including liver and kidney.

Ammonia

A small quantity of ammonia is formed in and absorbed from the gut, and is metabolized in the liver. There is a little ammonia in the peripheral blood of normal subjects – but analysis is difficult.

Up to about 350 µmol/l of ammonia nitrogen can be found in the blood in cases of liver failure particularly when there are neurological complications (p. 160) – analysis is of doubtful clinical value. Excess ammonia is formed because of gastrointestinal bleeding, and this is unable to be converted to urea by the damaged liver. After a porto-caval shunt the blood ammonia rises further, but sterilization of the gut prevents synthesis of ammonia.

Further reading

Balis ME. Uric acid metabolism in man. *Adv Clin Chem* 1976; **18**: 213–46.

Schriver CR, Rosenberg LE. *Aminoacid Metabolism and its Disorders*. Philadelphia: W.B. Saunders, 1973.

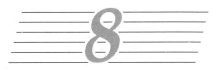

Plasma Proteins

Objectives

In this chapter the reader is able to

- revise the biochemistry and immunology of the plasma proteins
- study the factors controlling plasma albumin concentration
- study the causes of changes in the main immunoglobulin fractions
- study the causes of congenital and acquired changes in other plasma proteins.

At the conclusion of this chapter the reader is able to

- investigate a patient with hypoalbuminaemia
- understand the protein and related changes in multiple myeloma and other paraproteinaemias
- understand the protein changes in inflammation
- understand the clinical value of estimation of protein in plasma and of serum electrophoresis.

Introduction

Plasma contains over one hundred proteins with a great diversity of physicochemical characteristics and physiological roles. Most have a role to play in plasma or tissue fluids but some merely represent cellular or tissue proteins shed into the circulation as a result of degradative processes. However, while the functions of many of them are now known or suspected, there remains a

group, some of which are present at high concentrations in plasma, about whose function little or nothing is known.

Many diseases are associated with changes in the concentration, structure, or function of plasma proteins. Most often these changes result from the pathological processes of the disease but in some cases, such as genetic deficiencies, they may be the cause. Despite the enormous biochemical and physiological interest in the plasma proteins, their measurement in the laboratory only provides clinically useful information in a limited number of circumstances.

The laboratory investigation of plasma proteins

Electrophoresis

In a suitable alkaline buffer solution (usually pH 8.6) the serum proteins become $(sodium)^+$ $(proteinate)^-$. The ions of the different serum proteins have different mobilities in an electric field, and these depend on their net charge, size, and shape.

Simple electrophoresis on cellulose acetate or agarose gel is a useful initial investigation upon which the choice of specific protein measurements can be made. Some 12 to 13 groups of serum proteins can be assessed by electrophoresis; typical patterns are shown in Figs. 8.1 and 8.2. Variations in the density of bands allows an approximate assessment of the concentration of these proteins, while variations in their electrophoretic mobility

Fig. 8.1 Examples of electrophoresis of serum and plasma. **A** Bisalbuminaemia, no other abnormality in serum. **B** Fast albumin due to bilirubin binding, slightly raised γ-globulin level (increased polyclonal IgG) with β–γ fusion (increased IgA) in serum from a patient with cirrhosis. **C** Plasma from a patient with α_1-antitrypsin deficiency with early cirrhosis resulting in a polyclonal increase in IgG. **D** Low albumin, slow α_1-antitrypsin variant, decreased α_2- and increased γ-globulin in serum from a patient with chronic aggressive hepatitis. Modified with permission from Whicher JT. *Br J Hosp Med* 1980; **24**: 348–60

Fig. 8.2 Further examples of serum electrophoresis. **A** Nephrotic syndrome: prealbumin is visible; albumin is not noticeably decreased; there is a marked increase in the intensities of the α_2-zone and β-lipoprotein; and the γ-globulin reflects a hypercatabolic decrease in IgG secondary to the protein-losing state. **B** Simple acute-phase response with increased α_1- and α_2-globulins. **C** Paraprotein in a patient with myeloma: there is immune suppressions with a pale γ-area and decreased albumin; the split β-zone is due to a transferrin variant. **D** IgG paraprotein. Modified with permission from Whicher JT. *Br J Hosp Med* 1980; **24**: 348–60

reflect changes in charge due to alterations in structure or in the concentration of substances bound to the proteins. Electrophoretic separations should be interpreted in the laboratory; densitometric scans are of little value except for the quantitation of paraproteins, where they are the most reliable method.

Individual proteins can be identified on all electrophoretic separations by the application of specific antisera to the separation or a 'blot' made from it. The techniques are known as immunofixation and immunoblotting.

Immunochemical measurements

The quantitative measurement of some plasma proteins provides useful clinical information and this is listed in Table 8.1. Proteins present at concentrations above 1 mg/l can be measured by simple radial immunodiffusion, the Laurell rocket technique, nephelometry, or turbidimetry. Proteins present at lower concentrations are measured by techniques such as radioimmunoassay, fluorescence immunoassay, or enzyme immunoassay. There is wide variation in results achieved by different methods and in different laboratories. It is important to relate measurements to an appropriate reference range based on the same calibration material.

The quantitation of plasma proteins by assays based upon their function are now confined to the investigation of proteins with functional abnormalities undetectable by immunochemical or electrophoretic techniques.

Metabolism of plasma proteins

Synthesis

Most plasma proteins are synthesized in the hepatocyte, although there is increasing evidence for the concomitant production of

Table 8.1 Information gained from zone electrophoresis or specific plasma protein measurement in certain pathological processes

	Zone electrophoresis	Plasma protein measurement
Immune deficiency	Severe IgG deficiency visible as decreased γ-globulin. Other deficiencies not reliably detected	IgG IgA concentration IgM
Immune response	Hypergammaglobulinaemia. Oligoclonal responses in immune deficiency, autoimmune disease, and chronic infections. β–γ fusion due to increased IgA	Many patterns of IgA and IgM increases are of little use. IgA increases in cirrhosis and biliary obstruction, though other tests are more useful IgM increase in cord blood indicates intrauterine infection
Immunocytoma	Paraprotein in serum Detection of Bence Jones protein in urine	Paraprotein measurement for monitoring progress. β_2-Microglobulin measurement for monitoring progress Measurement of immunoglobulins other than paraprotein to assess immune paresis
Allergy	–	Total IgE Specific IgE
Inflammation	Acute phase increase in α_1 and/or α_2 bands (INSENSITIVE)	C-reactive protein increased
Complement activation	Decreased β_2-band in fresh EDTA plasma (UNRELIABLE)	C_3 and C_4 levels may be decreased Complement activation products detectable
Decreased hepatic protein synthesis	Decreased prealbumin and transferrin (β_1). Fall in haptoglobulin (α_2) occurs in liver disease; may be due to accompanying haemolysis (UNRELIABLE)	Decreased levels of albumin and retinol-binding protein or prealbumin
Poor nutrition	Decreased albumin, prealbumin and transferrin (β_1) (UNRELIABLE)	Decreased albumin, prealbumin, transferrin, and retinol-binding protein
Protein-losing states	Decreased albumin and transferrin (β_1): increased α_2 (α_2-macroglobulin) in selective protein loss such as occurs from the kidney (UNRELIABLE)	Albumin in plasma and in urine in nephrotic syndrome. IgG/albumin clearance ratio useful in childhood nephrotics
Intravascular haemolysis	Decreased haptoglobin	Decreased haptoglobin
Genetic variants		–
Albumin	Bisalbuminaemia.	
α_1-Antitrypsin	α_1-Band absent or of altered mobility. Normal α_1 with raised α_2 may represent heterozygous deficiency or vasculitis	Low α_1-antitrypsin
Caeruloplasmin	–	Low caeruloplasmin

some proteins in other tissues. Hepatic synthesis of many plasma proteins is controlled by specific regulatory mechanisms. For example, albumin synthesis depends upon the oncotic pressure in the hepatic extracellular fluid; synthesis of many proteins involved in inflammation is under control of humoral factors released from macrophages. The synthesis of some plasma proteins in the liver is very sensitive to the supply of amino acids. Several hormones have important effects, not only on the synthesis of proteins in the liver but also on their volume of distribution and catabolism.

Distribution

Proteins in the plasma pass continually from the vascular to the extravascular space. If venous constriction is prolonged, and maintained while blood is being collected, then the concentration of plasma proteins and protein-bound substances (e.g. calcium) may be raised by 10 to 15 per cent because water is lost from the plasma in the veins. Prolonged recumbency may lower the plasma protein concentrations by about 10 per cent, due to redistribution of water in the body.

Catabolism

Plasma protein breakdown probably occurs to a greater or lesser extent in most cells of the body. All capillary endothelial cells are capable of degrading plasma proteins during pinocytic transport across the cells; the amino acids so released are then used by tissues. This is the main mechanism of albumin catabolism. Those plasma proteins which contain carbohydrate side-chains, e.g. transferrin, are probably catabolized largely in the liver. Low molecular weight proteins and protein fragments produced by proteolysis are filtered through the renal glomerulus and reabsorbed and catabolized in the proximal tubules. Between 2 and 4 g of plasma proteins are filtered and broken down in this way daily. Several proteins, such as IgG and complement components, are broken down within macrophages as a result of forming complexes or cleavage products which are phagocytosed or pinocytosed following binding to surface receptors.

Total protein

The reference range for total protein, estimated in *serum*, is 62–80 g/l; this excludes fibrinogen, which is included in *plasma* proteins. The measurement of the total protein content of plasma may be used to assess degree of hydration of the patient and is required if the calculation of the total globulin is to be made. Total protein content is most commonly measured by the biuret technique which depends on a colour reaction between an alkaline copper reagent and the CO–NH peptide linkages.

Albumin

Physiology (Fig. 8.3)

Albumin is a single polypeptide chain with a molecular weight of about 66 000. It is synthesized in the liver where it amounts to 30 per cent of hepatic protein synthesis, though less than a third of hepatocytes appear to be synthesizing albumin at any one time. Albumin synthesis is sensitive to amino acid supply and thus nutritional state. In protein depletion with adequate energy albumin synthesis may be depressed by 60 per cent or more.

Albumin comprises more than half the total protein of plasma which represents about 40 per cent of the exchangeable albumin pool. The normal half-life of circulating albumin is 19 days.

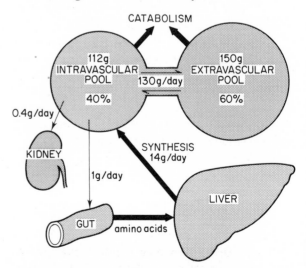

Fig. 8.3 Albumin distribution and metabolism. Quantities of albumin in g/day are approximate values for a 70 kg individual. Reproduced with permission from Whicher JT, Spence C. *Ann Clin Biochem* 1987; **24**: 572–80

Albumin acts as a binding protein for a wide range of substances in plasma forming a reservoir to buffer rapid changes in the free moiety. Calcium and fatty acids are of particular importance.

Albumin changes in disease

Hyperalbuminaemia
This occurs together with an increase in total protein and packed cell volume in dehydration.

Hypoalbuminaemia
This is usually due to a combination of an expanded extravascular pool, protein loss, and to a lesser extent decreased synthesis and increased endogenous catabolism.

Unless albumin synthesis ceases entirely, it will take some 10 days to 2 weeks for the plasma albumin level to fall below the reference range. This is due to the relatively long half-life, 19 days, of plasma albumin and to the fact that the absolute rate of catabolism falls with decreasing concentration. This is highlighted by the common observation that patients with paracetamol overdose (p. 242) and massive hepatic necrosis rarely show hypoalbuminaemia before they die 5 to 7 days later.

Albumin provides about 80 per cent of the plasma colloid osmotic pressure and decreased levels result in oedema which is almost always present with albumin levels below 20 g/l. The loss of intravascular volume associated with such oedema results in secondary aldosteronism (p. 212). Patients with hypoalbuminaemia have less sites available for drug binding and this may result in higher free levels of drugs with consequent toxic effects (p. 238). Similarly, neonates with hyperbilirubinaemia (p. 157) will be more susceptible to kernicterus if plasma albumin is low. In contrast, hypoalbuminaemia does not result in a disturbance of calcium balance as the free or ionized calcium is under rapid regulatory control from the parathyroid glands (p. 177). The fact that nearly 50 per cent of the plasma calcium is albumin-bound does however mean that in hypoalbuminaemia the total calcium measured will be low (p. 174).

Malnutrition
Albumin synthesis is sensitive to the dietary supply of amino acids and inadequate dietary intake is a cause of hypoalbuminaemia. However 24 weeks depletion of protein and energy sufficient to cause a 25 per cent loss in body weight is only accompanied by a 7 per cent fall in plasma albumin concentration. Thus although severe protein malnutrition such as kwashiorkor (p. 108), may result in plasma albumin levels of less than 20 g/l, it is probable that this only occurs over an extended period of time and is due in part to infection. Plasma albumin level is not a very reliable indication of nutritional status.

Liver disease
The plasma albumin is frequently low in liver disease but it must not be assumed that this reflects hepatic synthetic capacity and thus liver cell mass (p. 154). Only 15 to 20 per cent of hepatocellular mass is necessary to synthesize normal amounts of albumin. Hypoalbuminaemia in patients with normal or increased synthesis is due to an increased total exchangeable pool, probably accompanied by increased catabolism. In portal hypertension a significantly higher proportion than normal of newly synthesized albumin enters the hepatic lymph rather than the bloodstream and passes across the liver capsule into the ascitic fluid (p. 159). Also in chronic liver disease fluid retention results in an expansion of the extravascular pool.

Inflammation
Any form of tissue damage, such as myocardial infarction, trauma, surgery or infection, there is an increase in the plasma acute phase proteins (p. 99) and a fall in the plasma concentration of albumin, transferrin, prealbumin and retinol-binding protein (Fig. 8.4). The plasma albumin concentration usually falls by about 20 per cent over 2 to 3 days. Albumin synthesis falls by as much as 70 per cent and probably results

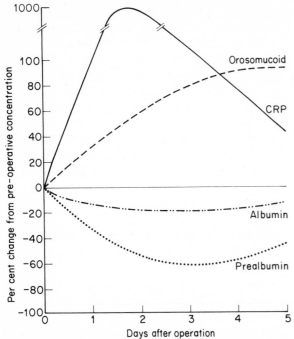

Fig. 8.4 The acute phase response to the trauma of uncomplicated surgery. C-reactive protein (CRP) and orosomucoid both increase in serum concentration, whereas albumin and prealbumin show a negative acute phase response

from a diversion of hepatic protein synthesis towards the acute phase proteins and away from proteins not involved in the inflammatory response. This does not however explain the rapid change in plasma concentration which results from alterations in capillary permeability and lymphatic return causing a shift of albumin from the intravascular to the extravascular pool. This acute phase response accompanies many complications and detracts from the value of plasma albumin measurement as a means of assessing decreased albumin synthesis or increased loss.

Analbuminaemia

This is a rare genetic defect, probably recessively inherited. Homozygotes have very low levels of plasma albumin (0.16–2.4 mg/l) although family members, assumed to be heterozygotes, have normal albumin levels presumably because 50 per cent of albumin synthetic capacity is more than enough to maintain normal plasma levels, perhaps as a result of feedback stimulation.

Genetic structural variants of albumin

Known as the paralbumins, these are of two kinds: those which show altered charge and thus electrophoretic mobility (e.g. bisalbuminaemia, Fig. 8.1) and those which have a tendency to polymerize.

Increased albumin loss

Many of the conditions giving rise to increased albumin loss are also associated with inflammation, accompanied by decreasing albumin synthesis and a shift of albumin into the extravascular pool.

Nephrotic syndrome

Glomerular damage may result in increased permeability of the glomerular basement membrane to plasma proteins (p. 122), giving rise to some of the lowest plasma albumin levels seen in any condition and may result in the oedema which characterizes the nephrotic syndrome. Plasma albumin concentrations of 5–10 g/l are not unusual in children. The degree of hypoalbuminaemia does not correlate well with the amount of proteinuria, and urinary albumin excretion is the most useful method of assessing healing of the glomerular lesion.

Gastrointestinal protein loss

This normally accounts for 2 to 15 per cent of albumin degradation. In many conditions this is increased, sometimes to as much as 35 per cent, and may result in hypoalbuminaemia. It is caused either by loss of inflammatory exudate in conditions such as Crohn's disease, ulcerative colitis, and coeliac disease (p. 170), or by leakage of lymph into the gastrointestinal lumen as in constrictive pericarditis, and lymphoma and carcinoma with lymphatic obstruction.

Burns

The fall in plasma albumin following thermal burns results from a combination of loss from superficial tissues, decreased synthesis associated with the acute phase response, and shifts in distribution from the intravascular to the extravascular compartments.

Other transport proteins

There are a number of proteins present in plasma, besides albumin, whose primary role appears to be the binding of other molecules. These proteins, like albumin, serve to transport substances which are relatively insoluble in plasma or to provide a pool of bound and biologically inactive molecules to buffer changes in the level of active free hormones or metals. In addition, toxic substances may be rendered inactive by protein binding. Many of the binding proteins are known to interact with specific cellular receptors which affect the metabolism of the bound ligand (Table 8.2).

Prealbumin and retinol-binding protein

These circulate in plasma as a complex which has a single binding site for tri-iodothyronine and thyroxine and carries about 20 per cent of the plasma concentration of these hormones. Retinol-binding protein binds retinol and the complex formation with prealbumin stabilizes this interaction thus providing the vitamin A transport system of plasma (p. 110).

Both prealbumin and retinol-binding protein show decreased plasma concentrations in association with both the acute phase response and decreased amino acid supply to the liver. Retinol-binding protein is probably the most sensitive indicator of nutritional deficiency (p. 108) and shows significant falls even after 24 h deprivation of protein and energy. For this reason it is widely used as a method of assessing the response to parenteral (p. 112) and other forms of nutrition where it shows a much more rapid response than albumin. It is however important to appreciate that in common with albumin, transferrin, and prealbumin, it is a negative acute-phase reactant whose synthesis falls in association with inflammation. This proves the major limitation in the use of such measurements to assess nutrition, as many of these patients have injury or infection resulting in an acute phase response.

Transferrin

This is the major iron transport protein of plasma, binding iron with such efficiency that only micromolar quantities of free iron remain in the plasma (p. 145). This may be of importance as an antimicrobial effect by restricting the availability of free iron to bacteria in tissue fluids. The clinical significance of transferrin and other iron-binding proteins is considered in Chapter 13.

Caeruloplasmin

This is a blue-coloured glycoprotein containing six copper atoms, synthesized in the liver. It may function as a copper transport

Table 8.2 Transport proteins

Protein	Substance bound or transported	Page
Albumin	Fatty acids	70
	Bilirubin	150
	Some drugs	238
	Metal ions such as Ca^{2+}	175
	Cu^{2+}	146
Transferrin	Fe^{2+}	145
Caeruloplasmin	Cu^{2+}	146
Thyroxine-binding globulin	T_3, T_4	200
Sex-hormone binding globulin	Testosterone, oestradiol,	221, 217
Transcobalamins	Vitamin B_{12}	144
Prealbumin ⎱	⎰ T_3, T_4	200
Retinol-binding protein ⎰	⎱ Vitamin A	110
Apolipoproteins	Lipids	68

protein or, in inflammation, as an oxygen-radical scavenger.

The most widely known genetic cause of low caeruloplasmin levels is Wilson's disease (p. 146).

Proteins of inflammation

Mechanisms in inflammation

Inflammation is a series of cellular, vascular, and humoral events resulting from any form of tissue damage which facilitates the phagocytosis of foreign material or dead host tissues. Many plasma proteins have key roles to play in mediating and regulating this process (Table 8.3). Inflammation is initiated by the activation of several mediator pathways of which the most important are plasma proteins. Low molecular weight compounds such as prostaglandins are also involved. Trauma may result in activation of the coagulation, kallikrein, kinin, plasmin and complement pathways. The interaction between these sytems results from the broad spectrum of proteolytic action possessed by a number of the component enzymes. This tangled network of proteases produces important inflammatory mediators which result in the cellular events of inflammation: vascular permeability, vasodilatation, chemotaxis and opsonization. All of these facilitate the arrival of macrophages and polymorphonuclear leucocytes and enhance the phagocytosis of tissue debris or foreign material such as micro-organisms. The process may be activated by antibody–antigen complexes or bacterial endotoxins activating complement directly. Several proteins also act to inhibit the proteases of the mediator pathways while others inhibit proteases released by phagocytosing leucocytes.

Inflammation results in several systemic responses (p. 231) which act to potentiate the cellular and biochemical events occurring in the tissues. The most well studied of these are fever, leucocytosis and the acute-phase response. Fever enhances antibody production, phagocytosis and bacterial destruction by accelerating specific enzymatic reactions. Leucocytosis provides increased numbers of phagocytic cells which are attracted from the bloodstream by chemotactic factors emanating from the site of inflammation. The acute phase responses (p. 231) which act to potentiate synthesis and thus plasma and tissue levels of many of the proteins involved in inflammation. It is a physiological mechan-

Table 8.3   Roles of plasma proteins in inflammation

Protein	Possible role	Acute phase response
Mediators		
Complement proteins	Opsonization	↑↑
	Chemotaxis	
	Vascular permeability	
Coagulation proteins	Clotting	↑↑
	Formation of matrix for repair	
Plasminogen	Activates many proteases	
	Breaks down fibrin	↑
C-reactive protein	Binds to many macromolecules activating complement. Acts as an opsonin	↑↑↑
Inhibitors		
Inhibitors in complement and coagulation pathways	Control mediator pathways	↑↑
α_1-Antitrypsin	Proteases from phagocytes	↑↑
Other protease inhibitors	Proteases from phagocytes	↑↑
Scavengers		
Haptoglobin	Scavenger haemoglobin	↑↑
Caeruloplasmin	May scavenge oxygen radicals	↑

ism to provide increased concentrations of these key proteins which may be consumed performing their functions at the site of inflammation. Fever and the acute phase response appear to be mediated by cytokines, including interleukin-1, derived from macrophages.

Acute phase protein synthesis is switched on very rapidly in the liver following the onset of inflammation. Within six hours much of the synthetic capacity of the hepatocyte is diverted towards synthesis and secretion of the most rapidly produced of these proteins.

The acute-phase proteins (Fig. 8.4)

The inflammatory proteins which show acute-phase behaviour, i.e. increase in plasma concentration following and during inflammation, are widely measured in the clinical laboratory as a means of diagnosing and monitoring a variety of inflammatory diseases. Individual proteins of this group are also of importance because changes in their structure or concentration may relate to other disease processes. The major acute-phase proteins are indicated in Table 8.3.

In general acute-phase protein measurements are more specific and sensitive as indicators of inflammation than erythrocyte sedimentation rate (ESR) or plasma viscosity. They may be used in the following clinical situations:

1 to indicate underlying organic disease when symptoms are equivocal, e.g. back pain, abdominal pain, joint pain;
2 to monitor the response of chronic inflammatory diseases to treatment, e.g. rheumatoid arthritis, polymyalgia, Crohn's disease;
3 to indicate intercurrent infection when microbiological diagnosis may be slow or unreliable, e.g. intra-abdominal infection following gastrointestinal surgery, septicaemia in leukaemics on cytokine therapy, meningitis in neonates.

The complement system

The complement system comprises a group of proteins which, following activation, interact with each other in a sequential fashion to produce biological effector molecules which facilitate the elimination of antigens, cells and particles by phagocytosis. Complement components are chemotactic for phagocytes, act as opsonins and cause vascular permeability. They may also result in lysis of cells. Antibody–antigen complexes and proteases activate the 'classical' pathway while bacterial cell surfaces (endotoxins) activate the alternative pathway. Complement is thus an important part of the antibody-mediated immune defence mechanism. However, its role extends far beyond this as it is a key inflammatory mediator system and is responsible for opsonization of bacteria in the absence of antibody.

α_1-Antitrypsin

Two systems of protease inhibitors exist in plasma, one comprising the specific inhibitors of the inflammatory mediator pathways, and the other serving to inhibit proteolytic enzymes released from macrophages and polymorphonuclear leucocytes during phagocytosis. α_1-Antitrypsin inhibits collagenase and elastase released from the neutral granules of polymorphonuclear leucocytes. α_1-Antichymotrypsin inhibits cathespin G from the same source. α_2-Macroglobulin is a broad-spectrum inhibitor able to inhibit serine, cysteine, aspartic and metalloproteases.

α_1-Antitrypsin, in common with most other plasma proteins, shows genetic polymorphism. Unlike many of the others however, several common variants of this protein appear to result in disease.

Some 30 different allotypes have now been described. The genotypes are designated by the prefix Pi (for protease inhibitor) and a letter. Two distinct disease processes are associated with the deficient allotypes of α_1-antitrypsin. The PiZZ variant results in liver accumulation of protein and cirrhosis (p. 158). PiZZ, PiSZ variants result in low plasma concentrations of α_1-antitrypsin and *chronic obstruc-*

tive pulmonary disease (COPD).

The lung is constantly exposed to protease release by alveolar macrophages and polymorphonuclear leucocytes phagocytosing inhaled debris. Under normal circumstances, the elastase and collagenase are adequately inhibited by α_1-antitrypsin in tissue fluids. In deficiency however, progressive proteolytic damage to the elastic tissue of the lungs results in emphysema with subsequent chronic bronchitis and the clinical picture of COPD. The incidence of the disease in the severely deficient phenotypes is variable and depends on the level of particulate inhalation, the frequency of lower respiratory tract infections, and in particular on cigarette smoking. Cigarette smoke has been shown to oxidize the thiol at the active centre of α_1-antitrypsin rendering the small amounts present functionally ineffective. In general about 50 per cent of PiZZ individuals are found to have COPD by the age of 30 years rising to 90 per cent at the age of 50 years. These severe genetic deficiencies of α_1-antitrypsin form a group of the commonest inborn errors of metabolism in Europeans.

Haptoglobin

Haptoglobin binds one molecule of haemoglobin forming a complex which is rapidly cleared from the circulation by the reticuloendothelial system and in particular the Kupffer cells of the liver. The plasma level of haptoglobin of 1–3 g/l is able to bind 0.75–1.75 g/l of haemoglobin (p. 139).

Decreased plasma haptoglobin occurs in any condition which is associated with significant intravascular haemolysis. The senstivity of plasma haptoglobin concentration to a haemoglobin load is exemplified by the fall in haptoglobin commonly seen in athletes after cross-country running. All forms of acute and chronic haemolysis may be associated with low haptoglobin levels and the protein is often undetectable. In the absence of inflammation and an acute phase response the plasma haptoglobin level is as sensitive as radiochromium–labelled red-cell survival for detecting intravascular haemolysis and thus provides a useful diagnostic test.

Tissue-derived proteins and oncofetal proteins

Some of the proteins present in low concentrations in plasma are cell membrane proteins shed into the blood during cell membrane turnover or as a result of cell death. A number of other trace proteins, the oncofetal proteins, are produced by tumours as a result of depression of genes coding for fetal proteins or proteins not normally produced by the tissue of origin of the tumour (p. 233).

β_2-Microglobulin

β_2-Microglobulin is a low molecular weight protein comprising a single polypeptide chain of 100 amino acids with a molecular weight of 11800. It is found in every body fluid and is synthesized by all nucleated cells. It is known to be identical to the B-chain of the HLA complex and is probably shed from the cell membrane into tissue fluids as a result of cell turnover. The main source of the plasma β_2-microglobulin is not clear although raised plasma levels are seen in most inflammatory conditions and in malignancies of the lymphoid system. It is catabolized in the kidney where it is freely filtered at the glomerulus with over 99 per cent of this filtered load being reabsorbed and catabolized in the proximal renal tubule (p. 122).

The proteins of immune defence

Immunoglobulins

The immune system can be divided into two functionally co-operative but developmentally independent pathways of lymphoid differentiation. T-lymphocytes derived from the thymus are a functionally diverse group of cells concerned with immune regulation and antigen elimination, whereas B-lymphocytes synthesize and secrete antibody.

The immunoglobulin molecules which mediate antibody activity have a remarkable structural heterogeneity and their synthesis is an adaptive response triggered by the antigenic configuration with which they interact. They have the capacity to complex with specific antigens and interact with both cells and other circulatory plasma proteins to produce a series of biological effector functions which results in the elimination of antigen, e.g. complement activation, binding to macrophages.

Immunoglobulin structure

All immunoglobulins consist of one or more basic units comprised of two identical heavy (H) chains, each of molecular weight about 50000, and two identical light (L) chains, each of molecular weight about 20000, joined together by a variable number of disulphide bonds. The *N*-terminal parts of both H- and L-chains contain the variable amino acid sequence (V region) which determines antigenic specificity, thus allowing each molecule to have two antigen combining sites. The remaining parts of the H-chains (constant or C region) have certain structural and thus antigenic differences which allow their classification. They also contain the effector sites which allow the molecules to interact with cells and complement.

Specific immunoglobulins

IgG is a monomer of the basic immunoglobulin unit and is present in high concentrations in all extracellular fluids. It accounts for 75 per cent of the plasma immunoglobulins and may be thought of as the antibody which protects the tissue spaces and, in particular, aggregates or coats small soluble proteins such as bacterial toxins. The newborn child has a high level of IgG of maternal origin which declines to a very low level by about six months postpartum (Fig. 26.1; p. 248).

The bulk of *IgA* synthesis occurs in plasma cells located beneath the mucosa of the gastrointestinal tract, the respiratory tract, the skin and in exocrine glands where it is produced as a dimer. It is present in colostrum where it protects the newborn infant from gastrointestinal infection.

Plasma *IgM* consists of a pentamer of basic immunoglobulin units and because of its very high molecular weight is largely confined to the vascular space. IgM is the first immunoglobulin to be secreted after stimulation of the B-lymphocyte to differentiate to form the plasma cell.

IgE is a monomeric immunoglobulin which is rapidly bound to the cell membranes of mast cells and basophils. The combination of antigen with this cytophilic antibody causes degranulation of these cells with release of kinins, histamine and prostaglandins which cause vascular permeability and smooth muscle contraction. Such phenomena are responsible for asthma and hay fever.

IgD together with IgM constitute the membrane receptor of the B-lymphocyte.

Immunoglobulin deficiency

Primary deficiencies

Primary genetic immunoglobulin deficiencies are rarer than secondary deficiencies. They are most often sought in children with recurrent infections or a combination of infections with allergy. They are, however, occasionally fortuitously recognized in the laboratory during serum protein electrophoresis performed for other purposes.

Decreased synthesis of most or all immunoglobulin classes has been described in a number of the familial syndromes.

Selective immunoglobulin deficiency may affect all classes but primary IgA deficiency is by far the commonest with an incidence of about 1/500 of the population. It is usually symptomless but may be associated with gastrointestinal, respiratory or renal infections. Affected people have a higher incidence of immune-complex disease.

The early diagnosis of immune deficiency is important if adequate treatment is to be instituted. Simple electrophoresis is inadequate as selective immunoglobulin deficiencies may be difficult to recognize; quantitative immunoglobulin measurements are essential.

Secondary deficiencies
Secondary deficiencies are more common than primary deficiencies and may occur in about 4 per cent of hospital patients.

Transient immunoglobulin deficiency in the newborn is important in premature babies. The majority of maternal IgG crosses the placenta in the last trimester of pregnancy and the baby's own IgG does not reach acceptable levels until 6 months after birth. Those babies born before 22-weeks gestation will have severe hypogammaglobulinaemia and those born before 34 weeks may develop it within two months.

IgG has the longest half-life of the plasma immunoglobulins (22 days) and thus any factors increasing immunoglobulin catabolism will affect IgG most. Protein loss results in an increased endogenous catabolism of most plasma proteins and while proteins synthesized in the liver also show a marked increase in synthesis, immunoglobulins do not. The result is a progressive decrease in IgG which may be reduced to very. low levels even despite small external losses, as for example in a selective glomerular proteinuria (p. 122).

Suppressed synthesis of immunoglobulins affects IgM most, then IgA and IgG least. The commonest cause is lymphoid neoplasia which may take months or years to manifest its effect. There is a very real risk of infection in this type of immune deficiency as B-cell proliferation is suppressed and the immune response to antigenic challenge is progressively lost.

Polyclonal hypergammaglobulinaemia

When an immune response occurs, whether due to infection, immune complex diseases, or autoimmune conditions, a polyclonal increase in plasma immunoglobulins is seen. In certain conditions the immunoglobulin classes respond in a selective manner and may provide some clinically useful information.

Immunoglobulin measurements are useful in diagnosing infection *in utero* and in the first six months of life. The rise in IgM after birth is due to the first antigenic challenges met by the infant. Intrauterine infection may give rise to IgM production before birth with high levels of cord blood IgM. This is useful in the diagnosis of congenital toxoplasmosis, rubella, cytomegalovirus, herpes simplex and syphilis.

The differential pattern of immunoglobulin response may be useful in liver disease. A very high plasma IgM is typical of primary biliary cirrhosis (p. 159). IgG is raised in chronic aggressive hepatitis (p. 158), while IgA is typically high in the macronodular Laennec type of cirrhosis, regardless of the cause.

IgE measurement has a role in asthma and allergy, particularly in children where high IgE levels are associated with extrinsic asthma and a good response to certain therapeutic regimes. The measurement of antigen-specific IgE gives similar information to skin tests in the identification of substances to which a patient is allergic.

Monoclonal hypergammaglobulinaemia

Immune stimulation usually results in a more or less heterogenous population of B-lymphocytes undergoing multiplication and differentiation to form plasma cells producing immunoglobulins directed against a wide range of antigenic configurations. This is because almost all macromolecular antigens have multiple antigenic sites. Not infrequently however, a raised γ-globulin may be of restricted heterogeneity due to the response of relatively few B cell clones to antigenic challenge. Such oligoclonal gammopathies show faint bands or zones in the gamma region on electrophoresis. Such restricted heterogeneity of immune response is a characteristic of chronic immune stimulation where there is progressive switching-off of B-cell clones leaving only those with the highest affinity receptors for the antigen still producing immunoglobulin. Occasionally, monoclonal immunoglobulin production results.

Malignant proliferation of a single clone of immunoglobulin-producing B-cells may also result in the production of a homogeneous population of immunoglobulin molecules with reference to class, sub-class, light-chain type and charge. Such 'paraproteins' form discrete bands on electrophoresis (Fig. 8.2).

The malignant proliferation of B-lymphocytes may be thought of as representing populations of cells which have undergone neoplastic transformation at various stages during the maturation process. The B-cell lymphomas and chronic lymphatic leukaemias are typified by small lymphocytes with little capacity for immunoglobulin synthesis except for small quantities of IgM. Some 15 per cent of such tumours produce paraproteins. *Waldenstrom's macroglobulinaemia* is a lymphoma comprising intermediate B-lymphocytes with the capacity to synthesize considerable quantities of IgM, producing high serum levels which often give rise to the hyperviscosity syndrome. Skeletal manifestations are rare and, like the lymphomas and chronic lymphatic leukaemia, there is anaemia and lymphadenopathy. *Myeloma* is a malignant proliferation of more or less mature plasma cells which most often secrete IgG and less commonly IgA and rarely IgD, IgM or IgE. The disease usually presents with bone involvement, pain or fracture, infection due to immune paresis and renal failure.

Benign paraproteins usually occur in the absence of any obvious predisposing factor but may be associated with the conditions which give rise to the oligoclonal gammopathies.

Laboratory investigations

The investigation of paraproteinaemia is one of the most important protein studies carried out in the laboratory. The aim of the investigation is to establish the monoclonal nature and type of the paraprotein, provide biochemical evidence of the likelihood of a malignant origin, and perform precise estimation of paraprotein for monitoring therapy.

The existence of a paraprotein must first be established by simple electrophoresis. Immunofixation or immunoelectrophoresis against monospecific antisera to H- and L-chains will enable identification and confirmation of monoclonality by the presence of a single class of H-chain and one type of L-chain.

The H-chain type of paraprotein is clinically relevant as its nature may allow a search for the appropriate type of B-cell tumour in a previously undiagnosed case. For example, an IgM paraprotein is most unlikely to be due to myeloma so that skeletal X-rays are unimportant but examining for enlarged lymph nodes is essential. In established myeloma the complications of the disease are very different with different immunoglobulin classes.

The presence of immunoglobulin fragments is one of the most important criteria of malignancy suggesting de-differentiation and failure of normal immunoglobulin synthesis.

Bence Jones protein (BJP) (monoclonal-free light-chain)

This is by far the most important of the fragments and its presence in urine (p. 127) is a strong indication of a malignant B-cell tumour. However, all plasma cells secrete a slight excess of light chains which pass through the renal glomerulus to be largely reabsorbed in the proximal tubule. Increased amounts of polyclonal light-chain may be detectable in the urine in polyclonal hypergammaglobulinaemia. It is thus essential to establish the monoclonality of the light-chains by immunofixation of adequately concentrated urine. It is important to look for BJP not only as an indication of malignancy but also in the investigation of a suspected B-cell tumour in the absence of a serum paraprotein, as some 20 per cent of myelomas have only BJP production from the tumour. Such tumours may be more de-differentiated and aggressive.

Bence Jones protein may damage the

renal tubule causing obstruction and 'myeloma kidney', and it may be responsible for amyloid formation.

Paraprotein measurement is important as the absolute plasma concentration provides some indication of the probability of malignancy, while a rising level is a strong indicator of a proliferating malignant clone. It is an excellent tumour marker (p. 233) and the level is useful for monitoring therapy of all types of B-cell tumour. Decreased levels of immunoglobulins other than the paraprotein is a common feature of malignant B-cell tumours. Their measurement is thus useful in assessing the probability of malignancy and in anticipating the complication of immune deficiency in known B-cell tumours.

The heavy-chain diseases

Some monoclonal B-cell tumours may produce only immunoglobulin H-chains. The most important of these, *α-heavy chain disease*, is associated with gut lymphomas in people predominantly of Mediterranean and Middle-eastern origin.

Cryoglobulins

These may be simple monoclonal immunoglobulins which precipitate in the cold. Many paraproteins have this characteristic when cooled to 4 °C but are likely to be clinically significant only if they precipitate above 22 °C.

They may also comprise immunoglobulin-anti-immunoglobulin complexes. These are most often monoclonal IgM with anti-IgG activity complexed to IgG (monoclonal rheumatoid factor) but may be polyclonal (polyclonal rheumatoid factor). In all types of cryoglobulin the aggregated immunoglobulin may activate complement and give rise to vasculitis.

If the diagnosis is suspected the blood must be collected and separated at 37 °C. If a precipitate then appears on cooling it may be washed in saline at 4 °C and subjected to immunofixation to establish whether it is monoclonal or polyclonal.

Protein analysis in other body fluids

Changes in the protein composition of urine (p. 122) and cerebrospinal fluid (p. 227) are described elsewhere. The detection of undigested albumin in meconium is used to investigate cystic fibrosis (p. 168).

Exudates and transudates

In pleural or ascitic fluid a transudate, being a plasma ultrafiltrate modified by circulatory changes, usually has a protein concentration less than 30 g/l (specific gravity <1.015): an exudate, caused by inflammation or malignancy, usually has a protein concentration more than 40 g/l (specific gravity >1.018). Such changes are unreliable, and cytology and culture are preferred.

Further reading

Haider M, Haider SO. Assessment of protein calorie malnutrition. *Clin Chem* 1984; **30**: 1286–9.

Whicher JT, Calvin J, Riches P, Warren C. The laboratory investigation of paraproteinaemia. *Ann Clin Biochem* 1987; **24**: 119–32.

Whicher JT, Spence C. When is serum albumin worth measuring? *Ann Clin Biochem* 1987; **24**: 572–80.

Plasma Enzymes

Objectives

In this chapter the reader is able to

- study the factors which influence plasma enzyme concentration.

At the conclusion of this chapter the reader is able to

- understand the relation between pathological processes and measurable changes in enzyme activity and concentration.

Classification

The enzymes found in plasma can be grouped into three types.

I Plasma-active
These act on substrates in plasma; the group includes the coagulation enzymes.

II Extracellular fluid-active
These are synthesized in cells close to their site of activity in the transcellular and extracellular fluid, into which they are secreted; the group includes the digestive enzymes.

III Cell-active
These are synthesized in the cells where they act; the group includes the enzymes of intermediary metabolism. Those enzymes found in the plasma mainly originate from the cytosolic and microsomal fractions of the cell. The cell:plasma gradient of enzyme activity is usually of the order of 10 000 : 1 to 1000 : 1, and the plasma half-life of these enzymes is usually 1 to 10 days, though there is wide variation.

Metabolism

The quantity of most enzymes in the blood plasma (except prothrombin) is low: for example, the concentration of creatine kinase is about 80 µg/l (1 nmol/l). The cell-active enzymes enter the plasma in small amounts as a result of the continuous normal ageing of cells, or due to diffusion through undamaged cell membranes. They leave the plasma through inactivation and catabolism, or rarely by excretion into the bile, small intestine, or urine. This normal steady state of the passage of enzymes from cells to extracellular fluid to disposal maintains the plasma concentration of most enzymes at a fairly constant level. The following factors may affect enzyme concentration

(i) altered synthesis of enzyme within the cells (e.g. drug induction, p. 160)

(ii) increased (or uncommonly decreased) amount of enzyme-forming tissue (e.g. neoplasia p. 232, resection)

(iii) altered cell permeability. Any 'damage' to a cell which causes an increase in the permeability of the cell membrane, even without actual necrosis, will allow enzymes to escape at a greater rate (e.g. exercise, p. 230)

(iv) an alteration in the rate of inactivation or of disposal of enzyme

(v) an obstruction to a normal pathway of enzyme excretion.

As a result of the operation of one or more of these factors there is generally a rise in the concentration of enzyme in the plasma, and this is usually detectable by current methodology (assuming unchanged inhibitors and activators) as an increase in enzyme activity – often measured in serum rather than in plasma as some anticoagulants may inhibit some enzymes. Changes in inhibitors or activators may be important: certain poisons act as enzyme inhibitors, and some vitamin deficiencies (p. 110) cause cofactor deficiencies and reduced enzyme activities. Immunoassays to measure enzyme concentration are available and more are being developed. They have particular value for assays such as that of trypsin in plasma, where the presence of natural antienzymes renders activity analysis meaningless.

Changes in disease

Plasma enzyme changes in disease are related in many ways to cell pathology. Different tissues contain a great number of different enzymes in various concentrations; following tissue injury plasma enzyme levels do not necessarily change in proportion to those in the damaged tissue. In severe generalized tissue damage, e.g. after heat stroke or cardiac arrest, high values for concentrations in plasma of almost all cell enzymes may be found. An increase in the plasma activity of any one enzyme is rarely diagnostic of damage to the cells of any one organ or tissue. For example, both myocardium and liver contain the three enzymes, aspartate transaminase, lactate dehydrogenase, and isocitrate dehydrogenase, in high concentration. Yet after a myocardial infarction the plasma aspartate transaminase and lactate dehydrogenase (but not isocitrate dehydrogenase) concentrations are increased; whereas after hepatocellular damage the plasma aspartate transaminase and isocitrate dehydrogenase are increased, and less so lactate dehydrogenase. Increased permeability of the damaged cell membrane affects the release of one enzyme more than another, and intracellular location of an enzyme is

important, cytosolic enzymes being released before organelle enzymes when a cell is damaged. Rates of inactivation and of disposal are not the same for all enzymes – in the above example 'heart' isocitrate dehydrogenase and 'liver' lactate dehydrogenase are relatively unstable. The different distribution and behaviour of the isoenzymes of the enzymes under consideration can explain many apparent paradoxes.

Isoforms and isoenzymes

Isoforms are different molecular forms of the same enzyme defined by its main catalytic activity. Isoenzymes are isoforms that are genetically determined. For example, CK-1 and CK-3 are isoenzymes, as are bone and intestinal alkaline phosphatase, whereas bone and liver alkaline phosphatase are isoforms. Common usage, followed in this book, is for the word isoenzyme to mean any multiple molecular form.

In clinical biochemistry two types of isoenzyme are important: when different tissues contain different forms of the enzyme (such as alkaline phosphatase, p. 180), and when different forms of the enzyme are present in all cells but not in the same proportion (such as lactate dehydrogenase, p. 133).

Isoenzymes are generally distinguishable by both biochemical and physical properties. They can usually be simply separated by electrophoresis, and then visualized by staining. Chromatographic or immunological separations may be used. Also they may often be distinguished by their different kinetic properties with related substrates, or by different sensitivities to temperature changes or to inhibitors.

Use of enzyme assays in clinical practice

Because of methodological variations, it is particularly important that results for enzyme assays be referred to the analysing laboratory's own reference range. The use

Table 9.1 Enzyme assays regularly used in clinical practice

Enzyme	Fluid	Disease	Page no.
Acetylcholinesterase	A	Neural tube defects	225
Acid phosphatase–total	P	Prostatic carcinoma	234
–'prostatic'	P	Prostatic carcinoma	234
Alanine transaminase	P	Liver disease	155
Alkaline phosphatase–total	P	Liver disease	155
	P	Bone disease	180
–isoenzymes	P	Liver disease	155
	P	Bone disease	180
	P	Malignancy	234
Amylase	P	Acute pancreatitis	166
	P	Salivary gland disease	162
	U	Acute pancreatitis	166
Angiotensin-converting enzyme	P	Sarcoidosis	188
Aspartate transaminase	P	Myocardial infarction	133
	P	Liver disease	155
Cholinesterase	P	Suxamethonium apnoea	229
	E	Insecticide poisoning	229
Creatine kinase–total	P	Skeletal muscle disease	229
	P	Myocardial infarction	132
–CK-2	P	Myocardial infarction	132
Glucose-6-phosphate dehydrogenase	E	Haemolytic anaemia	141
γ-Glutamyltransferase	P	Liver disease	156
Lactate dehydrogenase –total	P	Myocardial infarction	133
–'heart'	P	Myocardial infarction	133
Lipase	P	Acute pancreatitis	166
Lysozyme	P U	Leukaemia	234
Trypsin	J	Chronic pancreatitis	167

P, plasma (serum); A, amniotic fluid; E, erythrocyte; U, urine; J, pancreatic juice.

of enzyme assays in diagnosis is discussed elsewhere (Table 9.1).

Further reading

Lott JA, Wolf PL. *Clinical Enzymology*. New York: Field, Rich and Associates, 1986.

Wilkinson JH, ed. *The Principles and Practice of Diagnostic Enzymology*. London: Edward Arnold, 1976.

Nutrition, Vitamins and Trace Elements

Objectives

In this chapter the reader is able to

- revise the nutritional requirements for energy, protein, carbohydrate, fat, vitamins and minerals
- revise the biochemical function of the vitamins and trace elements.

At the conclusion of this chapter the reader is able to

- understand the pathophysiology and presentation of nutritional deficiencies
- investigate suspected deficiencies of vitamins and trace elements
- use the laboratory in the management of total parenteral nutrition.

Introduction

Adequate nutrition is essential for health; disease, poverty or ignorance can produce malnutrition. Nutritional requirements increase during pregnancy and lactation, in childhood and in certain hypercatabolic states. Recommended daily intakes of nutrients vary from country to country. Table 10.1 lists the current recommended UK daily intakes for the macronutrients (carbohydrate, fat and protein), organic micronutrients (vitamins) and inorganic micronutrients (minerals and trace elements).

Nutritional deficiency

Deficiency of a nutrient may arise due to

(i)   poor diet
(ii) poor absorption from the gastrointestinal tract (p. 170)
(iii) impaired metabolism, e.g. poor dihydroxylation of cholecalciferol in renal disease
(iv) increased requirements in pregnancy, lactation and growth
(v)   increased excretion.

Nutritional deficiencies will normally resolve when the diet is restored by supplementation and may manifest as subclinical deficiency (with depletion of body stores) or as an overt deficiency disease.

Figure 10.1 shows the series of changes which occur over time to produce a clinical disease with low dietary intake. Measurement of blood or tissue nutrients may not correlate well with a pathological state and therefore nutritional assessment should consider the whole patient and not just measured concentrations.

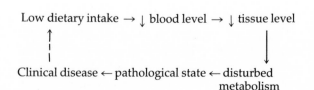

Fig. 10.1 The development of disease in nutritional deficiency

Table 10.1 Nutritional requirements (sedentary males aged 18–34 years). RDI is the recommended daily intake (UK)

	RDI	Comments
Energy	10.5 MJ	
Protein	63 g	
	11 per cent of total energy	
Carbohydrate	50 per cent of total energy	See Chapter 5 for discussion of inherited metabolic disorders of carbohydrate metabolism
Fat	No more than 34 per cent of total energy	See Chapter 6 for discussion of relation of heart disease to fat intake and metabolism
Vitamin A	750 µg (as retinol equivalents)	Deficiency disease: xerophthalmia
Vitamin D	None (with adequate sunlight)	See Chapter 16 for discussion of vitamin D metabolism
Vitamin E	No RDI (UK)	Only therapeutic use is in treatment of haemolytic anaemia of premature infant
Vitamin K	No RDI (UK)	See Chapter 14 for discussion of clotting factors
Vitamin B$_1$ (thiamin)	1.0 mg	Deficiency diseases: beriberi, Wernicke-Korsakoff syndrome
Riboflavin	1.6 mg	Deficiency disease: angular stomatitis
Nicotinamide	18 mg (as nicotinic acid equivalents)	Deficiency disease: pellagra
Vitamin B$_{12}$ (cyanocobalamin)	No RDI (UK)	See Chapter 13 for discussion of vitamin B$_{12}$ deficiency
Folate	300 µg	See Chapter 13 for discussion of folate deficiency
Vitamin C	30 mg (ascorbic acid)	Deficiency disease: scurvy
Calcium	12.5 mmol (500 mg)	See Chapter 16 for discussion of calcium and phosphate requirements and metabolism
Magnesium	No RDI (UK)	See Chapter 16 for discussion of magnesium requirements and metabolism
Iron	200 µmol (10 mg)	See Chapter 13 for discussion of iron requirements and deficiency and overload
Zinc	230–380 µmol (15–25 mg)	Deficiency disease not well established; depression and delayed wound healing, acrodermatitis enteropathica
Copper	>30 µmol (>2 mg)	See Chapter 13 for discussion of copper deficiency and overload
Manganese	45–90 µmol (2.5–5.0 mg)	No deficiency disease. Neurotoxic symptoms with overload
Chromium	1.0–3.8 µmol (50–200 µg)	Deficiency impairs glucose tolerance
Cobalt	25–65 µmol (1.5–4.0 mg)	Constituent of vitamin B$_{12}$
Iodine	0.8–1.1 µmol (100–140 µg)	See Chapter 18 for discussion of iodine deficiency
Molybdenum	1.6–5.2 µmol (150–500 µg)	No deficiency disease

Protein-energy malnutrition

Table 10.2 shows a classification of protein-energy malnutrition found in children of developing countries. There is growth retardation and increased susceptibility to infection (p. 80). Even with treatment, many children with marasmus and kwashiorkor die so early that detection is important. Simple anthropometric measurements (e.g. weight-for-height; head circumference; arm circumference) can quickly identify children at risk and are preferred to the slower biochemical indices

Table 10.2 Protein-energy malnutrition

Weight as percentage of local standard	Oedema present	Oedema absent
80–60	Kwashiorkor	Underweight
<60	Marasmic kwashiorkor	Marasmus

of protein malnutrition. Measurement of plasma proteins, particularly retinol-binding protein and prealbumin (p. 97) can be used to assess the efficacy of treatment.

Many deficiencies of vitamins, minerals and trace elements co-exist with protein-energy malnutrition and the clinical presentation of a severely malnourished patient might be complex.

Starvation

Adults adapt better to periods of low protein and energy intake as they do not have the extra requirements of growth. Starvation is characterized by a low resting energy expenditure (basal metabolic rate, BMR) fuelled by fat oxidation with conservation of muscle protein. Survival depends on the extent of fuel stores and the ability to conserve energy; thin men may die after 2 months of complete starvation, an obese woman can survive 6 months of therapeutic starvation if micronutrient needs are met.

Hypercatabolic states

After trauma (e.g. a road traffic accident), major surgery or extensive burns, a hypercatabolic state exists. Resting energy expenditure may double or increase further. If energy requirements are not met patients rapidly lose weight and may 'waste away'. The increased breakdown of fat and muscle protein is caused by increased circulating catecholamines, glucagon, and cortisol (p. 231). Treatment aims to promote a positive nitrogen balance with intravenous hyperalimentation (p. 112).

Micronutrient deficiency

Vitamin A

The active form of vitamin A in rhodopsin in the retina is retinal; vitamin A deficiency results in night blindness (an early symptom) and xerophthalmia which can progress to permanent blindness and is common in countries where rice is the dietary staple food. Xerophthalmia blinds about 500 000 young children annually worldwide, of whom about half die.

The vitamin is present in the diet as fat-soluble retinol or as β-carotene, which is hydrolysed in the intestine to form retinol. After absorption and esterification in the mucosal cells, vitamin A ester is transported in plasma bound to proteins (retinol-binding protein and prealbumin, p. 97). Fat malabsorption (p. 170) and protein deficiency (p. 80) can therefore lead to vitamin A deficiency.

Assessing vitamin A deficiency
The ophthalmological signs of even mild vitamin A deficiency are obvious so that biochemical assessment of its plasma levels is unnecessary in endemic regions. Plasma vitamin A concentrations are measured although it is not easy to relate values to tissue stores (Fig. 10.2).

Vitamin B$_1$

Vitamin B$_1$ (thiamin) deficiency may result in beriberi which has two forms: dry beriberi (a polyneuropathy) and wet beriberi (with oedema). Chronic alcohol abuse with poor nutrition may present as a peripheral nerve disorder indistinguishable from dry beriberi. This may progress to the *Wernicke–Korsakoff syndrome*, with ophthalmoplegia, nystagmus, ataxia and psychosis.

Thiamin pyrophosphate is an essential cofactor in oxidative decarboxylation but it is not clear how this biochemical feature relates to the clinical syndromes of thiamin deficiency.

Assessing thiamin deficiency
The best biochemical assessment of thiamin status is the measurement of red cell thiamin content but this is not widely available. Thiamin status can be specifically assessed by measuring the activity of erythrocyte transketolase before and after addition of thiamin pyrophosphate, a cofactor for the transketolase reaction.

Nicotinamide

Pellagra, the disease caused by nicotinamide deficiency, is characterized by dermatitis, diarrhoea and dementia, and is endemic in populations who eat maize. In developed countries, pellagra is occasionally seen in alcoholics and in patients with the malabsorption syndrome (p. 170).

Nicotinamide is used in the synthesis of NAD and NADP, the pyridine nucleotides which accept hydrogen in cellular metabolism, and are essential for glycolysis and oxidative phosphorylation. Nicotinic acid is the precursor of nicotinamide and may be derived from the diet or synthesized from tryptophan.

In the carcinoid syndrome, tryptophan is metabolized to hydroxyindoles and not to nicotinic acid and pellagra may develop. Hartnup disease (p. 90) is a rare inherited disorder of neutral amino acid transport with decreased intestinal tryptophan uptake and nicotinic acid deficiency may result.

Assessing nicotinamide deficiency

Plasma nicotinamide can be measured using microbiological or chromatographic assays which are sensitive to the low levels found in pellagra. Chemical methods which detect the urinary metabolites of nicotinic acid have been used but are relatively poor in assessing the response to therapy.

Vitamin C

Vitamin C (ascorbic acid) deficiency is common, particularly in old people living alone or in institutions but rarely presents as frank scurvy. In the UK, 1 per cent of people aged 70 or more are vitamin C deficient. Deficiency produces perifollicular haemorrhages and gingivitis and these features may be related to poor collagen synthesis. Ascorbic acid is required for the hydroxylation of lysine and proline, for carnitine synthesis and for catecholamine synthesis.

Assessing vitamin C deficiency

The biochemical confirmation of sub-clinical vitamin C deficiency is not easy. The *ascorbic acid saturation test* is popular because it is simple and corrects any deficiency which is present. The patient takes ascorbic acid orally (5.7 μmol (1 mg)/kg body weight) every day until at least 0.4 mmol (70 mg) is excreted in the 8 h overnight urine; this occurs within 3 days in a normal subject and may take more than a week if the patient is deficient.

Ascorbic acid can be measured in plasma but this is a misleading marker of vitamin C status. Measurement of leucocyte or 'buffy layer' (leucocytes and platelets) ascorbic acid is a better marker of tissue saturation, which is less influenced by recent intake and reflects long-term nutritional status.

Zinc

Severe zinc deficiency is seen in the rare acrodermatitis enteropathica, in which there is a defect in intestinal zinc absorption. Milder forms may develop in patients receiving total parenteral nutrition and in hypercatabolic states. The symptoms of zinc deficiency include dermatitis and delayed wound healing.

Zinc is essential for the function of a number of enzymes including carbonate dehydratase, alkaline phosphatase, lactate dehydrogenase and DNA polymerase.

Assessing zinc deficiency

There are no body stores of zinc and plasma levels are the most convenient assessment of zinc status. Zinc is bound to albumin, α_2-macroglobulin and transferrin; blood samples for zinc analysis should be obtained without venous stasis.

Chromium

Gross chromium deficiency has only occurred after prolonged total parenteral nutrition but a sub-clinical deficiency may exist in some patients with non-insulin-dependent diabetes mellitus. Glucose tolerance (p. 59) improves with chromium supplementation.

Total parenteral nutrition

Patients with short bowel syndrome, intestinal fistulae, intra-abdominal sepsis, pancreatic abcess or fistula or pseudocyst require total parenteral nutrition (TPN). A mixture of glucose (p. 47), amino acids (p. 84), vitamins and inorganic salts in water is infused into a central vein, usually continuously.

Hypercatabolic patients (p. 110) need a high energy intake and this is sometimes termed 'intravenous hyperalimentation' (IVHA). The administration of large amounts of glucose ('dextrose') can cause reactive hypoglycaemia (p. 58) and central vein thrombosis. *Intralipid* and *Travmulsion* are emulsified triglyceride and are concentrated energy sources but tend to 'sludge' in catheters. A 500 ml bottle of glucose (50 per cent) supplies 4.18 MJ but has an osmolality of 3800 mmol/kg H_2O. A 500 ml bottle of *Intralipid* (20 per cent) supplies the same amount of energy at an osmolality of 330 mmol/kg H_2O.

TPN regimes vary and should be tailored to the individual requirements of each patient. A person recovering from gastrointestinal surgery will probably require 2 to 3 days TPN, supplying (per 24 h) 6–8 MJ in 2–3 l fluid containing amino acids, glucose and fat. A patient with burns, sepsis and fever may require 10 to 14 days TPN, supplying (per 24 h) 10–15 MJ in 3–4 l fluid containing amino acids, glucose and more fat.

Total parenteral nutrition may also be used in patients with acute pancreatitis or inflammatory bowel disease and in patients receiving chemo- or radiotherapy. Its use has been advocated in patients with weight loss (>10 per cent ideal weight) before operation.

The aims of nutritional support are to promote a positive nitrogen balance (p. 82), to prevent further tissue breakdown and to improve healing and to prevent sepsis. Patients can be quickly mobilized after operation.

Monitoring

Careful clinical monitoring is essential for patients receiving parenteral nutrition and there are computer programs (designed by the manufacturers of parenteral solutions) to assist in this. External catheters require meticulous care to avoid the problems of infection, occlusion, breakage and air embolism.

Fluid status should be assessed clinically and biochemically by monitoring plasma and urine urea and electrolytes. Mild hyponatraemia (p. 28) is common. Amino acids are infused to promote protein synthesis; an increase in plasma urea may indicate that amino acids are being diverted into the urea cycle (p. 81) rather than used anabolically. Renal function should be checked daily with measurement of plasma urea and creatinine (p. 128). Hyperglycaemia (p. 53) is common and daily monitoring of plasma glucose is essential. Insulin is often infused to promote an anabolic state, and shifts potassium from the extracellular fluid. Plasma potassium levels provide a limited assessment of potassium status (p. 29). Hypophosphataemia (p. 182) is commonly seen. Liver function tests are often measured twice a week; prolonged total parenteral nutrition sometimes produces abnormalities in liver function. The biochemical changes resemble those of a mild cholestasis due to fat deposition.

Nutritional status is best assessed by a combination of tests: body weight, anthropometric measurements, nitrogen balance (p. 81), plasma protein measurements (p. 97), and haematological tests. Plasma magnesium (p. 189) should be measured weekly and plasma zinc (p. 111) twice a month. Sophisticated formulations make vitamin deficiencies rare in patients receiving total parenteral nutrition.

Disorders of excess

Obesity

Obesity rarely has a metabolic component. It is a recognized risk factor for the development of coronary artery disease (p. 75).

Vitamin toxicities

Toxicities of the water-soluble vitamins (vitamin B_1, riboflavin, nicotinamide, cyancobalamin, folate and vitamin C) are rare as an excess can readily be eliminated.

The body stores fat-soluble vitamins (A, D, E and K) and so deficiencies of these vitamins take a long time to develop. However, toxicity may result from enthusiastic ingestion of vitamin tablets. Vitamin D toxicity, resulting in hypercalcaemia is described on p. 179.

Vitamin A toxicity can occur acutely in children; symptoms include headache, vomiting and peeling of skin. The symptoms disappear if intake stops. Chronic vitamin A toxicity has been reported in adults and children. There is hepatosplenomegaly, dry skin, bone erosion and weakness, and fasting plasma retinol is usually greater than 3.5 μmol/l (reference range 1–3 μmol/l).

Trace metal poisoning

Industrial or environmental exposure to mercury, cadmium or lead can produce renal damage, evidenced by aminoaciduria (p. 90) and secondary porphyrinuria (p. 143) and elevated urine β_2-microglobulin (p. 122). Iron (p. 146) and copper (p. 146) are also potentially toxic.

Patients undergoing haemodialysis for renal failure (p. 122) are vulnerable to exposure from a number of toxic agents, including copper (p. 146) and aluminium. Dialysis encephalopathy is now thought to be due to high concentrations of *aluminium* in dialysis fluid prepared from tap water. Patients on haemodialysis also receive aluminium from the binding agent aluminium hydroxide given to decrease phosphate absorption from the gastrointestinal tract. Early features of aluminium toxicity include general malaise, vomiting and weight loss. These are also common symptoms of uraemia so measurement of plasma aluminium and dialysis fluid aluminium is important in patients receiving chronic haemodialysis. Plasma aluminium is less than 1 μmol/l in health; there is a risk of dialysis dementia if plasma aluminium exceeds 7 μmol/l. Lower concentrations have been implicated in the development of anaemia and osteodystrophy (p. 187) in patients undergoing chronic haemodialysis.

Further reading

Clayton BE. Clinical chemistry of trace elements. *Adv Clin Chem* 1980; **21**: 147–76.

Marshall WJ, Mitchell PEG. Total parenteral nutrition and the clinical chemistry laboratory. *Ann Clin Biochem* 1987; **24**: 327–36.

Wills MR, Savory J. Aluminium poisoning: dialysis, encephalopathy, osteomalacia and anaemia. *Lancet* 1983; **ii**, 29–34.

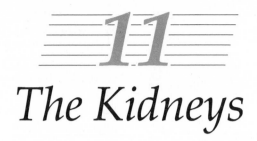

The Kidneys

Objectives

In this chapter the reader is able to

- revise the physiology of renal excretory and other functions
- study the principles of tests for clearance and for other alterations of renal function
- study the biochemical changes in the main groups of renal diseases, including the effects of drugs and relation to treatment.

At the conclusion of this chapter the reader is able to

- understand the abnormal biochemistry produced by different types of altered glomerular and tubular function
- understand the principles and applications of examination of the urine
- use the laboratory to investigate a patient with proteinuria
- use the laboratory to investigate a patient with suspected primary or secondary alterations of renal function
- understand the causes of renal calculi, and investigate a suspected case.

Pathophysiology

The formation of urine

Glomerular filtration

In a healthy adult about 650 ml of plasma (1200 ml of blood) pass through the glomeruli every minute, and about 125 ml of glomerular filtrate is formed. Water passes freely from the plasma through the glomeruli and small diffusible ions and molecules are present in the glomerular filtrate at about the same concentration as in the plasma. Substances of a molecular weight greater than about 10 000 do not pass freely through the glomeruli and are present in the glomerular filtrate at progressively lower concentrations than in plasma as their molecular weight increases. The basement membrane of the glomerulus acts as a molecular sieve.

The filtration of proteins is also affected by their charge. The surface of the basement membrane contains negatively charged glycosaminoglycans (principally heparan sulphate) which repel negatively charged proteins and prevent their filtration. For these reasons less albumin (highly negatively charged) appears in the filtrate than would be expected for its size.

In man excretion of the end products of metabolism is also not wholly by filtration.

Tubular reabsorption and excretion

The renal tubules conserve water and adjust the concentration of soluble constituents of the body using both passive and active transport from the glomerular filtrate.

Sodium
Reabsorption of sodium occurs throughout the tubule.

(a) Seventy per cent of the filtered sodium is reabsorbed in the proximal tubule by an active transport mechanism. This produces an electrochemical gradient along which negatively charged chloride ions pass and an osmotic gradient along which water passes. Sodium reabsorption at this site depends on adequate availability of chloride.

(b) Sodium is reabsorbed throughout the tubule in exchange for hydrogen-ions. In the proximal tubule this results in the reclamation of filtered bicarbonate while in the distal tubule there is net generation of bicarbonate (p. 38).

(c) In the distal tubule sodium is reabsorbed in exchange for potassium and hydrogen-ions which compete for a transport system which is stimulated by aldosterone. Secretion of this hormone is controlled by renal blood flow and thus plasma volume and forms an important homeostatic mechanism for adjusting sodium and thus water content of the body (p. 19).

Potassium

This is almost all reabsorbed in the proximal tubule by an active transport mechanism. Urinary potassium is derived from the distal tubule where potassium and H^+ are excreted into the tubule in exchange for sodium reabsorption under the influence of aldosterone. The effect of this competition between potassium and H^+ is that if H^+ is in short supply, as in alkalosis, more potassium will be lost in the urine. The converse is true in acidosis. Similarly hypokalaemia, with less available potassium, will result in excessive H^+ loss and the development of alkalosis.

Water

This is reabsorbed in the proximal tubule along the osmotic gradient produced by sodium and potassium reabsorption. This accounts for about 80 per cent of the filtered water, leaving the tubular fluid iso-osmotic with plasma but greatly reduced in volume. Differential reabsorption of water and solute occurs in the loop of Henle creating a hyper-osmolar environment in the renal medulla and producing a hypo-osmolar

urine. This then enters the collecting ducts which pass down into the hyper-osmolar medullary tissue. The duct cells are impermeable to water unless ADH (p. 195) is present when water passes from the lumen into the blood along an osmotic gradient. In this way the urinary osmolality can be varied between about 40 and 1400 mmol/kg according to the water intake.

Proteins

About 8 g of protein per day passes into the glomerular filtrate (about 4 g of this is albumin) at a concentration of about 40 mg/l. Most of this is reabsorbed by pinocytosis in the proximal tubule though a small amount is passed in the urine (Fig. 11.1). Normal urine contains 40–120 mg/24 h of protein, about half of which is derived from the plasma and the remainder is derived from the tubules and lower urinary tract.

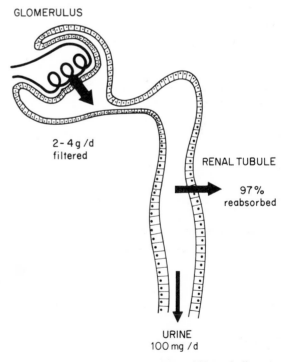

Fig. 11.1 The renal reabsorption of filtered albumin

Other solutes

Glucose, urate and amino acids are actively reabsorbed in the proximal tubule by specific, energy-requiring, saturable transport mechanisms. Phosphate is partially reabsorbed in the proximal tubule by a mechanism which is inhibited by parathyroid hormone and its presence in the urine is important for buffering. Calcium is reabsorbed throughout the nephron by a mechanism which is stimulated by parathyroid hormone and inhibited by loop diuretics such as frusemide. Urate is secreted into the distal tubule. (Salicylates and thiazide diuretics first inhibit secretion and at higher concentrations inhibit reabsorption.) Urea is partly reabsorbed by passive diffusion but the majority remains in the tubular fluid while small amounts of creatinine are secreted into the tubules. A normal adult excretes about 1200 mmol of solute per day of which about 700 mmol are ions and the rest mainly urea.

The urine that is finally secreted has an entirely different composition from the glomerular filtrate from which it is derived (Table 11.1).

Table 11.1

	Daily excretion	
Constituent	Glomerular filtrate	Urine
Water	180 000 ml	1500 ml
Sodium	20 000 mmol	150 mmol
Albumin	4 g	0.04 g
	(60 µmol)	(0.6 µmol)
Urea	900 mmol	400 mmol

Foreign substances
Substances such as inulin and *p*-aminohippuric acid (PAH) are used in studies of renal function. Inulin in the plasma, after being excreted into the glomerular filtrate, passes through the tubule without either secretion or reabsorption; no endogenous substance behaves exactly in this way (Fig. 11.2(c)). PAH is excreted into the tubule, as well as passing into the glomerular filtrate, and the renal plasma is virtually freed ('cleared') of PAH in its passage through the nephron unit (Fig. 11.2(e)); the 8 per cent which is not cleared has passed through the kidney tissue that is not excretory.

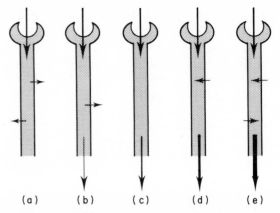

Fig. 11.2   Simplified diagram showing different ways in which the renal tubules can handle substances freely filtered through the glomeruli. (a) Glucose – virtually completely reabsorbed. (b) Urea – partly reabsorbed. (c) Insulin – unaltered. (d) Creatinine – partly secreted into the tubules. (e) *p*-Aminohippuric acid – wholly excreted into the tubules

Clearance

The different types of excretion can be expressed quantitatively by using the concept of clearance. The clearance of any substance from the plasma is, in theoretical terms, the volume of plasma which a given volume of urine (usually a 1 min excretion) 'clears' of that substance. It is calculated (as ml/min, or sometimes as ml/s) as

$$\frac{\text{urine concentration} \times \text{urine volume (ml/min)}}{\text{plasma concentration}}$$

The units of concentration are irrelevant, as long as they are the same for plasma and for urine – they are now usually expressed as mmol/l.

In practice the kidneys do not clear one unit volume of plasma completely of an excreted substance; hence clearance can be more conveniently defined as the minimum volume of plasma which is needed to provide the quantity of a substance which is excreted in the urine in 1 min (or in 1 s). The renal clearance of any substance may be measured by comparing the urinary excretion of that substance over a given period with its average concentration in the plasma during that period, and the more constant is the plasma concentration the more reliable is the result. The average clearance, in adults, of glucose (assuming absence of glucose from the urine) is 0, of urea is 75, of inulin is 125, and of PAH is 650, all expressed as ml/min. These figures may be corrected to standard surface area, 1.73 m², and surface area is used as the conventional standard of comparison because it correlates reasonably well with the functional mass of the kidneys.

Because of the way in which it is excreted by the normal kidney, the clearance of inulin (and sometimes of ^{51}Cr-EDTA) is taken as a measure of the glomerular filtration rate, namely 125 ml/min. The clearance of PAH is taken as a measure of the effective renal plasma flow, namely 650 ml/min. These are all exogenous substances that require intravenous infusion. The filtration fraction (the proportion of the plasma that is filtered at the glomeruli, normally about 20 per cent) can be calculated as inulin clearance/PAH clearance × 100.

It is possible, by measurement of PAH excretion at high plasma PAH levels, to calculate a factor termed the tubular excretory maximum for *p*-aminohippuric acid (Tm_{PAH}). This is a measure of proximal tubular secretory function. By measurement of glucose excretion at high plasma glucose levels, a factor termed the tubular reabsorptive maximum for glucose (Tm_G) can be calculated; this is a measure of proximal tubular reabsorptive capacity though it is not independent of the glomerular filtration rate. All these clearance investigations are research procedures and, because they require infusion, not suitable for routine clinical work.

The simple measurement of endogenous creatinine clearance is often used as an estimate of glomerular filtration rate. It gives slightly higher results than inulin clearance as creatinine is secreted by the tubules at all levels of renal function. However in general the results of creatinine clearance determination are proportional to the true glomerular filtration rate until renal function becomes grossly impaired. Urea clearance measures principally, but not wholly, glomerular filtration, and gives a result lower (by about 30 per cent) than the glomerular filtration rate because urea is partly reabsorbed.

Such concepts and calculations assume that all nephrons have identical functional capacity, though this is not true in health or in disease.

Threshold

The threshold of a given constituent of the plasma is that concentration in the plasma above which, assuming normal glomerular and tubular function, it is excreted in the urine. The threshold of glucose is about 10 mmol/l. As the plasma concentration of glucose is normally below this, glucose can be called a threshold substance. Tubular reabsorption of glucose removes from the glomerular filtrate practically all the glucose that is filtered through the glomeruli at plasma glucose levels below 10 mmol/l by a saturable active transport mechanism. The threshold level of urea is zero, i.e. urea is excreted in the urine however low its concentration in the plasma, and urea can be called a non-threshold substance. The threshold of any substance may be altered by physiological or pathological changes in the renal plasma flow, the glomerular permeability, or the tubular reabsorptive capacity.

Other functions of the kidney

The main function of the kidney is the maintenance of the *milieu interieur* by changes in the rate of excretion of the different constituents of the plasma (including water).

Investigation of the changes which take place in the homeostatic and excretory powers of the kidney in disease is the principal purpose of renal function tests. Other properties of the kidney must not be forgotten. The juxtaglomerular apparatus produces the enzyme renin, which acts on angiotensinogen in plasma to form the vasoconstrictor substance angiotensin, which is also the most potent stimulator of aldosterone secretion (p. 207). The kidney produces a specific stimulus to erythrocyte production, erythropoietin (p. 143) and converts 25-hydroxycholecalciferol to 1,25-dihydroxycholecalciferol (p. 178). The tubular cells have independent metabolic activities. The distal tubules produce ammonia from glutamine and amino acids, and hydrogen-ions from carbonic acid, for exchange with sodium; their functions in the control of acid–base balance are discussed in Chapter 4.

Biochemical changes in renal disease

Renal damage and renal function

The effects of renal impairment depend to a great extent on whether the impairment is mainly of glomerular function or mainly of tubular function: all nephrons are not usually impaired to the same extent.

Glomeruli

Damage to glomerular function leads to a reduction in the glomerular filtration rate. Prerenal disorders such as haemoconcentration or a fall in the peripheral arterial pressure, or passive venous congestion of the kidney, reduce the filtration pressure, hence there is a fall in the glomerular filtration rate: postrenal obstruction also reduces glomerular filtration by back-pressure. This fall, whether due to prerenal or postrenal causes or to renal disease, leads to retention of excretion products produced by normal metabolism and cell turnover. If excretion fails to balance production, plasma levels of urea, creatinine, urate and phosphate rise.

If the proximal tubular cells are unaffected they will absorb a normal total amount of water and electrolytes thus reducing urine volume. If there is dehydration and plasma hyper-osmolality ADH will be secreted and water will be reabsorbed in excess of solute forming a concentrated urine. Otherwise even normal nephrons will form dilute urine. If plasma volume and blood pressure are low (as in prerenal

disorders) aldosterone secretion will be maximal and sodium reaching the distal tubules will be reabsorbed in exchange for potassium and H^+ producing a urine low in sodium. The reduced amount of filtered sodium results in decreased distal tubular exchange for H^+ and potassium with acidosis and hyperkalaemia.

In renal diseases with azotaemia, if there are residual functional glomeruli, the high urea in the filtrate will result in an osmotic diuresis through these nephrons with failure of the tubules to adequately reabsorb the water and solutes. If there are sufficient nephrons left polyuria will result.

Pathological damage to the basement membrane of the glomeruli allows both plasma and erythrocytes to leak through the affected glomeruli: there is therefore both proteinuria (more severe with membranous lesions) and a haematuria (more severe with proliferative lesions). The nephrotic syndrome is used to describe the clinical syndrome with oedema due to hypoalbuminaemia resulting from proteinuria.

Tubules

Damage to tubular function leads to failure of reabsorption and to loss of renal compensation for changes in body fluid volume, osmotic pressure, and acid–base status. The constituents of glomerular filtrate which are affected may be many, and include water, electrolytes, protein, and many non-ionized substances. In this case large volumes of dilute urine are passed. Excessive amounts of sodium, potassium and bicarbonate are lost and hydrogen ions cannot be excreted. This results in volume depletion, hypokalaemia and acidosis. Alternatively, renal tubular syndromes may affect only one or a few reabsorbable substances.

It is possible to contrast renal insufficiency with renal failure. Renal insufficiency may be considered to be present when the plasma levels of excreted end-products are still normal, whilst in renal failure (usually when clearances have fallen below 50 per cent) these plasma concentrations, e.g. of urea, are above normal.

Acute oliguric renal failure

Prerenal failure

This is caused by any major decrease in renal perfusion, such as circulatory failure as in shock. Glomerular filtration falls, and there is oliguria. The urine often contains a trace of protein and less than 10 mmol/l of sodium as a result of decreased renal perfusion stimulating aldosterone secretion (p. 207). If the plasma is hyper-osmolar, as in dehydration, then the urine will be concentrated with a urine/plasma osmolality ratio above 1.5. If the plasma is hypo-osmolar, as in Addisonian crisis, the urine will be dilute despite oliguria. The plasma urea concentration rises rapidly, between 7 and 20 mmol/l every 24 h as the reduced amount filtered is largely reabsorbed, whereas creatinine, not being reabsorbed, shows much less increase in plasma concentration. In addition, concomitant tissue breakdown, if present, provides an increased level of urea.

When blood pressure and hydration are returned to normal urine output will increase and the metabolic abnormalities will return to normal. If this does not occur or if the patient is well hydrated and normotensive it is likely that renal damage is present.

Acute tubular necrosis

This is caused by prolonged renal ischaemia, and may follow circulatory failure or by a variety of toxins (including incompatible blood transfusion) producing acute tubular necrosis. Decreased glomerular filtration, and possibly tubular obstruction by debris, contribute to the renal failure. In the first phase there is anuria or marked oliguria, and any urine that is passed has an osmolality similar to that of plasma, and contains more than 30 mmol/l of sodium. The urine also has an apparently high specific gravity because of the high protein content; however the corrected specific gravity is about 1.010. There is a profusion of all types of casts, and the urine may contain haemoglobin or myoglobin if this high tubular concentration of the pigment is the cause of the disorder. The clinical and biochemical features of uraemia rapidly develop; there may also be features of tubular damage such as aminoaciduria. Water overload and oedema may occur if intake greatly exceeds output either intravenously or by mouth. A common problem in the differential diagnosis of acute oliguria is to distinguish between prerenal oliguria and acute tubular necrosis. This can usually be done from a clinical history, blood pressure and apparent hydration of the patient, and laboratory tests are of limited value. If renal perfusion is slow due to hypovolaemia, aldosterone secretion is maximal and in the presence of functioning tubules urinary sodium will be less than 30 mmol/l. Measurement of urinary osmolality or urea is less valuable as the urine will only be concentrated if ADH secretion is stimulated by hyperosmolality which it will not be in haemorrhage, acute myocardial insufficiency and Addisonian crisis.

Should the patient recover, with or without dialysis, there is a diuretic phase, partly because the recovering tubules have a low reabsorptive power. In this phase there may be a polyuria of 3–5 l per day, continuing mild proteinuria, and loss of sodium and potassium. Return of concentrating ability and fall of plasma urea heralds recovery. Water, sodium, and potassium balance must be carefully monitored, by plasma and urine analyses, throughout the course of the disease.

Acute glomerulonephritis

In the acute phase of glomerulonephritis there is obstruction and rupture of glomeruli with oliguria, haematuria (a 'smoky' urine), and proteinuria of up to about 5 g/24 h. Moderate numbers of casts are present in the urine. Glomerular filtration is impaired but renal plasma flow is unaltered: there is a low filtration fraction. Tubular function is slightly impaired. Retention of sodium and water leads to dilution of the extracellular fluids, and this dilution in combination with general capillary damage gives rise to oedema. The plasma albumin level and the total protein are decreased by this dilution. Hypertension is common. The condition may progress to anuria, azotaemia, acidosis, and hyperkalaemia, whilst uraemic symptoms may or may not be present.

The onset and degree of recovery may be assessed by examination of the urine for protein, and quantified by plasma creatinine (or clearance) measurements. Persisting nephritis is accompanied by a proteinuria of up to 0.5 g/24 h, and occasionally by haematuria. Proteinuria disappears when recovery is complete.

Chronic renal failure

Compensated chronic renal failure

Chronic bilateral renal disease, due to various pathological causes, leads to renal failure as the disease progresses. The concentrating power of the kidney is lost and this proceeds until only a urine of fixed osmolality (about 300 mmol/kg) and specific gravity (1.010) can be formed. There is an osmotic mild polyuria resulting from the effect of the increased urea in the glomerular filtrate of the remaining functional nephrons (more marked at night) which leads eventually to dehydration. There is progressive decrease in glomerular filtration rate and the renal failure is no longer termed compensated when the plasma urea rises above normal. This occurs when glomerular filtration falls below about 50 per cent, depending somewhat on dietary protein. The other plasma non-protein nitrogen constituents, particularly creatinine and uric acid, also rise. Proteinuria is rarely above 5 g/24 h as protein can only be lost through functioning glomeruli. Protein excretion may even fall as the disease progresses. Excretion of casts is variable.

Metabolic acidosis develops because of retention of the hydrogen-ions of acid phosphates and sulphates and of organic acids, and also because of failure of the

damaged tubules to produce hydrogen-ions and ammonia. The high plasma phosphate concentration and failure to metabolize 25-hydroxycholecalciferol (p. 118) are usually associated with a fall in the plasma ionized calcium concentration, which can cause secondary hyperparathyroidism. Demineralization is seen and 'renal rickets' can develop in children; in adults various types of osteodystrophy, aggravated by acidosis, may be seen (p. 187). The hypocalcaemia does not usually lead to tetany because of the counteracting acidosis (p. 175). As a rule there is a moderate degree of potassium retention, especially when there is oliguria; and excessive urinary loss of sodium which leads to sodium depletion. Potassium deficiency is occasionally seen. Glucose tolerance is often impaired. Plasma amylase is increased due to retention. The usual lipid abnormality is a Type IV hyperlipidaemia (p. 74) due to increased synthesis of triglycerides, but an increase in plasma cholesterol (Type IIb) may develop.

Chronic pyelonephritis

In this type of chronic renal disease tubular damage predominates. Concentrating power is therefore lost early and there is polyuria, whilst the plasma urea and creatinine may be still normal; later all features of chronic renal failure develop. The urine contains many leucocytes but very little protein, generally less than 2 g/24 h.

Uraemia (end-stage renal failure)

As renal failure progresses and glomerular filtration falls below about 10 per cent of normal, the clinical syndrome of uraemia begins to appear. The patient shows symptoms of irritation of the gastrointestinal tract, mental and neurological disorders, haematological and vascular changes and muscular twitching, and has a foetid or ammoniacal odour of the breath. These symptoms, and the eventual death in coma, are only slightly due to the raised level of urea in the plasma, for the effects of a raised plasma urea alone are a diuresis, headache and sedation, and possibly gastrointestinal irritation (due to conversion of urea to ammonia). Hypertension, anaemia and circulatory failure, and sodium depletion with dehydration, acidosis, hypocalcaemia, and potassium retention, may all play a part. Phenols, guanidines, indoles, abnormal amino acids, and undetermined 'toxic retention products' including 'middle molecules' of molecular weight 500–5000 (but not creatinine), have all been blamed as the cause of the symptoms.

Postrenal obstruction

If obstruction to the outflow of urine is prolonged, due for example to prostatic enlargement or to spreading carcinoma of the cervix, the patient may become uraemic from the effects of the back-pressure, and may have tubular damage leading to sodium loss. Unless the obstructive cause leads to bleeding, the only urine abnormality may be a trace of protein. The level of the plasma urea or creatinine can be taken as a measure of the degree of obstruction. When slow decompression of the urinary tract is performed before prostatectomy, a levelling-out of the progressive fall in the plasma creatinine may be taken as an indication that surgery should proceed.

Renal tubular syndromes

Disorders of the renal tubules, whether congenital or acquired, affect one or many of the functions of the tubule – namely reabsorption of protein and amino acids (p. 89); reabsorption of glucose; reabsorption of water and electrolytes; production of ammonia and hydrogen ions. When there are congenital tubular transport defects, there are often parallel intestinal transport defects.

Of the many proximal tubular defects, renal glycosuria (without other abnormalities) is not uncommon (p. 61), and there can be specific loss of phosphate causing a rickets-like disturbance (p. 187).

Fanconi syndrome (p. 90)
This includes disorders that combine generalized aminoaciduria and loss of glucose, phosphate, urate, potassium, and protein of low molecular weight; often there is an acidosis. The proximal tubules may show pathological damage. Many congenital disorders (e.g. galactosaemia, glycogen storage diseases, cystinosis) give rise to abnormal metabolites which damage the proximal tubule, but the most important causes of the Fanconi syndrome are nephrotoxicity from drugs (e.g. aminoglycoside antibiotics) and metabolic poisons such as mercury, lead and cadmium.

Cystinuria
There is diminished reabsorption of the related basic amino acids cystine, ornithine, arginine, and lysine: in homozygotes the 24 h excretion of cystine may be increased from the normal 0.05 mmol to higher than 2 mmol, and calculi form because cystine is relatively insoluble.

Renal tubular acidosis
There is a distal tubular defect of failure of ion-exchange with consequent hyperchloraemic acidosis (and failure to excrete a urine more acid than pH 6.0) and eventual osteomalacia. There is urinary loss of calcium and phosphate, sometimes nephrocalcinosis, and also of potassium causing hypokalaemia. In the rarer proximal tubular acidosis, often seen in a Fanconi syndrome, the primary disorder is failure to reabsorb bicarbonate. Other types have been identified.

Ureteric transplantation

The ureters may be transplanted into the colon or into an isolated loop of ileum. In either case severe hyperchloraemic acidosis may develop. This is due to differential reabsorption of urinary chloride more than of urinary sodium from the bowel, and possibly also to renal tubular damage from pyelonephritis. Potassium deficiency is often present. Urea and excess ammonia may also be reabsorbed from the bowel, and there can be mild uraemic symptoms.

Haemodialysis

The treatment of chronic renal failure by repeated dialysis requires close and specialized biochemical control, but anomalous biochemical ill-effects may nevertheless develop. Phosphate deficiency may be seen. Osteodystrophy can worsen, possibly due to toxicity from aluminium in dialysis fluid or antacids, and metastatic calcification is a risk. Over-rapid dialysis produces a low extracellular osmotic pressure: the disequilibrium syndrome involves cellular overhydration due to urea being too rapidly removed from the ECF, but still tending to remain in the cells, with a consequent osmotic imbalance. If the plasma creatinine is normal whilst the plasma urea continues to rise, this reflects increased protein intake or catabolism, and not ineffective dialysis.

Proteinuria and the nephrotic syndrome

A functional way of classifying proteinuria is as glomerular, tubular, overflow, and nephrogenic.

Glomerular

When there is glomerular damage the negative 'charge barrier' of glycosaminoglycans in the glomerular basement membrane is impaired first, allowing increased filtration of albumin. This typically occurs when damage is minimal, as in early diabetic nephropathy where it may be used as an indicator of reversible renal damage. It is also characteristic of the 'minimal change' lesion of childhood glomerulonephritis where massive albuminuria of up to 40 g/24 h may be seen. The glomerular damage in this condition is however easily healed and it carries excellent prognosis when treated with steroids.

More severe damage to the glomerular basement membrane results in destruction of the collagen matrix and loss of the molecular sieving capacity with the appearance in the urine of high molecular weight

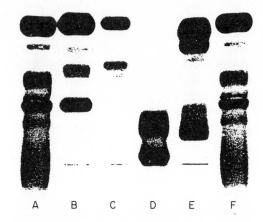

Fig. 11.3 Electrophoresis of concentrated urine compared with normal serum. **A** Normal serum. **B** Glomerular proteinuria with albumin, α_1- and α_2-globulins, and transferrin: the fast α_2-zone results from the passage of haptoglobin molecules into the urine of a patient with a haptoglobin variant. **C** Tubular proteinuria: relatively small albumin band; split α_2-zone due to the presence of α_2-microglobulins; trace of transferrin with β_2-microglobulin in the β_2-position just anodal to serum C3. **D** Bence Jones proteinuria: two dense bands of Bence Jones protein in the γ-region. **E** Fictitious proteinuria due to addition of egg white by the patient; none of the bands has the same mobility as those in serum. **F** Normal serum. Modified with permission from Whicher JT. *Br J Hosp Med* 1980; **24**: 348–60

proteins such as transferrin (90 000) and IgG (150 000).

Albuminuria and hypoalbuminaemia causing oedema is known as the nephrotic syndrome. It is invariably due to glomerular damage with albuminuria ranging from 5 to 40 g/24 h. Secondary impairment of tubular function may occur due to lysosomal enzyme release as a result of massive protein reabsorption in the proximal tubules.

Tubular

In renal tubular damage there is an excess in the urine of low molecular weight proteins such as β_2-microglobulin (11 800) which are normally filtered in relatively large amounts and largely reabsorbed in the tubule. Tubular proteinuria does not exceed about 4 g/24 h unless there is concomitant glomerular damage. Tubular damage often gives rise to the Fanconi syndrome but proteinuria is probably the most sensitive indication of early damage from drugs and heavy metals.

Overflow

If there is increased production of low molecular weight protein which enters the plasma it will be filtered and reabsorbed in the proximal tubule until the reabsorptive capacity is saturated; it will then 'overflow' and appear in the urine in increased amounts. Bence Jones protein (p. 103), haemoglobin (from haemolysis), and myoglobin (in crush injury) behave in this way.

Nephrogenic

Proteins may enter the urine from the urinary tract itself. Plasma protein exudation causes proteinuria in cystitis and nephritis and local production of mucoproteins may occur in carcinoma of the bladder. In addition bacteria and pus cells may break down in stored urine to release protein.

Clinical causes of proteinuria

Proteinuria is an important indication of renal disease in which it is almost invariably present. It may indicate renal damage in conditions such as hypertension and pre-eclampsia or it may result from primary renal conditions such as glomerulonephritis and pyelonephritis. The proteinuria of severe anaemia is due to renal anoxia, and that of heart failure is due to anoxia and to congestion. The often transient proteinuria of fever, exercise and of cerebral vascular accidents may be from secondary 'toxic' glomerular damage. Slight proteinuria may often be found in severe malignant disease. The 'benign' proteinuria which occasionally occurs in pregnancy, and 'orthostatic albuminuria', have been thought to be due to mechanical pressure on the renal veins which causes renal vascular congestion, but may be due to other causes of altered renal circulation. Orthostatic proteinuria may be found in many presumably healthy young men, especially with lordosis, at routine medical examination; in this condition, in contrast to patients with glomerulonephritis, a morning urine sample passed on waking is free of protein, and erythrocytes are never found in excess. In all these types of prerenal proteinuria the proteinuria rarely exceeds 2 g in 24 h, and erythrocytes and casts are scanty.

The nephrotic syndrome

The urinary proteins in this condition are those of a molecular weight of less than about 200 000 and are comprised mainly of albumin. The amount of albumin versus high molecular weight proteins present in the urine gives some indication of the nature of the damage to the glomerular basement membrane and the extent and selectivity of the protein leakage can be assessed by differential clearances (p. 127). The proteins lost in the urine are often decreased in the plasma and this change with an increase in the pre-β and β-lipoproteins, α_2-macroglobulin and fibrinogen gives the characteristic electrophoretic pattern (Fig. 8.2; p. 92). Plasma iron (bound to transferrin), copper (bound to caeruloplasmin), total calcium (bound to albumin) and protein-bound hormones, are decreased. The low plasma albumin gives rise to oedema which tends to develop when the proteinuria exceeds 10 g/24 h. The decreased blood volume which results from fluid loss to the extravascular compartment gives rise to secondary aldosteronism and sodium retention, exacerbating the oedema. Haematuria, decreased glomerular filtration rate and rising urea only occur when there are complications. The cause of the considerable increase in plasma lipid fractions and α_2-globulins is related to the hypoalbuminaemia and is due to increased liver synthesis of several proteins including the apolipoproteins. There is often lipaemia and the plasma cholesterol level may reach 25 mmol/l.

Renal calculi

The components of renal calculi comprise low molecular weight crystalloids which make up most of the stone, and high molecular weight matrix substances which are partly mucoprotein. A calculus cannot form unless at some time the urine was saturated in respect of the crystalloids of the calculus.

The largest number of calculi consist either of calcium oxalate, or of mixtures of calcium phosphate and magnesium ammonium phosphate, sometimes with calcium carbonate or calcium oxalate – these are whitish. The aetiology of most of these calcium-containing calculi is unknown. Abnormalities such as a continually concentrated urine (e.g. due to excessive sweating by unadapted Europeans in the tropics), bacterial infection (particularly when this makes the urine alkaline), or 'stasis' (due to congenital abnormalities or acquired obstruction) are often predisposing factors: the contribution of initiators and inhibitors of crystallization is uncertain. Calcium calculi are less soluble in alkaline urine. Hypercalciuria is present in many cases, and excess gut absorption of calcium (e.g. idiopathic hypercalciuria, p. 188) may often be the cause. Renal tubular acidosis produces hypercalciuria and an alkaline urine. Of the many causes of hypercalcaemia with hypercalciuria (p. 181), primary hyperparathyroidism is probably the most important specific disease as the calculi may be the presenting feature (p. 185). In osteoporosis (p. 185) there can be hypercalciuria with a normal plasma calcium.

Oxalate crystals may also arise from a rare inborn error of metabolism, primary hyperoxaluria. In hyperuricaemia, usually associated with gout (p. 86), uric acid calculi (which are brown) are common; these are less soluble in acid urine. Cystine calculi (which are yellow) are usually the presenting feature of cystinuria.

Biochemical investigations
Any stones already passed by the patient should be analysed for the constituents named above. Essential investigations on the patient's plasma are for calcium, phosphate, and alkaline phosphatase, for urate, and also for urea and bicarbonate. A 24 h urine is examined microbiologically, and chemically for cystine, calcium, and often oxalate. Further investigations may be necessary to establish the cause of any hypercalcaemia (p. 181).

Other calculi

Prostatic calculi
These contain calcium phosphate and carbonate, but no oxalate.

Bladder calculi
These are usually renal calculi that have passed through into the bladder and enlarged. They may originate in the bladder in infected urine, as calcium–magnesium–ammonium phosphate.

Renal function tests

Renal function tests have two main purposes. Either they detect possible renal damage in a patient who has a disorder that may involve the kidneys, or they determine the degree of functional damage of kidneys that are known to be diseased. Examination of the urine for proteins, cells and casts checks for an 'active lesion', whilst clearance studies and related tests investigate loss of function. Once renal damage has been detected, renal function tests may reveal the principal site and degree of the disturbance in the nephron, but rarely the cause of the renal injury. About two-thirds of the renal tissue must be functionally damaged for renal function tests to show any abnormality, and renal failure develops when there is inability to maintain homeostasis. A person with only one healthy kidney will show a normal response to renal function tests. As with liver function tests, partial damage to most of the nephrons (as in nephritis), with the healthy remainder overworked, is more likely to show disturbed renal function than will complete destruction of some nephrons when the major remainder of the kidney remains healthy (as in carcinoma of the kidney). Even if renal function appears to be satisfactory when the patient is taking a normal dietary load, dynamic tests for adaptability of the kidney to abnormal circumstances may reveal failure of function when there is renal insufficiency.

Simple examination of the urine

Volume

The normal 24 h urine volume of an adult is between 750 and 2000 ml. This depends on the fluid intake (which is usually a matter of habit) and on the loss of fluid by other routes (primarily sweating which, in absence of fever, depends on physical activity and on the external temperature). A marked alteration in the output of urine may be a prominent sign in disease of the kidneys.

Oliguria develops also in any non-renal disease in which there is a decreased glomerular filtration rate due to deficient intake of water, or excessive loss of fluid by other routes, for example by haemorrhage, or as diarrhoea and vomiting. Polyuria is a characteristic sign of chronic renal insufficiency due either to tubular damage or osmotic diuresis through the residual nephrons. Polyuria of low osmolality is also found in diabetes insipidus, in hysterical polydipsia, or after mobilization of fluid from ascites or oedema. Polyuria occurs as an osmotic diuresis in any disease where there is an increased excretion of metabolites, notably in diabetes mellitus.

The minimal 24 h output of urine needed to remove the waste products of normal metabolism is about 500 ml. A patient may be said to have oliguria when the urine volume is below 400 ml in 24 h, and anuria when the 24 h urine volume is below 100 ml, but these terms are loosely used.

Quantitative measurements of urinary volume are of limited value unless measurements are also made of fluid intake and of fluid loss by other routes. The 12 h day output and the 12 h night output should be measured separately. Normally the day urine is of greater volume than the night urine. The night urine equals or may exceed the day urine in severe glomerulo-tubular disease (p. 120), if there is a disturbance of intestinal absorption (p. 170), or in Addison's disease (p. 212).

Urine concentration: osmolality and specific gravity

Osmolality is the physiologically significant measure of urine concentration. However, this analysis requires laboratory apparatus, whereas measurement of specific gravity (which depends on the mass of solutes present and not on their osmotic activity) can be done in the side-room. Osmolality and specific gravity are usually affected in disease in the same direction, but because of variation in the nature of the solutes the one value cannot be calculated from the other.

In health urine contains between about 1400 and 400 mmol of solutes per 24 h; the maximum and minimum values over that period are about 1000 and 300 mmol/kg. The normal specific gravity (correctly called relative density) of a pooled 24 h urine sample is between 1.025 and 1.010; the maximum and minimum values are usually about 1.030 and 1.005. Under normal circumstances the urine concentration varies inversely with the urine volume. The concentration of urine is highest in the first morning specimen (overnight urine), and is lowest in a specimen passed an hour after much fluid has been taken. A constant specific gravity throughout day and night of about 1.010, or osmolality of about 300 mmol/kg, being the values of protein-free plasma, occurs in severe chronic renal disease. Disorders associated with oliguria usually produce a concentrated urine but only if ADH secretion is stimulated. Polyuria tends to lead to a urine of low concentration. In diabetes mellitus there is polyuria with urine of high concentration: even when the specific gravity of the urine has been corrected for the presence of glucose (p. 257) the specific gravity of the urine is still raised because of the high concentration of salts in the urine. A correction must also be applied when interpreting the urine specific gravity in the presence of marked proteinuria (p. 257), whilst protein has a negligible effect on osmolality. Oliguria with a low specific gravity (after correction for the proteinuria) and low osmolality occurs in acute tubular necrosis because the tubules do not concentrate the limited amount of glomerular filtrate.

pH

On a normal mixed diet the urine is usually acid, generally varying in pH between about 5.5 and 8.0. A vegetarian diet, which causes a tendency to alkalosis (p. 34), thereby produces an alkaline urine. The pH of the urine in disease may reflect both the acid–base status of the plasma, and the function of the renal tubules. It may also be grossly altered by bacterial infection of the urinary tract, or deliberately by acid- or alkali-forming drugs.

Appearance

If no coloured abnormal constituents are present, then the higher the concentration of urine the deeper is its colour. The rate of excretion of the normal urinary pigments ('urochromes') is constant, and a pale urine has a low specific gravity, a dark urine has a high specific gravity.

Coloured urines occur in certain diseases or metabolic disorders, and after the administration of many drugs (Table 11.2).

Table 11.2

Colour of urine	Direct cause	Indirect cause
Red-brown	Haemoglobin/methaemoglobin myoglobin	Intravascular haemolysis Crush syndrome
Red	Rifampicin	Antibiotic therapy
	Phenindione	Anticoagulant therapy
	Beetroot	Food
Reddish-purple	Porphyrins	Erythropoietic porphyria
Reddish-purple (on standing)	Porphyrins	Acute intermittent porphyria
Pinkish-brown (on standing)	Urobilin	Haemolytic anaemia
Orange (green fluorescence)	Eosin	Colouring agent, e.g. in sweets
	Riboflavin	Vitamin therapy
Yellow	Mepacrine	Malaria therapy
	Tetracyclines	Antibiotic therapy
Green-yellow	Bile pigments	Cholestatic jaundice
Green-blue	Pyocyanin	*Ps. aeruginosa* infection
	Methylene blue	Colouring agent
Blue (especially on standing)	Indigo compounds	Indicanaemia in intestinal disease or suppuration
Purple	Phenolphthalein (in alkaline urine: the urine becomes clear on acidification)	Purgatives
Brown-black (on standing)	Melanin	Malignant melanoma
	Homogentistic acid	Alkaptonuria (inborn error of metabolism)
		Ochronosis associated with phenolic poisoning
Black	Iron sorbitol	Parenteral iron therapy
Cloudy	Bacteria and leucocytes	Urogenital tract infection
	Bacteria	In vitro infection
	(in acid urine) Urates	Usually normal
	(pink) Oxalates	
	(in alkaline urine) Phosphates	Usually normal
Smoky	Erythrocytes	Glomerular damage or slight urinary tract haemorrhage

Smell

Urine which is infected with Gram-negative organisms often has a distinctive unpleasant smell. In addition, urine infected with urea-splitting organisms has an ammoniacal smell. If urine which had a normal odour on arrival at the laboratory develops such a smell, this indicates bacterial decomposition and the specimen is unfit for most chemical analysis. Certain drugs, for example paraldehyde, impart a typical odour, as does the rare maple syrup urine disease (p. 89).

Protein

The commercial strip tests, which are colour reactions based on the protein error of indicators, are popular because of their convenience (p. 257). They are simple, do not require clarification of the urine, and are very roughly quantitative; but may give false weak positives in alkaline urine. They are relatively insensitive to proteins of neutral charge, such as Bence Jones protein and β_2-microglobulin.

Differential urinary protein excretion

The differences in protein excretion between mild and severe glomerular damage and in tubular damage have led to the measurement of the clearance ratio of various proteins to determine the nature of the underlying lesion. Thus the albumin/IgG clearance ratio is used to identify 'minimal change', steroid responsive, glomerulonephritis in children (the picture of predominant albumin excretion is often referred to as 'selective proteinuria', i.e. it is selective for albumin). The β_2-microglobulin/albumin clearance ratio is used to determine tubular damage where there will be a higher clearance of β_2-microglobulin relative to albumin than in other forms of proteinuria.

It is important to appreciate that the quantity of albumin in the urine is unrelated to the nature of the underlying lesion in glomerulonephritis and that it may be used to monitor the response to therapy in the short term. In the long term decreasing albuminuria may reflect a falling GFR in chronic renal failure and thus be very misleading. In diabetes however the presence of only small amounts of albumin in the urine, 'microalbuminuria', is an indication of reversible damage. By the time albumin is detectable by albumin sticks the damage is irreversible.

Casts

The tubules secrete an α_1-glycoprotein called Tamm-Horsfall protein, of molecular weight about 80 000. In the presence of albumin it comes out of solution in gel form as casts. Various types of casts have different inclusions; e.g. granular casts contain degenerated tubular cells.

Mucoproteins

These may be found in urine when there is disease of the lower urinary tract, or may be derived from semen, when spermatozoa will be present in the urinary deposit, or from vaginal discharge. Mucoprotein is precipitated from urine in the cold on adding 33 per cent acetic acid dropwise.

Bence Jones protein

The low molecular weight protein is a free monoclonal immunoglobulin light chain and is synthesised in excess in multiple myeloma and related neoplasms (p. 103). Electrophoresis of concentrated urine is the most sensitive test; and Bence Jones protein may also be detected by layering urine on concentrated HCl (Bradshaw's test). The classical test for Bence Jones protein is that it precipitates when acidified urine is heated to 40–50 °C (whereas normal urinary protein does not begin to precipitate until 60 °C) and redissolves on heating the urine to boiling point, to reappear on cooling, at about 70 °C: this now is only of historical interest. Indicator strip tests for proteinuria are relatively insensitive to Bence Jones protein owing to its neutral or positive charge.

Haemoglobin and haemoglobin derivatives

Haemoglobin has a threshold at about 1 g/l plasma: haemoglobin released into the plasma is first bound to haptoglobins; when these are saturated the remaining free haemoglobin dissociates into subunits and is filtered through the glomeruli (p. 114). These are proteins and give the normal tests for urinary proteins and can be detected and identified by spectroscopic and chemical examination.

Formed elements

The microscopical examination of fresh urine for erythrocytes, other cells, and casts is an important part of the tests of renal function: the finding of more than an occasional leucocyte, erythrocyte, or granular cast points the way to further investigations. Leucocytes indicate infection, erythrocytes glomerular rupture or haemorrhage in the renal tract and granular casts tubular damage, especially acute tubular necrosis. Collection for a 12 h period permits degeneration of cells, and a 2 h morning collection is preferred.

The commercial strip tests for free haemoglobin in urine (which utilise its peroxidase activity) are also a test for erythrocytes (p. 259).

Crystals

In urine crystals are usually not pathological. Uric acid and calcium oxalate may be found in health in acid urine, and phosphates in alkaline urine. However cystine crystals are pathological, and are an indication of the inborn error metabolism, cystinuria (p. 121).

Glomerular function

Urea

Urea is derived from dietary protein and endogenous protein catabolism (p. 84). Increased production occurs on high protein diets or after gastrointestinal haemor-

rhage and when there is increased tissue breakdown as in starvation, trauma and inflammation. The capacity of the normal kidney to excrete urea is high and in the presence of normal renal function urea levels rarely rise above normal despite increased production. A plasma urea concentration above 15 mmol/l almost certainly indicates renal impairment. In the absence of increased urea production, plasma urea does not usually rise above normal until GFR has fallen by at least 50 per cent. The plasma urea is the most useful test of 'renal excretory function', as it correlates well with the clinical consequences of retained metabolic products (uraemia) in renal insufficiency. Thus a patient with a GFR of 30 ml/min and a urea of 40 mmol/l following major surgery will suffer the effects of uraemia and require appropriate treatment, whereas another patient with chronic renal failure on a low protein diet with a similar GFR may have a urea of 10 mmol/l and be clinically well. Knowledge of the GFR itself is of little value in managing these patients, the plasma urea is far more useful.

Creatinine

The plasma creatinine level is less affected by diet and tissue breakdown than is the plasma urea, though severe muscle wasting results in lower plasma creatinine levels and meat meals may increase it. While the independence of the plasma creatinine level of exogenous altering factors may be an advantage in that plasma creatinine levels more closely reflect the GFR, it has the disadvantage of being less sensitive than urea to renal impairment when tissue breakdown provides an increased load of urea. However, plasma creatinine is the more useful for following the progress of renal deterioration over a long period of time as it is less affected by non-renal factors. Plots of the reciprocal of plasma creatinine show a linear deterioration of renal function in many patients with renal disease and may be used to predict when dialysis will be necessary.

Creatinine clearance test

The value of this test is that of a roughly quantitative measure of glomerular function when simpler tests have already demonstrated renal impairment. Although it is often so performed, the test is not usually suitable, because of lack of sensitivity, as the first diagnostic test for impairment of renal function. The creatinine clearance may be normal when early renal damage has been demonstrated by (tubular) failure to concentrate urine in the water deprivation test, or by the presence of proteinuria – as in hypertension. This test may be done over 4 h, but a 24 h period is recommended. The results are independent of the rate of urine flow.

Method

A careful and accurate 24 h collection of urine is made. At some time during the day (but not within 1–3 h after a large meal) a blood sample is taken for plasma creatinine analysis; this and the whole 24 h urinary collection are sent to the laboratory.

Interpretation

Endogenous creatinine clearance is a rough measure of the glomerular filtration rate and is normally 100–130 ml/min (1.7–2.1 ml/s) in an adult of normal size. Correction is necessary for surface area (p. 117) in children, or in adults of abnormal build.

Values below 90 ml/min (corrected to normal surface area) are indicative of diminished glomerular filtration rate. The test has particular value in the general assessment of renal function in cases when plasma analyses are invalid, e.g. after dialysis, or when the plasma urea (but not the plasma creatinine) has been lowered by a low protein diet. Because there is considerable tubular secretion of creatinine when the plasma creatinine is high, the test is not then quantitative for glomerular filtration rate. Difficulty with accurate collection of 24 h urine output renders this test less useful than it might be, and it is probable, that a single plasma creatinine measurement is as useful for monitoring the progress of renal disease.

The infusion of amino acids increases GFR and this has been used as a dynamic test of renal functional reserve.

Tubular function

The response of these tests of tubular reabsorption is impaired early in tubular damage, or in any severe renal disease with a fall in glomerular filtration rate. The tests are invalid if the patient is receiving diuretics, or on a very low protein diet.

The presence of tubular damage may be inferred from the presence in the urine, in excess, of substances normally largely reabsorbed by the tubule. Low molecular weight proteins such as β_2-microglobulin, amino acids, and glucose may all be tested for very simply and such investigations should precede the use of more complex tests.

Urine concentration test

The simplest screening test is to measure the osmolality of every urine specimen passed over a 24-h period of normal activity. If the osmolality of any sample exceeds 800 mmol/kg, or the specific gravity is above about 1.020, then concentrating activity is unimpaired.

Vasopressin test

This is less unpleasant for the patient than is full water deprivation, and depends only on renal tubular function.

Method

The patient has nothing to drink after 18:00. At 20:00, five units of vasopressin tannate is injected subcutaneously. All urine samples are collected separately until 09:00 the next day with the patient taking normal food and drink.

Alternatively 2 µg of the synthetic analogue, *DDAVP* (desmopressin), is injected intramuscularly, or 40 µg given intranasally, at 09:00 without overnight fluid restriction, and all urine samples collected for the next 12 h.

Interpretation

Satisfactory concentration is shown by at

least one sample having a specific gravity above 1.020, or an osmolality above 700 mmol/kg (reached between 5 and 9 h in the *DDAVP* test). The test may be combined with measurements of plasma osmolality: the urine/plasma osmolality ratio should reach 3, and values less than 2 are abnormal.

Water deprivation tests (24 h)

Although this test is simple and sensitive, it is unpleasant for the patient, and many investigators prefer a vasopressin test. However this test differs in that it depends both on the posterior pituitary response to water deprivation, and on the renal tubular response to antidiuretic hormone. It is therefore also used in the differential diagnosis of psychogenic polydipsia and diabetes insipidus (p. 195). The test is contraindicated if there are biochemical or clinical signs of renal failure.

Method
Day before test. No fluid is permitted after breakfast until the conclusion of the test, and normal meals are otherwise taken.

Day of test
After waking the patient empties his bladder, and the urine is kept. Further samples are collected at 60 min and 120 min.

Interpretation
If any of the three specimens has an osmolality above 900 mmol/l, or a specific gravity (corrected for protein) above 1.025, the renal concentrating capacity is unimpaired and the ADH response is normal.

Urine dilution (water load) test

This simple test of measuring the rate of excretion of a water load is no longer performed as it is very insensitive for alteration of renal tubular function.

Urinary acidification test

This procedure tests the ability of the renal tubules to form an acid urine and to excrete ammonia. It is useful if there is doubt whether a patient's acidosis (confirmed by plasma analysis) is due to a prerenal cause, or to kidney damage as in renal tubular acidosis.

Method
The patient fasts from midnight until the conclusion of the test. At zero time, the patient empties the bladder completely and the urine is collected.

The patient takes 0.1 g (1.9 mmol) of ammonium chloride/kg body weight and drinks a litre of water – a standard dose of 5 g is sometimes used. In children the dose should be proportional to the body surface area.

At 2 h, 4 h and 6 h, complete urine specimens are collected – the laboratory may require use of special containers.

Interpretation
In a normal subject the urine will be acidified to pH 5.3 or less, and will contain more than 1.5 mmol of ammonia per hour, in at least one of the specimens. If there is marked damage to the renal acidifying powers, the pH of the later specimens of urine will be unaltered from that of the resting specimen, and less than 0.5 mmol of ammonia per hour will be excreted. The pH results are more significant than the ammonia results, as 3 days are needed for full development of extra ammonia ion excretion.

There is a more sensitive 5-day test: this requires the patient to be in hospital and is rarely needed.

Further reading

Broadus AE, Thier SO. Metabolic basis of renal stone disease. *New Engl J Med* 1979; **300**: 839–45.

Evans DB. Acute renal failure. *Br J Hosp Med* 1978; **19**: 597–604.

Parfrey PS. Proteinuria. *Br J Hosp Med* 1982; **27**: 254–8.

Payne RB. Creatinine clearance: a redundant clinical investigation. *Ann Clin Biochem* 1986; **23**: 243–50.

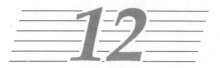

The Cardiovascular System

Objectives

In this chapter the reader is able to

- study the pathophysiological effects of myocardial infarction
- study the biochemical effects of heart failure
- study the metabolic causes of hypertension.

At the conclusion of this chapter the reader is able to

- use the laboratory in the investigation of myocardial infarction
- investigate a patient with hypertension.

Myocardial infarction

Enzyme assays in plasma are widely used in the investigation of myocardial infarction and are abnormal at some time in at least 95 per cent of cases; they are not necessary in a clinically typical case with, for example, an unequivocal electrocardiogram. In a limited number of cases an 'urgent' assay (p. 253) may be valuable for diagnosis; in many others a sample taken on admission, but analysed routinely, may be used for monitoring in comparison with later samples. A second rise, in such cases, can be important confirmation of a second infarction. In general, the higher and longer is the rise in plasma enzyme activity, the greater is the extent of myocardial damage, and usually the poorer is the prognosis. Attempts have been made, by assays

repeated at short intervals (especially of CK), to calculate the amount of enzyme released from the myocardium and to quantify the damage, but this depends also on the site of the infarct and can give misleading results.

The cardiac enzymes

The enzymes that have been most used are creatine kinase (CK), aspartate transaminase/aminotransferase (AST), and lactate dehydrogenase (LD) – and their 'cardiac' isoenzymes. The muscle protein myoglobin has also been employed but is too sensitive to minor degrees of *skeletal* muscle damage.

The biochemical pathogenesis of myocardial infarction is considered elsewhere (p. 75).

Creatine kinase
This is present in high activity in cardiac and skeletal muscle and brain, and is absent from liver and erythrocytes.

Two dimeric subunits B ('brain') and M ('muscle') give rise to three isoenzymes BB, MB, and MM – now called CK-1, CK-2, and CK-3. CK-1 (CK-BB) is found mainly in brain and thyroid, and is rarely measured. In skeletal muscle most enzyme is CK-3 (CK-MM), with about 3 per cent being CK-2 (CK-MB), whilst in cardiac muscle about 30 per cent of the CK is CK-2. In health CK-1 (from both cardiac and skeletal muscle) is usually more than 95 per cent of the total CK in plasma. When cardiac muscle is damaged, a significant proportion of the increased plasma CK is therefore CK-2, in contrast to the usual pattern after skeletal muscle damage when there is an increase largely in CK-3. In addition, CK-3 has a longer half-life in plasma than has CK-2. Separate assay of mitochondrial CK, and of subunits of M, is at present useful only for research.

Aspartate transaminase

This is present in high activity in cardiac muscle, skeletal muscle, kidney, and liver (p. 155).

Lactate dehydrogenase

This is widely distributed in the tissues, the highest activity being found in kidney, skeletal muscle, liver, cardiac muscle, erythrocytes, and malignant tissue; a slight non-specific rise in total LD occurs in most forms of widespread organic disease.

Two tetrameric subunits H ('heart') and M ('muscle') give rise to five principal isoenzymes, LD-1 to 5 (H_4 to M_4), all normally detectable in plasma. In myocardium and in erythroid cells the electrophoretically fast-moving LD-1 predominates, and in liver (and also skeletal muscle) LD-5 predominates. Both after myocardial infarction and in hepatitis there is an increase in total LD, but in myocardial infarction this is mainly LD-1 whereas in hepatitis it is mainly LD-5. Separate assay of the 'cardiac' or 'heart-specific' (but also 'erythroid') LD-1 and LD-2 is useful. This can be done by a wide variety of methods, including the preferential reaction of H-sub-units with the substrate analogue oxobutyrate which gives rise to the name 'hydroxybutyrate dehydrogenase: HBD' – this is confusing as it implies the existence of an independent enzyme.

Diagnostic enzyme patterns

The use of specific enzymes in the investigation of a case of suspected myocardial infarction depends on

(a) the time course of their release from infarcted tissue, which is a property of their molecular size and shape, and of their location in the cells; and on their rate of disposal from the plasma;

(b) whether alterations in plasma enzyme activity can result from confusing or complicating clinical conditions.

This is summarized in Table 12.1 which shows model changes, though there is wide variation in the responses of individual patients.

In practice most clinical problems can be covered by estimation of total plasma CK if the patient is seen early, in the first 24 h, and of 'cardiac' LD if the patient is seen late, after about 24 h. If the diagnosis is

Table 12.1 Typical changes in plasma enzymes after serious, but non-fatal, myocardial infarction

Plasma enzyme	Time of initial rise above upper reference limit (h)	Time of peak rise (h)	Peak enzyme value as multiple of upper reference limit	Time of return within reference range (days)	Conditions with raised enzyme values that may cause problems in diagnosis
Total CK	6	24	×10	3	Skeletal muscle damage (p. 229); cardiac surgery
CK-2 (CK-MB)	4	15	×15	2	Severe skeletal muscle damage; cardiac surgery
AST	12	24	×6	5	Acute hepatitis (p. 159); severe skeletal muscle damage
'Cardiac' LD	12	36	×6	12	Haemolysis, especially from an artificial heart valve or pulmonary infarction: renal infarction
Total LD	24	24	×4	10	As for 'cardiac' LD, and in hepatitis and any major tissue damage

uncertain, or the time of infarct doubtful, both assays should be done. If there is still doubt, then assays may be repeated 12 h and 24 h later. Estimation of CK-2, or of the individual LD isoenzymes, is required only in special cases, particularly for very early diagnosis (CK-2) which may be needed for therapy with streptokinase or tissue plasminogen activator. Also complicating conditions (such as hepatic involvement, or skeletal muscle damage from recent surgery or intramuscular injection) may be raising enzyme values and there then is a problem in differential diagnosis. AST assays are now less often used in cardiology though popular in some centres; total LD is too non-specific.

Angina pectoris does not give abnormal results. Cardiac arrest and congestive heart failure lead to a prolonged rise in enzyme activities, due to secondary damage to liver and skeletal muscle and consequent enzyme release, and probably also to delayed disposal of enzyme. After pulmonary infarction an increase in plasma LD, from both erythrocytes and liver, sometimes is seen. Changes in primary liver disease are described on p. 155, and in skeletal muscle disease on p. 229.

Hypertension

Essential hypertension

About 95 per cent of cases are essential hypertension. These have no regular pattern of changes in hormone secretion or other measurable biochemical variables unless there is secondary renal functional damage or heart failure. It is generally accepted that there is usually an alteration of sodium flux, with a high intracellular sodium and a low sodium efflux rate constant (a measure of output from cells by the sodium pump), though its relation to pathogenesis is controversial. Such measurements can be done on leucocytes or erythrocytes; though very important for research, they have no current place in diagnosis and management.

Secondary hypertension

Some cases of hypertension are secondary to an identifiable hormonal or other metabolic cause. These are important, because once the primary cause has been suspected clinically, and identified by appropriate investigations, successful treatment is often possible.

Renin–angiotensin system (p. 208)

Excess production of angiotensin, sufficient to cause hypertension, may arise from excess renin.

Renal artery stenosis
Renal ischaemia is responsible for excess renin production. For diagnosis it may be necessary to assay renin in plasma from selective catheterization of renal veins.

Renin-producing tumours of the kidney
These patients have secondary aldosteronism and very high plasma renin values.

Serious renal and renovascular disease
This can be unilateral or bilateral, with abnormalities of the usual renal function tests (p. 124), and may lead to renin overproduction. Pre-eclampsia may be a particular instance (p. 220). Here plasma urate is raised earlier than is urea or creatinine.

Catecholamines

Chromaffin tumours
These produce excess adrenaline and noradrenaline, whether the tumour type is phaeochromocytoma, or more rarely a neuroblastoma (p. 215).

Secondary conditions
The hypertension that is sometimes associated with stress is ascribed to excess secretion of catecholamines. The hypertension that sometimes develops in acute porphyria is probably catecholamine-mediated.

Aldosterone

Primary aldosteronism (Conn's syndrome) (p. 211)

This is usually due to a single adenoma, which can be removed surgically.

Idiopathic adrenal hyperplasia (bilateral nodular)

This condition usually shows greater changes in plasma renin and aldosterone than does Conn's syndrome. However, differential diagnosis may depend on aldosterone assays in both adrenal veins.

Other adrenocortical hormones

Cushing's syndrome (p. 209)

Hypertension is a feature, whether the condition is endogenous, or due to exogenous factors.

Congenital adrenal hyperplasia (p. 211)

Hypertension is a feature of the 11-β and the 17-α hydroxylase deficiencies, probably due to excess deoxycorticosterone.

Other metabolic abnormalities

The hypertension that sometimes results from oral contraceptives (p. 217) is related to their oestrogen content, whilst the occasional hypertension of pregnancy is multifactorial. Although hypertension is seen in many cases of hypercalcaemia, and is therefore related to the plasma calcium level, the cause of the frequent hypertension of primary hyperparathyroidism is unknown.

Heart failure

Chronic heart failure

Whatever the initial cause, secondary changes in other systems give rise to a consistent pattern of biochemical changes.

Kidney

Decreased renal perfusion gives rise to a fall in glomerular filtration rate. There is proteinuria, and a rise in plasma urea and creatinine.

Liver

There is a slight rise in plasma transaminases and in bilirubin concentration, and bromsulphthalein excretion is impaired at an early stage.

Electrolytes

The pathogenesis of the changes, primarily from altered renal function, is complex. Generally, there is retention of water, and, to a lesser extent, of sodium with slight hyponatraemia, and secondary hyperaldosteronism. Plasma potassium changes are variable, but hyperkalaemia develops if secondary renal damage becomes severe. Treatment, particularly with diuretics, will greatly modify these responses, which therefore require careful biochemical monitoring.

There may be a mild acidosis, with both metabolic and respiratory components (p. 40), depending on the relative contributions of right and left heart failure.

Acute heart failure

Secondary hypoxic damage to the liver will produce rises in transaminases, and jaundice is common: a raised alkaline phosphatase and γ-glutamyltransferase may be found.

Acidosis is often severe, with a combined respiratory component from pulmonary oedema, and metabolic component including hyperlactataemia (p. 61). Hypoxia and a low Po_2 will depend on the degree of loss of alveolar gas exchange.

Further reading

Lee TH, Goldman L. Serum enzyme assays in the diagnosis of acute myocardial infarction. *Ann Intern Med* 1986; **105**: 221–33.

Marks V. Hypertension. In: Williams DL, Marks V, eds. *Biochemistry in Clinical Practice*. London: William Heinemann Medical Books, 1983: 479–86.

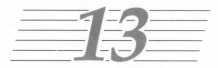

The Haemopoietic System

Objectives

In this chapter the reader is able to

- revise the biochemistry of haemoglobin synthesis and degradation
- revise the physiology of iron absorption and circulation
- study the factors that influence erythropoiesis.

At the conclusion of this chapter the reader is able to

- understand the biochemical basis of the pathological effects of the abnormal haemoglobins
- understand the biochemical basis, presentation, and investigation of the porphyrias
- use the laboratory for the biochemical investigation of lead poisoning
- use the laboratory for the biochemical investigation of vitamin B_{12} and folate deficiency
- investigate iron deficiency and overload
- investigate copper deficiency and overload.

Chemistry of erythrocytes

The circulating erythrocyte has a life-span of about 120 days: metabolic decay, and changes in composition, begins after about 100 days. The erythrocyte contains about 66 per cent water, and 33 per cent haemoglobin. The average electrolyte composition is Na^+ 7 mmol/l, K^+ 100 mmol/l,

Cl^- 70 mmol/l, pH 7.2, and the main difference in ionic composition from muscle cells is the high concentration of chloride (p. 18). Because of the relatively lower water content of erythrocytes, their total concentration of diffusible substances such as glucose and urea is less than in plasma: hence analyses of whole blood for glucose (p. 51) and urea (p. 84), and for many other substances, do not give the same results as analyses of plasma.

Haemoglobin

Haemoglobin synthesis (Fig. 13.1)

Succinate (as succinyl CoA) and glycine combine in the haemopoietic organs, using pyridoxal phosphate as co-factor: 5-amino-laevulinate (ALA) is produced under the influence of ALA-synthase, which is the principal rate-controlling enzyme for the overall synthesis of haemoglobin. Two ALA molecules condense to form one molecule of porphobilinogen, a substituted mono-pyrrole, and four porphobilinogen molecules then condense to form uroporphyrinogens of series I and III, which are cyclic tetrapyrrole (porphyrin) isomeric compounds. Uroporphyrinogen I is the precursor of other porphyrins, but plays no further part in haem synthesis. Uroporphyrinogen III is the precursor of the porphyrin III series, and is converted to coproporphyrinogen III and then via protoporphyrinogen to protoporphyrin IX. This chelates iron(II) (ferrous iron) to form

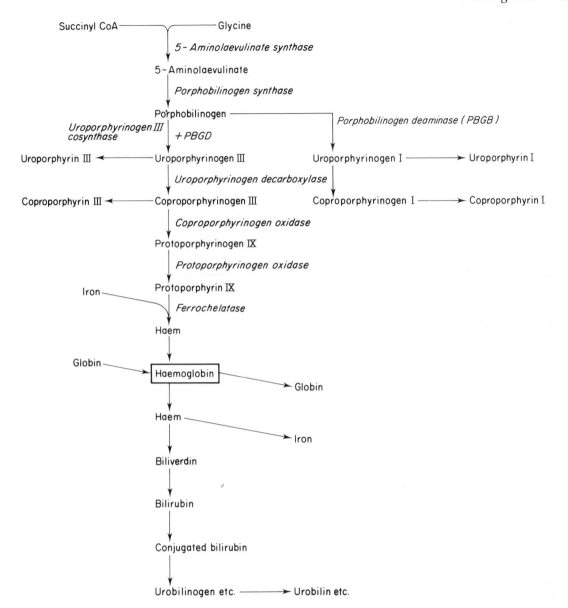

Fig. 13.1 The principal steps in the synthesis and degradation of haemoglobin, with the enzymes indicated in the synthetic pathway

haem (Fig. 13.2). Haem inhibits both synthesis and activity of ALA synthase in the liver, though the precise inhibitory mechanism in the erythroid cells is uncertain; this exerts a negative feedback control over the synthesis of porphyrins and haemoglobin.

Each molecule of haem combines with one globin polypeptide chain, of two types, α or β. An intact haemoglobin molecule comprises four haem molecules with two α chains and two β chains, with a total molecular weight of about 68 000. Erythrocytes also contain a small amount of free protoporphyrin.

Haemoglobin catabolism (Fig. 13.1)

In the reticuloendothelial system erythrocytes are destroyed and the liberated

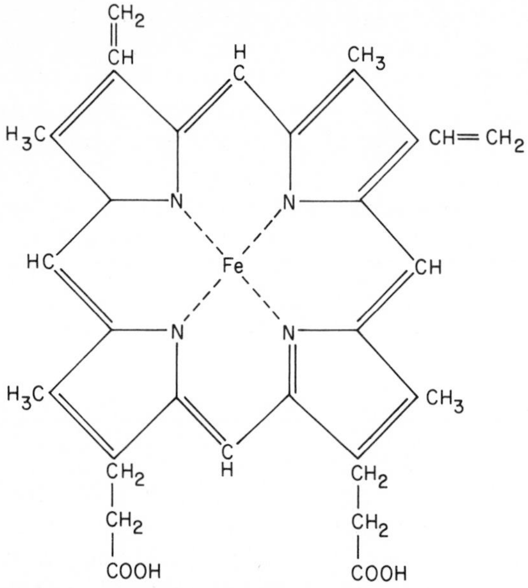

Fig. 13.2   Biochemical structure of haem

haemoglobin is degraded. Some haem is also released in the marrow during erythroblast maturation or from dead cells of ineffective erythropoiesis, or from non-haemoglobin haems, and likewise degraded. Globin is separated from haem, and hydrolysed to amino acids. The porphyrin ring is then opened and the iron is removed, with the formation of the straight chain compound biliverdin, and carbon monoxide. Biliverdin is converted to bilirubin by reduction. The iron (p. 145), and the amino acids of the globin, are retained and re-utilized; the pyrrole rings enter the plasma as unconjugated bilirubin and are eventually excreted. There are other minor pathways producing dipyrroles.

The normal adult male contains about 800 g of haemoglobin (reference range in blood 130–180 g/l), of which about 7 g are produced and destroyed daily. In women the total body haemoglobin is about 600 g (reference range in blood 115–165 g/l).

Haemoglobin derivatives

Oxyhaemoglobin
Haemoglobin without oxygen (deoxy-haemoglobin) is mauve; fully oxygenated haemoglobin, with each haem + globin pair taking up 2 atoms of oxygen, is yellow-red; 1 g of haemoglobin takes up 1.34 ml of oxygen. The symbol for oxyhaemoglobin should thus be HbO_8, but HbO_2 is conventional.

Carboxyhaemoglobin
Carbon monoxide binds to haemoglobin 200 times more avidly than does oxygen. Therefore in the presence of carbon monoxide (from smoke due to fires, from imperfect combustion of coal or paraffin, or present in car exhaust gas or coal gas – but not natural gas, resulting from heavy cigarette smoking) carboxyhaemoglobin (haem-CO-globin, HbCO) is preferentially formed. Symptoms develop when about 20 per cent of the oxyhaemoglobin has been replaced; above 70 per cent there is unconsciousness and death. Carboxy-haemoglobin is cherry-red, especially in dilute solution. Quantitative assay of car-boxyhaemoglobin is usually made by differential spectrophotometry owing to its different absorption spectrum from haemoglobin: this does not detect the traces produced during normal haemoglobin catabolism, nor the slight excess present in haemolytic disease.

Methaemoglobin
This is haematin-globin, containing $Fe^{III}OH$ (symbol Hi): methaemoglobin, an oxidized form of haemoglobin, cannot carry oxygen for respiration. In normal metabolism haemoglobin is cycled by auto-oxidation and reduction through methaemoglobin, though less than 1 per cent of it is so present at any one time.

Methaemoglobin is brown, and methaemoglobinaemia can be suspected by the colour of the patient and of the diluted blood, and diagnosed by differential spectrophotometry. An appearance of 'cyanosis' develops when about 15 per cent of the haemoglobin (2.5 g/dl), and there are symptoms of anoxia when more than 30 per cent of the haemoglobin, is present as methaemoglobin. Congenital methaemo-globinaemia is rare, being due either to lack of the recycling methaemoglobin reductases, or to the presence of an abnormal haemoglobin (Hb M) which easily converts to methaemoglobin. Acquired methaemoglobinaemia may be caused by a number of oxidizing drugs; by nitrites which are produced in the intestine from excess nitrates, used as a food preservative, or in drinking water polluted by industry, or by agricultural fertilizers (infants being particularly susceptible); by aniline and related compounds via skin absorption, especially in industry.

Sulphaemoglobin
This is of uncertain structure, related to methaemoglobin, and unless of the rare Fe^{II} variety, cannot carry respiratory oxygen. Sulphaemoglobinaemia is usually produced by the same drugs as cause methaemoglobinaemia, in the presence of in vivo (intestinal) hydrogen sulphide which completes the chemical reaction. Conversion of about 5 g/dl of the haemoglobin causes 'cyanosis'. Sulphaemoglobin is also brown: diagnosis of its presence requires spectrophotometry and chemical tests.

Glycated haemoglobin
Haemoglobin can bind to glucose to form derivatives that are stable for the life of the erythrocyte. The concentration of glycated haemoglobin A_1, the major component being HbA_{1c}, reflects the integrated glucose concentration to which the erythrocyte has been exposed over about the previous two months, and in health does not exceed about 8.5 per cent of the total haemoglobin (p. 55).

Myoglobin
This oxygen-carrying molecule consists of a monomeric haem + globin (different from that of haemoglobin), containing one Fe^{II} atom, with a molecular weight of about 17 000. It is present in skeletal and cardiac muscle where it acts as an oxygen carrier, and it is released in any condition when there is rapid destruction of muscle fibres.

Because of its low molecular weight it is rapidly cleared from plasma and presents as myoglobulinuria (red-brown urine), and this is a sensitive index of muscle cell damage even from violent exercise. Myoglobin in urine can be diagnosed chemically or immunologically but does not react with simple tests for haemoglobin. Severe myoglobulinuria may lead to acute renal tubular obstruction if accompanied by oliguria.

It is possible to detect myoglobin in serum by immunoassay within a few hours of a myocardial infarction, but this test is not as sensitive or specific as measuring creatine kinase (p. 132).

Haptoglobins
These are specific α_2-globulins that bind haemoglobin at the globin: there are several haptoglobins with a complex pattern of genetic differences. The function of haptoglobins is to conserve iron: after intravascular haemolysis they bind haemoglobin up to about 1.25 g/l of plasma, and only above that concentration does free haemoglobin appear in the plasma where it is degraded, and released haem is bound to haemopexin; further haem is oxidized and bound as methaemalbumin. Haptoglobin bound to haemoglobin is taken up mainly in the liver; the haptoglobin is degraded and the iron is saved.

A low plasma haptoglobin concentration is found after repeated or major intravascular haemolysis. As haptoglobins are synthesized in the liver, they are reduced in chronic liver disease in parallel with albumin. A high plasma haptoglobin concentration is non-specific, occurring as part of an acute-phase reaction (p. 100).

Haemoglobin remaining in the plasma is in part oxidized to methaemoglobin: globin is split off, leaving haem and haematin.

Haemopexin
This is a β_1-glycoprotein that binds remaining haem.

Methaemalbumin
This compound is haematin + albumin. It is brown, and its presence in plasma is always abnormal. Methaemalbumin is formed following severe intravascular haemolysis,

after the haptoglobins and haemopexin are saturated. Other causes of methaemalbuminaemia are bleeding into the abdominal cavity or acute haemorrhagic pancreatitis; pancreatic digestion converts haemoglobin to haematin, which is absorbed and bound to plasma albumin. It is identified spectroscopically, before or after the addition of ammonium sulphide (Schumm's test); the haem–haemopexin complex also gives a positive Schumm's test.

Haemoglobinaemia and haemoglobinuria

Intravascular haemolysis from a wide variety of causes liberates haemoglobin into the circulation, and accounts normally for about 10 per cent of the breakdown of erythrocytes. If this is at a rate greater than the removal capacity of the above binding systems, then free haemoglobin, usually less than 50 mg/l, can be detected in the plasma. Haemoglobin is filtered through the glomeruli as an α–β dimer, and can be reabsorbed and metabolized in the tubules. When the reabsorptive capacity of the tubules is overloaded at a plasma concentration of more than about 300 mg/l, haemoglobinuria can be detected, and some haemoglobin is oxidized to methaemoglobin – the urine is brown.

Haemoglobin in urine accompanied by erythrocytes is usually of renal or postrenal origin; however, massive excretion of haemoglobin (as other protein, p. 122) may itself cause renal tubular obstruction. In some forms of chronic haemoglobinaemia, especially in paroxysmal nocturnal haemoglobinuria, the brown insoluble iron storage compound haemosiderin (an iron(III) hydroxide–protein complex related to ferritin), derived from the tubular metabolism of haemoglobin, is deposited in the tubules, and some may be found in a spun urine deposit.

Commercial tests are available (p. 259) for the detection of haemoglobin in urine: they utilize the peroxidase activity of haemoglobin.

Abnormal haemoglobins

The study of different haemoglobins due to genetic variants in the globins has provided important insights into genetics, and more recently into molecular biology, since, by a knowledge of the small chemical changes in the globin, it has become possible in many cases to predict both the abnormal biochemical properties of the abnormal haemoglobin and the changes in the patient, and to deduce the nature of the primary change in the DNA.

There are also variant myoglobins, not apparently related to muscle disease.

As well as the α and β chains of normal Hb A ($\alpha_2\beta_2$), γ and δ globin chains are regularly found in adults. Hb A_2 is $\alpha_a\delta_2$, and constitutes about 2.5 per cent of the haemoglobin of an adult. Hb F (fetal haemoglobin) is $\alpha_2\gamma_2$, and constitutes less than 1 per cent of the haemoglobin of an adult, though 75 per cent at birth.

The haemoglobinopathies

Haemoglobinopathies are conveniently classified into two main groups.

In the first group one or more amino acids are altered in the α or β globin chains, giving rise to the formation of an *abnormal haemoglobin*. More than 100 clinically relevant forms have been described: there is also a group of abnormal haemoglobins with high affinity for oxygen, producing erythrocytosis, and other rarities. With some, such as Hb S (of sickle cell anaemia) which is the commonest and best-known of these haemoglobinopathies, presence of the abnormal haemoglobin can give rise to deformation of the cells, anaemia, and other symptoms. In Hb S, as an example, the α chains are the normal type as in Hb A, but the glutamic acid at position 6 of the β chains is substituted by valine.

In the second group there is deficient formation of normal haemoglobin, and these constitute the *thalassaemias*. In α-thalassaemia, α chain formation is deficient, with production of the abnormal β_4 (Hb H) or γ_4 (Hb Bart's): the most severe homozygous (major) form is incompatible with life but there is a milder homozygous (minor) variety, Hb H disease. In β-thalassaemia the deficiency of β-chain formation leads to some compensatory increase in Hb A_2 and Hb F. The heterozygous state is known as the thalassaemia trait.

The haemoglobinopathies are described in detail in haematology texts.

Congenital haemolytic anaemia

Biochemically these are of two main groups.

Membrane defects

In these conditions, of which the commonest is hereditary spherocytosis, there is primary alteration of the erythrocyte membrane proteins and a consequent abnormality in the sodium pump. The fundamental causes have not been elucidated. The abnormal erythrocytes are destroyed excessively in the spleen, leading to anaemia and jaundice.

Enzyme deficiencies

Glucose-6-phosphate dehydrogenase deficiency

This is a relatively common group of disorders with multiple enzyme variants, especially in Negroes, South Chinese, and Mediterranean people, and may protect against malaria. Glucose-6-phosphate dehydrogenase (G6PD) is the enzyme responsible for the initial deviation of glucose into the pentose phosphate pathway (p. 48) to form 6-phosphogluconate; this pathway provides $NADPH_2$ in the erythrocyte for the conversion of oxidized to reduced glutathione which is essential for maintaining haemoglobin in the reduced state. The enzyme deficiency may cause haemolysis *per se*, though the mechanisms are uncertain, but haemolysis chiefly occurs after exposure of the erythrocyte to a wide variety of drugs and other agents, e.g. primaquine, broad beans (favism), and certain infections. The cells are deficient in reduced glutathione and thus accumulate methaemoglobin: haemolysis, dark urine, and jaundice are present. This deficiency may also produce neonatal jaundice.

Several screening tests are available but definite diagnosis is made by assay of the enzyme in erythrocytes; in homozygotes enzyme activity is reduced to less than 15 per cent of normal.

Other enzyme deficiencies

These are rarer, the most frequent being of pyruvate kinase, and are not related to the ingestion of drugs or other sensitizers.

Porphyrins

Biochemistry

The porphyrin precursors (Fig. 13.1) are part of the biosynthetic pathway of the haemoproteins. The classification of the porphyrins into uro-, copro-, and protoporphyrins, of series I and III, depends on the nature and spatial distribution of the substituents on the ring system.

Porphobilinogen is a colourless chromogen which can be oxidized to a porphyrin mixture for identification: it also yields a specific reddish pigment with Ehrlich's aldehyde reagent (p. 259). Porphyrins impart a characteristic dark red colour ('port wine') to urine when they are present in large quantities, and they give a pink fluorescence in ultraviolet light. Identification and quantitative estimation of all the individual porphyrins and precursors is a research procedure.

The excretion of porphyrins by a healthy adult is mainly coproporphyrins in the urine (less than 0.3 µmol/24 h), and protoporphyrins in the faeces. ALA and porphobilinogen are excreted in the urine, but not in the faeces.

Clinical disorders

Porphyrias

These conditions are primary inborn metabolic disorders of porphyrin metabolism. They are all due to specific deficiencies of enzymes of the pathway of haemoglobin synthesis in the liver or bone marrow: variable removal of feedback control by haem causes accumulation of precursors

Table 13.1   Summary of biochemical findings in porphyrias and lead poisoning

	Urine	Faeces	Erythrocyte
Congenital erythropoietic porphyria	↑ Uroporphyrin ↑ Coproporphyrin	↑ Coproporphyrin	↑ Uroporphyrin ↑ Protoporphyrin
Acute intermittent porphyria	↑ Porphobilinogen ↑ ALA		
Hereditary coproporphyria	↑ Coproporphyrin ↑ ALA	↑ Coproporphyrin	
Porphyria variegata	↑ Coproporphyrin ↑ ALA	↑ Protoporphyrin	
Erythropoietic protoporphyria		↑ Protoporphyrin	↑ Protoporphyrin
Lead poisoning	↑ ALA ↑ Coproporphyrin		↑ Protoporphyrin

behind the block (p. 134). Different enzyme defects lead to different patterns of changes in porphyrin excretion (Table 13.1).

Congenital erythropoietic porphyria

The metabolic defect in this very rare, but striking, disorder is deficiency of uroporphyrinogen III co-synthase, with an increase of porphobilinogen deaminase leading to excessive synthesis in the bone marrow of principally the unphysiological Type I uroporphyrin. The urine is coloured red by the porphyrins, as may be the teeth and bones; there may be a thousand-fold increase in total urinary porphyrins. The porphyrins in the skin cause severe solar photosensitivity as they absorb light energy which damages the tissues. Faecal porphyrin excretion is also high.

Acute intermittent porphyria

This is associated with increased ALA-synthase activity in the liver from feedback induction, secondary to porphobilinogen deaminase deficiency later in the metabolic pathway. This leads to excess synthesis and urinary excretion of ALA and porphobilinogen, and also of some preformed porphyrins; erythrocyte uroporphyrinogen I is low.

During acute episodes of the disease, which may be precipitated by oral contraceptives, barbiturates, alcohol or many other drugs, or by infection, there may be a 50-fold increased excretion of the porphyrin precursors; during clinical remission excretion may return almost to normal. The

nervous system is sensitive to the excess porphyrin precursors; there are variable psychiatric and neurological symptoms, and particularly attacks of acute abdominal pain probably caused by autonomic dysfunction. There is no photosensitivity. It is therefore important, in all clinically suspicious cases, to test the urine for porphobilinogen: during acute episodes the urine, clear on passing, darkens on standing after acidification. A low plasma sodium may be due to inappropriate secretion of antidiuretic hormone because of moderate increase of porphyrin precursors.

Hereditary coproporphyria

This is due to deficiency of coproporphyrinogen oxidase and has similar but milder symptoms caused by a moderate increase of porphyrin precursors.

Porphyria cutanea tarda

This is due to uroporphyrinogen decarboxylase deficiency, and is aggravated by alcoholism which is causing liver disease. This variety has cutaneous symptoms, and increased urinary uro- (and sometimes copro-) porphyrins are found during attacks.

Porphyria variegata

This is caused by protoporphyrinogen oxidase deficiency, is mainly found in South Africa, and has cutaneous and abdominal symptoms. During the acute phase excess porphyrin precursors, and often porphyrins, are present in the urine and faeces, whilst during latent phases excess porphyrins are found only in the faeces.

Erythropoietic protoporphyria
Deficiency of ferrochelatase leads to protoporphyrin accumulation in erythrocytes, plasma, and faeces. There is a photosensitive rash, and often liver disease as protoporphyrin is hepatotoxic. Urinary porphobilinogen and porphyrins are normal.

Porphyrinurias

In these secondary conditions the excess porphyrin in the urine (usually less than 1.5 μmol/24 h, which is insufficient to colour the urine) is almost always coproporphyrin III; the porphyrinuria is caused by another disease that is not a primary disorder of porphyrin metabolism. Porphyrinuria of about 1.0 μmol/24 h is consistently found, due to overproduction in the bone marrow, in blood disorders associated with excess haemolysis, in liver disease (particularly in cirrhosis, especially alcoholic, p. 158), and in poisoning from aromatic compounds and heavy metals, particularly lead.

Lead poisoning
This is cumulative, from a variety of environmental causes: it may present with anaemia, colic, neuritis, or psychiatric features – but not photosensitivity.

Excess lead interferes with haem synthesis by multiple enzyme inhibition, and there is altered haemopoiesis which produces stippled and nucleated erythrocytes. In early lead poisoning (with a blood lead of 4–5 μmol/l), the best screening test is detection of an increased erythrocyte zinc protoporphyrin, also with decreased ALA dehydratase: urinary coproporphyrins and ALA are also increased. These analyses need a specialized laboratory, and special care to avoid contamination when taking samples for blood lead.

The control of erythrocyte development

Erythropoietin

This is a glycoprotein produced mainly by the kidneys, in response to hypoxia: it acts on and is utilized by the stem cells in the bone marrow. Pure erythropoietin, produced by recombinant DNA technology, is now available for therapeutic use. Its assay in plasma or urine is possible as a research procedure. It is not detectable in the plasma of normal subjects, but can be found in chronic anaemia or after acute haemorrhage.

In polycythaemia vera, erythropoietin production is very low due to negative feedback, whilst in polycythaemia due to carcinoma of the kidney (and occasionally to other tumours and other renal diseases), there is an inappropriate autonomous continuing production of erythropoietin and failure of feedback.

Vitamin B$_{12}$

The vitamin B$_{12}$ group comprises a set of complex molecules, all of which contain cobalt (Co^{II}) in a corrin (porphyrin-like) ring, linked to a nucleotide. Vitamin B$_{12}$ acts as a multiple coenzyme: its deficiency causes megaloblastic anaemia, probably by interfering with methionine synthesis and folate metabolism. The biochemical basis of the neurological lesions of vitamin B$_{12}$ deficiency is not clear.

The normal dietary intake is 5–30 μg daily, of which less than 5 μg is absorbed. Vitamin B$_{12}$ is absent from plant foods, so vegans are eventually liable to develop deficiency. All vitamin B$_{12}$ in nature is originally synthesized by micro-organisms, but vitamin B$_{12}$ so synthesized in the human colon is not absorbed. The adult requirement is about 2 μg daily, and as body stores are about 3 mg (of which some 50 per cent is in the liver), 3 to 5 years are required free of dietary vitamin B$_{12}$ to develop deficiency.

Intrinsic factor is a glycoprotein, produced by the parietal cells of the stomach, and its synthesis is deficient in pernicious anaemia. It binds vitamin B_{12} (the original 'extrinsic factor'), and the resultant complex is absorbed into the villi of the terminal ileum, where the vitamin B_{12} is slowly split off and enters the circulation. About 1 per cent of a large oral dose of vitamin B_{12} can be absorbed in the absence of intrinsic factor.

Vitamin B_{12} in plasma

Vitamin B_{12} circulates bound to specific transport proteins (transcobalamins): the reference range for plasma vitamin B_{12} is 150–750 pmol/l, measured by competitive protein binding – though microbiological assay is also used.

Vitamin B_{12} deficiency

The principal causes are dietary deficiency (relative in pregnancy), lack of intrinsic factor, and gastrointestinal disease.

Investigation of the cause of a low plasma vitamin B_{12} (less than 80 pmol/l), with the appropriate haematological changes of a megaloblastic anaemia, often requires measuring radioactive vitamin B_{12} absorption in the absence and presence of added intrinsic factor. A urinary excretion (Schilling) test is popular if whole body counting is not available.

Schilling test

Method

After an overnight fast the patient empties his bladder. The patient takes 1 μg (37 kBq, 1 μCi) of (^{57}Co or ^{58}Co) B_{12} by mouth, and has an intramuscular flushing injection of 1 mg non-radioactive vitamin B_{12}. All urine passed in the next 24 h is pooled and sent to the laboratory.

If pernicious anaemia is suspected the test is repeated after four or five days, with an additional dose of 50 mg intrinsic factor orally taken with the dose of radioactive vitamin B_{12}.

Interpretation

In healthy subjects, 10 to 33 per cent of the dose of radioactive vitamin B_{12} is excreted in the urine in 24 h. In dietary deficiency, there is normal excretion. In pernicious anaemia, less than 5 per cent of the dose is excreted, while in malabsorption up to 10 per cent may be found. In pernicious anaemia, but not in malabsorption, normal absorption and excretion are restored when the test is repeated with added intrinsic factor. Renal insufficiency depresses excretion of vitamin B_{12} and invalidates the test.

Other tests

Measuring the ability of the stomach to excrete hydrochloric acid after stimulation (p. 163) used to be an important part of the investigation of megaloblastic anaemia and is still occasionally useful – presence of free hydrochloric acid negates the diagnosis of pernicious anaemia. It is possible to measure, in serum, antibodies to parietal cells and to intrinsic factor.

The oxidation of methylmalonyl CoA to succinyl CoA requires vitamin B_{12} as co-enzyme. The normal urinary excretion of methylmalonic acid, 30–60 μmol/24 h, is increased up to 4 mmol/24 h in most cases of untreated vitamin B_{12} deficiency; the assay is complex, but the investigation is sometimes useful.

Folate

The parent compound is folic acid, otherwise known as pteroylglutamic acid, and contains a pteridine double ring, *p*-aminobenzoic acid, and glutamic acid. The various dietary folates are converted to methyl tetrahydrofolate during absorption. This active form enters intracellular metabolism and is converted to the folate co-enzymes, which function for transfer of single carbon units in amino acid interconversion and in the synthesis of purines and pyrimidines. Its exact role in erythrocyte maturation is unknown, though its deficiency causes megaloblastic anaemia, probably through interference with DNA synthesis. Vitamin B_{12} is required for normal folate metabolism.

The normal daily dietary intake of folates

from plant and animal food is about 500 μg. The normal requirement is about 50 μg/24-h, and this is much greater in pregnancy; the body stores are about 5 mg, and 20 weeks without folate intake are required to develop deficiency. Folate is absorbed throughout the upper small instestine.

Folate in blood

The reference range for plasma folate is 5–45 nmol/l, and for erythrocyte folate is 200–1000 nmol/l, usually measured by microbiological assay, or alternatively by competitive protein binding.

Tests for folate deficiency in megaloblastic anaemia, usually nutritional (absolute; or relative as in pregnancy), or due to malabsorption (p. 170) or due to drugs which impair utilization, are less satisfactory than for vitamin B_{12}; the plasma folate slowly falls to less than 3 nmol/l, and the erythrocyte folate to less than 150 nmol/l. Plasma values fall first, at a sub-clinical stage of deficiency: erythrocyte values represent body stores – in a full study both should be measured.

Iron

Intake and absorption

The normal daily intake on a mixed diet is 10–20 mg (200–400 μmol), mainly in complexes such as myoglobin. For its absorption the presence of gastric hydrochloric acid and other factors, and possibly of ascorbic acid for reduction to Fe^{II}, is desirable: phytate and phosphate reduce the availability of iron for absorption in the same way as for calcium (p. 186). About 10 per cent (1–2 mg) is normally absorbed just to compensate for iron loss: as 20–25 mg of iron daily is needed for haemoglobin synthesis, most of this is obtained from recirculated iron (p. 138). Iron is absorbed, mainly as ferrous ions (Fe^{2+}), into the mucosa of the upper small intestine. There it is absorbed into the portal blood or is bound as the soluble storage product ferritin, which is a complex of iron(III)

hydroxide, phosphate, and the protein apoferritin. The mechanism by which apoferritin controls the rate of iron absorption is uncertain. More iron is absorbed when there is iron deficiency, or when erythropoiesis is increased.

Circulating iron

The iron is then transferred to the specific β_1-globulin, transferrin (siderophyllin), of molecular weight 80 000, and thus transported for haemoglobin and other synthesis. The normal plasma transferrin concentration is about 2 g/l, and plasma has a total iron-binding capacity of 45–75 μmol/l. In plasma the concentration of free iron, in equilibrium with iron-transferrin, is negligible, and the transferrin is about one-third saturated with iron; the amount of unsaturated transferrin is termed the unsaturated iron-binding capacity. The reference range for plasma iron is 14–34 μmol/l in men, and 11–30 μmol/l in women. There is a marked circadian rhythm, with a variation of about 7 μmol/l: highest values are at about 08:00, and lowest at 21:00.

Iron distribution

The main function of iron is acting as the metal component of haemoglobin and myoglobin, and of iron-containing enzymes (cytochromes, flavoproteins) of the electron transport system. The total body iron of an adult male is 3–4 g, and of a woman 2.5–3.5 g: about 65 per cent is as haemoglobin, 25 per cent as storage iron in the reticuloendothelial system (about equal parts of ferritin and haemosiderin), about 10 per cent as other tissue 'essential' iron (myoglobin, iron-containing enzymes, cytochromes), and only 0.1 per cent as plasma iron.

Iron is extremely well conserved. Men lose only about 0.5–1.0 mg of iron daily, mainly in the faeces, with 0.1 mg in urine and 0.2 mg in shed skin. Women lose in addition 15 mg at each menstrual period (30 ml blood) and 500 mg at each pregnancy: women are therefore at greater risk of going into negative iron balance. A 'unit' of blood given by a donor contains about 250 mg of iron.

Abnormalities of plasma iron concentration

The concentration is low in iron-deficiency anaemia, whether due to absolute or relative insufficient intake, malabsorption, or blood loss from any site – there is an accompanying increased erythrocyte protoporphyrin (p. 137). Low values are also found, with anaemia, in most chronic inflammatory diseases and infections.

Plasma iron concentration is high when the marrow cannot utilize iron, in megaloblastic anaemia, in thalassaemia, and in anaemias associated with abnormal haemoglobin and haemolysis: high values are found in severe hepatitis due to release from liver cells, or after oral overdose with iron.

In any full study of iron turnover, plasma total iron-binding capacity should be measured at the same time as plasma iron: it is high in iron-deficiency anaemia and in pregnancy, whereas it is low in anaemias of chronic infection. The concentration of transferrin (like that of other binding proteins) is decreased in protein malnutrition (p. 97) and by urinary loss in the nephrotic syndrome, and increased by hormonal contraceptives.

Iron stores

Reticuloendothelial accumulation, or deficiency, may be determined by histochemistry of bone marrow (or liver biopsy) for haemosiderin. This is reflected by the plasma ferritin (reference range 15–250 μg/l), which correlates with total body iron stores. In iron-deficiency anaemia the concentration is usually less than 10 μg/l, and low values will be found before the haemoglobin falls. In iron overload it may exceed 1000 μg/l, but raised values are also found in acute liver disease, and in many non-specific chronic disorders.

Haemochromatosis

The primary defect in this inborn error of metabolism is probably both of iron storage and of iron transport: iron absorption is excessive. The plasma total iron-binding capacity is low and is fully saturated, with a plasma iron usually less than 45 μmol/l. Serum ferritin is increased, and haemosiderin is widely deposited in tissues and can be detected in cells of a urine deposit: the total body iron may be 20–40 g. Iron in the liver may cause hepatomegaly and cirrhosis, and combined deposition in skin and pancreas cause 'bronze diabetes'. There is often hypogonadism.

Secondary haemochromatosis (haemosiderosis) can result from iron overload, particularly due to repeated transfusion but occasionally orally; serum ferritin assay may be used to monitor iron stores. Usually this deposition is mainly in the reticuloendothelial system and is asymptomatic, but hypoparathyroidism may develop.

Copper

The known biochemical functions of copper are in the electron transport system, and possibly in the synthesis of haemoglobin. The reference range for plasma copper is 13–24 μmol/l, almost all of which is bound to caeruloplasmin, a specific α_2-globulin (molecular weight 150 000) whose plasma concentration is 0.3–0.6 g/l. Less than 1.5 μmol/24 h of copper are lost in the urine.

Copper deficiency, with anaemia, may result from severe malnutrition or improper intravenous feeding. The plasma copper may be less than 7 μmol/l, and plasma caeruloplasmin less than 0.2 g/l.

A low plasma caeruloplasmin results from urinary loss in the nephrotic syndrome, or from malnutrition; and a high value (sometimes with a green plasma) may be due to hormonal contraceptives or is occasionally seen in late pregnancy and primary biliary cirrhosis.

Wilson's disease (hepatolenticular degeneration)

In this congenital metabolic disorder the primary defect is probably intrahepatic, with impaired hepatobiliary excretion of copper: the role of the impaired synthesis of caeruloplasmin is uncertain. Plasma copper is low, 6–9 μmol/l; caeruloplasmin less than 0.3 g/l; and urinary copper is increased to about 8 μmol/24 h. Copper deposition in the brain and liver cause the mental and hepatic symptoms, and in the cornea produces the Kayser–Fleischer ring. Deposition in renal tubules may produce a Fanconi syndrome, and the resulting aminoaciduria may be diagnostically useful (p. 90).

Further reading

Cavill I, Jacobs A, Worwood M. Diagnostic methods for iron status. *Ann Clin Biochem* 1986; **23**: 168–71.

Hindmarsh JT. The porphyrias – recent advances. *Clin. Chem* 1986; **32**: 1255–63.

Hoffbrand AV, Pettit JE. *Essential Haematology*. 2nd edn. Oxford: Blackwell Scientific Publications, 1984.

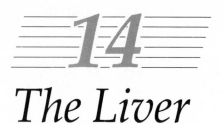

The Liver

Objectives

In this chapter the reader is able to

- revise the physiology of hepatic excretory and metabolic functions
- study the biochemical changes in the main hepatobiliary diseases, including the effects of drugs and the relation to treatment.

At the conclusion of this chapter the reader is able to

- understand the relation between different types of alteration of liver functional and structural integrity and the various groups of 'liver function tests'
- understand the pathology of jaundice, and its relevance to the investigation of a patient with jaundice
- understand the causes of gall-stones and investigate a suspected case
- use the laboratory in the investigation of suspected hepatobiliary disease.

Functions of the liver and their investigation

The liver is uniquely placed for handling dietary compounds in that it receives all the blood from the gut via the portal system and it is responsible for the synthesis of many metabolically important compounds from diet-derived precursors and for their interconversion. It is also responsible for the excretion or metabolism of toxic compounds both from the systemic circula-

tion and the portal blood. The principal functions of the liver may be summarized.

1. Major metabolites

The liver is the centre of metabolic activity for interconversion and synthesis of carbohydrate, protein and lipid.

Carbohydrate

The liver takes up glucose from the portal and systemic circulations without a requirement for insulin. Sugars and carbon residues from protein and fat are converted to glycogen and stored as carbohydrate reserve, being reconvertible to glucose. This reserve is small and will only last for a matter of hours. Glucose can be converted to lipid and after entry into the tricarboxylic acid cycle (TCA cycle), into ketones. These important energy-providing molecules are normally produced from fatty acids entering the liver when glucose is in short supply but when there is a large amount of glucose entering the liver, as in diabetes, ketones may be produced from it.

Protein

Albumin and most other proteins including coagulation factors are synthesized in the parenchymal cells. Normal albumin synthesis is about 10 g/24 h, and this represents about 30 per cent of the total protein synthetic capacity of the liver. Amino acids derived from the catabolism of protein are deaminated, the nitrogen residues (and ammonia from the gut) being converted to urea.

Lipid

The liver contains a store of triglyceride, some being derived from endogenous synthesis. Cholesterol and from it bile salts, are synthesized. Cholesterol released from the liver in VLDL provides, via LDL, most of the requirement of this compound by all cells for membrane synthesis. Cholesterol and other lipids are esterified, and vitamin D is hydroxylated. Bile salts are secreted into the biliary tract. The liver acts as a central site for the conversion of carbohydrate to triglyceride for secretion in the blood as VLDL and storage in fat. In addition fatty acids released from adipose tissue during starvation may be converted to triglyceride for restorage or to ketones for energy.

2. Detoxification

The liver detoxicates many metabolic products, hormones, drugs and toxins, often prior to their excretion in the urine. The detoxication process involves a chemical change and/or conjugation principally with glucuronic acid, glycine, or sulphate.

3. Excretion

The liver excretes many natural and foreign substances into the biliary tract. The parenchymal cells of the liver (hepatocytes), which comprise 60 per cent of its mass, are responsible for the conjugation of bilirubin and for its excretion in the bile. IgA from the blood, is also excreted in the bile where it protects the gut from certain bacteria.

4. Storage

The liver stores a variety of compounds, including iron, vitamin B_{12} and vitamin A.

5. Immunology

The Kupffer cells (specialized macrophages) take part in the overall activities of the reticuloendothelial system.

Investigation of function

When the liver is diseased, one or more but not necessarily all of its functions are impaired. Disruption of the normal liver architecture results in increased pressure in the portal system: portal hypertension. Under such circumstances, and when plasma albumin levels are low, a transudate forms across the liver capsule and ascites develops. The 'liver function tests' are tests of derangement of individual or related functions of the liver (or of secondary derangements elsewhere in the body), and there can be no test for 'liver function' as a whole. Many so-called liver function tests are in fact reflecting damage to hepatocytes or biliary epithelial cells rather than their function. It may be possible to extend a conclusion drawn from a single test to an appreciation of the activities of the liver as a whole, because many tests give similar abnormal results in particular diseases of the liver.

The results of liver biopsy are not necessarily comparable with the results of chemical tests, as many measured functional changes are not mirrored by visible structural changes in the liver cells and *vice versa*. In addition, histopathological changes are rarely uniform throughout the liver in disease.

The adult liver has considerable functional reserve. An isolated part may be removed or severely damaged by a localized disease (for example by carcinoma), and if the remainder is healthy, liver function may remain apparently normal when tested biochemically in the resting state – and there can be regeneration of functional cells. On the other hand, in a disease such as infective hepatitis, in which there is diffuse damage to the majority of liver cells, detectable derangement of liver function is always present.

The metabolism of bile pigments

Erythrocytes at the end of their life-span are destroyed in the reticuloendothelial system. This amounts to about 1 per cent of the total haemoglobin per day. The protein is catabolized in the lysosomes and the porphyrin ring is opened to form bilirubin (p. 138). Iron is released and becomes bound to transferrin: it is not excreted but enters the iron stores or is used for further haemoglobin synthesis. Most of the bilirubin is derived from haemoglobin, though about 20 per cent comes from the breakdown of tissue cytochromes, myoglobin and other haem proteins, and some from erythrocyte precursors destroyed in the bone marrow (ineffective erythropoiesis). Bilirubin, which in the free form is lipid- and not water-soluble, circulates in the plasma in a water-soluble form bound to albumin. In adults this form accounts for almost all the bilirubin found in plasma, and because it is bound to albumin it is not filtered at the renal glomerulus, and being no longer lipid-soluble cannot cross cell membranes, for example into brain cells. If bilirubin production increases beyond the capacity of albumin to bind it, free bilirubin entering the plasma passes rapidly into cells and may damage brain cells in certain parts of the brain causing kernicterus. In the liver this (unconjugated) bilirubin enters the hepatocytes by receptor-mediated uptake and is there conjugated primarily with glucuronic acid by a mechanism involving bilirubin uridyl diphosphate (UDP) glucuronosyltransferase. The pigment excreted in the bile is the water-soluble bilirubin diglucuronide, usually referred to as conjugated bilirubin. Bile also contains cholesterol and bile salts, which together with bilirubin must be present in the correct proportion to remain soluble. Failure of bile salt synthesis results in precipitation of bile components particularly cholesterol and blockage of small bile ducts.

The liver of an adult has the reserve capacity to conjugate and excrete 5 to 10 times its normal load of bilirubin, which is about 500 µmol/24 h. The enzymes responsible for conjugation are not fully active at birth (for example full activity of UDP glucuronosyltransferase takes three weeks to develop), and even less so in prematurity, so the neonatal liver barely has the capacity to excrete its normal bilirubin load, and this load may be increased due to excessive breakdown of erythrocytes. Jaundice before 24 h of age is abnormal, but a moderate hyperbilirubinaemia (<80 µmol/l) within the first week may not be pathological ('physiological jaundice') and it is well within the capacity of plasma albumin to render it water-soluble.

Excretion of bile pigments (bilirubin and urobilinogen)

Conjugated bilirubin is secreted into the biliary caniliculi whence it enters the bile duct and passes to the intestines where it is deconjugated. In the large intestine it is reduced by bacterial action to various pigments and pigment precursors including urobilinogen (this is a collective name given to a group of colourless chromogens one of which is stercobilinogen, though other terminology is used). Most of the urobilinogen is excreted in the faeces where it is oxidized by the air to the pinkish-brown urobilin pigments. Urobilin, with

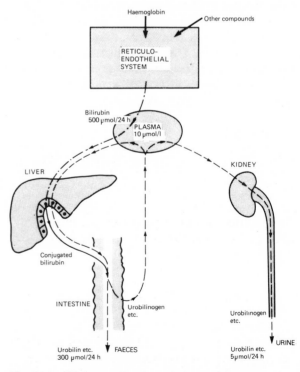

Fig. 14.1   Diagram of main pathways of the origin, circulation and excretion of bilirubin and principal related compounds in a normal adult

many other compounds both known and unidentified, forms the colouring matter of faeces; stercobilin, which is strictly one of the compounds of urobilin, is sometimes used as an alternative name for the urobilin group of pigments. A small fraction of the urobilinogen is absorbed into the portal circulation, and in the liver some of this urobilinogen is re-excreted into the bile, whilst the remainder is excreted by the kidneys. When urine is exposed to air, urobilinogen is oxidized to urobilin, though this makes up a negligible part of the colouring matter of normal urine. Most of the pigments that produce the colour of urine are unidentified, and they are known collectively as urochrome (p. 126).

There is no bilirubin in the faeces of a normal adult. In the newborn, bilirubin is found in the faeces and there is no urobilinogen in the faeces or urine, as the bacterial flora necessary for conversion of bilirubin to urobilinogen takes some months to develop fully. Bilirubin is found in the faeces of adults whose gut has been sterilized by antibiotics.

Biliverdin, a green oxidation product of bilirubin and intermediate in haemoglobin breakdown (p. 138), has little importance in the study of human liver disease. Figure 14.1 summarizes the normal metabolism of bilirubin in an adult.

Amniotic fluid

Bilirubinoid pigments are released into the amniotic fluid in small amounts when red cell breakdown has become severe in cases of isoimmunized pregnancy, particularly rhesus incompatibility. When measured, at about 32 weeks, the result can be used as a guide for early induction of labour or for intrauterine transfusion.

Plasma bilirubin and the van den Bergh reaction

Bilirubin (unconjugated) and conjugated bilirubin, which are both bound to protein (mainly albumin), can be distinguished chemically in plasma by their rate of reaction with diazotized sulphanilic acid to form azobilirubin (the van den Bergh reaction). Conjugated bilirubin reacts rapidly and a mauve colour appears within a few minutes (positive direct van den Bergh reaction). Unconjugated bilirubin does not give this immediate colour (negative direct van den Bergh reaction), but a colour develops after adding alcohol, caffeine or other special reagents (the indirect van den Bergh reaction). It is rarely necessary, except in certain types of haemolytic jaundice, to measure both bilirubin fractions. The presence of conjugated bilirubin in the plasma is indicated by the presence of bilirubin in the urine. In the investigation of most cases of jaundice the total plasma bilirubin gives sufficient information.

The reference range for plasma total bilirubin in adults is 3–15 μmol/l, and normal plasma, containing only a small proportion of conjugated bilirubin, does not give a positive direct van den Bergh reaction.

Bilirubin is slowly destroyed by ultraviolet or blue light and phototherapy may be used for treatment of neonatal hyperbilirubinaemia.

In neonatal jaundice where other pigments such as carotenes, which may interfere, are not present a direct measurement of the yellow colour of plasma may be used to measure bilirubin. This is the principle employed in commercial bilirubinometers (p. 261).

Jaundice

Jaundice can be detected clinically by orange-yellow colouration of skin and sclera when the plasma total bilirubin exceeds about 35 μmol/l. When jaundice is receding bile pigments may remain in the skin and the patient appear more jaundiced then the plasma total bilirubin level would warrant.

No single classification of jaundice is satisfactory for all purposes. It is possible to consider primarily (a) the anatomical site of the pathological lesion causing the jaundice (prehepatic, hepatic, posthepatic), or (b) the pathological causes (infective, toxic, etc) or (c) the nature of the alteration in bilirubin metabolism and transport.

Jaundice and altered bilirubin metabolism

Haemolytic causes

In haemolytic jaundice the rate of production of bilirubin is greater than the rate at which liver cells can excrete bilirubin. In adults, the plasma bilirubin rarely exceeds 80 µmol/l, and there is no excess conjugated bilirubin unless there is concomitant liver damage or pigment stones obstructing the biliary tract. In infants, haemolytic disease of the newborn and delayed formation of conjugating enzymes may lead to a plasma bilirubin in excess of 350 µmol/l. Kernicterus develops because the excess bilirubin is soluble in the lipid of the basal ganglia of the brain. Administration of sulphonamides may displace enough bilirubin from its albumin-binding sites to produce kernicterus at lower bilirubin levels.

Hepatocellular causes

Abnormalities at a hepatocellular level may be a defect of transport of bilirubin into the cell, defective conjugation or defective excretion into the bile canaliculi. Cholestasis, or reduction of bile flow, may be due to the latter in liver necrosis (e.g. infective hepatitis), or as a specific failure of excretion, or posthepatic obstruction.

Of the genetic failures of bilirubin metabolism the commonest is *Gilbert's syndrome*, a group of conditions affecting 1 to 5 per cent of the United Kingdom population (familial non-haemolytic hyperbilirubinaemia) in which, because of deficiencies of the transport mechanism, there is a fluctuating benign mild jaundice due to non-conjugated bilirubin. In the *Crigler-Najjar syndrome* there is congenital deficiency of UDP glucuronosyltransferase. There are other rare inherited conjugated hyperbilirubinaemias.

In hepatocellular damage, failure to excrete bilirubin into the biliary calculi leads to an increase in plasma conjugated bilirubin; there is jaundice and plasma total bilirubin may exceed 300 µmol/l.

Cholestatic causes

When cholestasis predominates, and especially when the cause is extrahepatic obstruction, the plasma total bilirubin (almost all conjugated) may exceed 500 µmol/l, and the patient may appear greenish-yellow due to the presence in plasma and skin of a little biliverdin. Kernicterus does not develop because the excess conjugated bilirubin is water-soluble and is therefore not deposited in the basal ganglia. Intrahepatic cholestasis is commonly caused by drugs, toxins and hepatocellular damage. It results from a disturbance of bile salt metabolism rendering the components of bile insoluble so that they form a precipitate which blocks the biliary canaliculi.

Bile pigments in the urine in disease

Bilirubin

No bilirubin can be detected in normal urine. Bilirubin (unconjugated) is not excreted by the healthy kidney because of its low water solubility and of its firm binding to protein, so that in haemolytic jaundice, when there is only a high plasma bilirubin, none can be detected in the urine – hence the old name for adult haemolytic anaemia, 'acholuric jaundice'. Conjugated bilirubin, being water-soluble and with some of it more loosely bound to protein, is readily excreted, and 'bilirubin' found in the urine is always in the conjugated form. When there is a high plasma conjugated bilirubin, this pigment can be detected in the urine when the plasma total bilirubin level exceeds about 30 µmol/l, and the froth (due to excess bile salts) of shaken urine appears yellow when the plasma bilirubin level exceeds about 50 µmol/l, though the threshold is variable.

Urobilinogen

A small amount of urobilinogen can be detected in fresh normal urine (p. 259), though these semiquantitative tests are insensitive and of little diagnostic value. In haemolytic jaundice more bilirubin passes to the intestines where an increased quantity of urobilinogen is formed. Much of this urobilinogen is absorbed, and excess urobilinogen is excreted in the urine. In the preicteric and recovery stages of infective hepatitis, and sometimes in cirrhosis without jaundice, excess urinary urobilinogen is found, presumably due to impaired ability of the liver cells to re-excrete urobilinogen.

In severe hepatocellular or obstructive jaundice less bilirubin reaches the intestine, little urobilinogen is formed, and urobilinogen is absent from the urine. Reappearance of urobilinogen in the urine is a sign of recovery from cholestasis. If posthepatic obstruction is due to malignancy and is complete, urobilinogen is constantly absent, whereas if it is due to a stone and is incomplete, bilirubin may occasionally pass into the intestine and urobilinogen be found in the urine.

Bile pigments in the faeces in disease

In severe cholestatic jaundice, or due to oral antibiotics which alter the intestinal flora, faecal urobilinogen excretion is greatly diminished. The quantity excreted also relates to the completeness of posthepatic obstruction, faecal urobilinogen and urobilin being often undetectable (clay-coloured stools) when the obstruction is complete due to a tumour, and appearing when there is incomplete obstruction.

Summary of changes in bile pigment metabolism

The results found in investigation of bile pigment metabolism in the principal types of jaundice are summarized in Table 14.1. Haemolytic anaemia is associated with characteristic disturbances of bile pigment metabolism provided that it is uncomplicated by secondary liver damage. Tests based on other aspects of disturbed liver function must be used to avoid the differentiation of hepatocellular jaundice from obstructive jaundice, and for the diagnosis and investigation of liver disease in the absence of jaundice.

Carbohydrate metabolism in disease

Although the liver maintains the normal blood glucose concentration (p. 47), obvious changes in carbohydrate metabolism are seen only in severe disease. When there is acute necrosis of the liver, hypoglycaemia usually develops. In chronic liver disease the capacity of the liver to convert glucose and other sugars to glycogen for storage is reduced though hypoglycaemia is not usually seen.

Protein metabolism

Changes in general protein metabolism, apart from alteration in plasma proteins

Table 14.1 Bilirubin changes in disease

Disease (example)	Plasma		Urine		Faeces
	Total bilirubin	Excess conjugated bilirubin (direct van den Bergh)	Urobilinogen	Bilirubin	Urobilinogen
Normal state	Present	–	Present	Absent	Present
Haemolytic (spherocytosis)	↑	–	Increased	Absent	↑↑
Hepatocellular (infective hepatitis)	↑↑	↑	Variable	↑	Low
Obstructive (carcinoma of pancreas)	↑↑↑	↑↑	Absent	↑↑	Absent

and enzymes, are only significant in severe liver disease. If liver damage is both acute and massive, as in acute hepatic necrosis, conversion of the amino acids to urea is greatly reduced, and the plasma and urine amino acid levels rise. The plasma urea concentration may be below 2.0 mmol/l.

The ammonium ions that are absorbed into the portal vein from the gut are normally almost completely metabolized by the liver, and little ammonia is present in peripheral blood (p. 90). When there is severe hepatocellular disease or cirrhosis, blood ammonia is increased. This is due to portal blood bypassing healthy liver cells in a collateral circulation (which may be marked after a porto-caval shunt), and to impaired liver cell metabolism.

Plasma proteins

In chronic liver disease, when large numbers of parenchymal liver cells have been destroyed, synthesis of albumin may be impaired. However, low albumin levels in liver disease are often due to other factors, such as an increased volume of distribution in ascites and increased metabolism (p. 95). Newly synthesized albumin is lost in hepatic lymph into the ascitic fluid, thus, in the presence of ascites, the plasma concentration of albumin provides no indication of functional liver cell mass. Albumin synthesis in hypoalbuminaemic patients with cirrhosis may thus be low, normal or increased and plasma albumin concentration is of no use in assessing prognosis. The plasma concentrations of some other plasma proteins that are synthesized in the parenchymal cells of the liver may also be reduced. However, the immunoglobulin levels are often raised. IgG and IgM are increased due to autoimmune reactions which are a common feature of most chronic liver diseases. IgA is raised due to failure of biliary excretion from the plasma together with local production by plasma cells in the liver. Different patterns of raised immunoglobulins may be seen in different types of liver disease but are probably insufficiently constant to be of clinical value.

Clotting factors

A low plasma fibrinogen may be found when there is extensive parenchymal cell damage, and the plasma concentration of prothrombin and of most other clotting factors is also reduced, giving a prolonged prothrombin time (see haematology texts). Alterations in blood coagulability must therefore be borne in mind if liver biopsy is proposed for the diagnosis of chronic liver disease – measurement of the prothrombin time and clotting time are essential preliminaries to liver biopsy.

Synthesis of prothrombin, and of several other clotting factors, depend upon the amount of vitamin K_1 that is reaching the liver cells, as well as on the functional state of those cells. In obstructive jaundice, absence of bile salts from the intestine causes diminished absorption of vitamin K_1 and the prothrombin time is therefore prolonged. Intramuscular injection of vitamin K_1 will restore the prolonged prothrombin time to normal in 24 h in a case of obstructive jaundice; it will not affect a prolonged prothrombin time which has been caused by hepatocellular damage, as there is then a defect in synthetic capacity for clotting factors.

Enzymes

Enzyme assays can be used principally in three different ways in the assessment of liver disease. Some enzymes synthesized in the liver, e.g. cholinesterase, show a fall in their plasma activity when there is hepatocellular damage though such measurements are no longer used. Some membrane-bound enzymes of the biliary epithelial cells of the canaliculi such as alkaline phosphatase show a rise in their plasma activity when there is cholestasis. Many enzymes which are present in high concentration in liver parenchymal cells, e.g. asparate transaminase, show a rise in their plasma activity when there is active hepatocellular damage.

Alkaline phosphatase and related enzymes

The alkaline phosphatases are a group of cytosolic or cell membrane enzymes able to hydrolyse organic phosphates in an alkaline environment. *In vivo* they are responsible for ATP hydrolysis and are frequently found associated with cell membrane 'pumps'. Plasma alkaline phosphatase activity is made up of constituents from several different tissues. These isoenzymes can be separated by electrophoretic techniques based upon differences in their charge due to carbohydrate side-chain variations in the enzymes from different tissues. In normal plasma most of the activity is derived from the hepatocytes and some from osteoblasts. However, in pathological states raised levels of alkaline phosphatase may be derived from hepatocytes, osteoblasts, intestinal epithelial cells, placental trophoblast, and some tumours. The reference range in adults is 30–130 U/l: 3–13 King-Armstrong units/dl (see p. 180 for sex variation, and p. 249 for age variation). Levels are higher during phases of bone growth (osteoblast-derived) and during pregnancy (trophoblast-derived). Subjects with 'secretor' status may show raised levels of intestinal alkaline phosphatase after fatty meals and in inflammatory conditions of the gut and liver. In liver disease a raised plasma alkaline phosphatase, particularly to more than 180 U/l (and usually in association with a raised plasma bilirubin), provides an indication of extrahepatic or intrahepatic biliary obstruction, e.g. in primary biliary cirrhosis. The increase is due mainly to stimulation by the cholestasis of excess enzyme synthesis in the liver cells lining the bile canaliculi which is then secreted into the liver sinusoids. The part played by possible impaired secretion into the bile and 'regurgitation' into the sinusoids is controversial. Moderate increases, generally to about 150 U/l, are characteristically found in the later stages of viral hepatitis when cholestasis due to altered bile salt secretion becomes the predominant pathological change. A raised plasma alkaline phosphatase with little increase in plasma bilirubin is also seen when there are primary or metastatic malignant deposits in the liver and a similar increase may be found in early cirrhosis. An increased plasma alkaline phosphatase is an early sign of cholestatic liver damage due to certain drugs such as chlorpromazine. The reason why alkaline phosphatase is raised in the absence of bilirubin is that bilirubin entering the blood due to local obstruction can be taken up in other areas of normal liver tissue and secreted; alkaline phosphatase however cannot and the plasma level rises.

In children or adolescents the physiological increase in alkaline phosphatase due to bone growth may mask changes due to hepatobiliary disease. There may also be possible confusion of increased bone and liver alkaline phosphatase when there is cirrhosis with osteomalacia, or multiple metastases.

The related enzyme 5'-nucleotidase is generally increased in plasma in the same hepatobiliary disorders as is alkaline phosphatase, but is unaltered in bone disease. It is now rarely measured as alkaline phosphatase isoenzymes can be identified with ease.

Transaminases (aminotransferases)

Active hepatocellular damage is reflected by increased plasma levels of aspartate transaminase (AST), reference range 11–35 U/l, and alanine transaminase (ALT), reference range 5–40 U/l. In general, somewhat higher values of plasma alanine transaminase, which is solely cytoplasmic, than of aspartate transaminase (cytoplasmic and mitochondrial) are found in acute viral hepatitis when cell membrane damage predominates. Somewhat lower values are seen in cirrhosis, malignancy and hypoxia where cell death occurs. The differences are not usually great and it is probably not worth measuring both enzymes as a routine for clinical diagnosis.

In viral hepatitis the transaminases rise above normal during the prodromal period.

Peak values (of about 500–2000 U/l) are found at the time of maximum illness and the value returns to normal in about four weeks unless subacute liver disease develops, when levels become persistently elevated. A similar but less marked increase with values rarely above 300 U/l usually occurs in nonicteric hepatitis and in glandular fever. Hepatocellular damage attributed to drug hypersensitivity may be shown by a continuing rise in plasma transaminase on repeated testing following administration of the drug. Alcohol raises the plasma transaminase in alcoholics but not in normal subjects. Moderately raised plasma transaminase values, usually between 50 and 300 U/l, are found in cirrhosis in proportion to the degree of active cell damage, but unrelated to coma or loss of liver cell mass. In malignant disease involving the liver, and in obstructive jaundice, the plasma transaminase values are usually moderately raised owing to hepatocellular damage, but rarely exceed 300 U/l. AST is also found in myocardium, being raised in myocardial infarction (p. 131) or following open cardiac surgery, and in erythrocytes, being raised in autoimmune or *in vitro* haemolysis. Destruction of large amounts of skeletal muscle as following road traffic accidents may also release the enzyme causing raised plasma levels. In these circumstances, it is unsuitable in the diagnosis or monitoring of liver disease.

γ-Glutamyltransferase

This enzyme provides a sensitive indication of most hepatobiliary disorders. In cholestatic disease it behaves like alkaline phosphatase, with particular sensitivity for hepatic metastases but there is no change in osteoblastic bone disease. In hepatocellular disease changes are similar to those of the transaminases.

Increased liver synthesis and plasma levels of this enzyme result from microsomal enzyme induction by drugs, the most important of these being alcohol in the chronic drinker. It is the most sensitive indication of hepatocellular damage in such patients. Contrary to earlier expectations it is not a useful indication of alcohol abuse.

Other enzymes

Other enzymes are raised in hepatocellular damage but experience has shown that their measurement adds nothing in clinically useful information to those already discussed.

Lipid metabolism

Bile salts

The liver synthesizes, per 24 h from cholesterol, about 1.3 mmol (0.5 g) of bile acids: these are principally cholic acid and chenodeoxycholic acid, conjugated with glycine and taurine. The bile salts are excreted into the intestine where they are essential for the adequate absorption of fats (p. 66) and of vitamin K and other fat-soluble vitamins; bacterial reduction produces deoxycholic acid and lithocholic acid respectively. Only a small quantity of bile salts is lost in the faeces, most being reabsorbed in the terminal ileum and resecreted in the bile. In obstructive jaundice or severe hepatocellular damage the flow of bile salts to the intestine is reduced and there may be steatorrhoea (p. 170).

Bile salts cannot be detected in normal urine. The historic Hay's test depends on the property of bile salts, excreted as sulphates, to lower surface tension; it is very insensitive and has no clinical value. The place of the recently introduced assay of plasma bile acid concentration as a test for cholestasis is not yet established. A raised fasting plasma bile acid concentration is a sensitive but non-discriminatory indicator of hepatobiliary damage. Bile salt clearance tests are a further refinement.

Other lipids

Although the liver is active in many metabolic processes involving cholesterol and other lipids, the alterations which occur in disease do not form useful liver function tests because of lack of both sensitivity and of specificity.

In cholestasis, whether due to drugs, the obstructive phase of hepatitis, or as post-hepatic obstructive jaundice, the plasma free cholesterol level is greatly increased due to failure to excrete cholesterol in the bile and subsequent incorporation of cholesterol in the VLDL particle. There is some increase in plasma ester cholesterol and in the phospholipids; lipoprotein X, an abnormal complex of albumin, apolipoprotein B and cholesterol, is always present. When there is parenchymal cell damage the free cholesterol level is variable depending on a balance between retention and diminished synthesis and there is a marked fall in the ester cholesterol (due to decreased levels of the liver-derived enzyme lecithin cholesterol acyl transferase (p. 70) and usually in the phospholipids. A low total plasma cholesterol is found in acute hepatic necrosis, or in the terminal stages of chronic hepatitis when VLDL secretion fails.

In biliary cirrhosis and obstruction there is a marked increase of all plasma lipid fractions including the phospholipids, and the increase in β-lipoproteins (p. 67) may be identified by electrophoresis; free fatty acids are often also increased. The biochemistry of fatty deposition in the liver (p. 77), and of cholesterol in relation to gallstones (p. 161), are discussed elsewhere.

Hepatic detoxication

Although the liver conjugates a great many metabolic products besides bilirubin, liver function tests utilizing only this principle are not at present used.

Hepatic transport and excretion

Porphyrins are excreted in the bile as well as in the urine. In many types of liver disease particularly in acute hepatitis and cirrhosis and in obstructive jaundice, biliary excretion of porphyrins is diminished and excess coproporphyrins can be found in the urine. Photosensitivity may result from skin deposition.

The liver removes many administered organic compounds from the plasma by uptake into parenchymal cells at a rate which depends on the plasma flow to the liver and the functional capacity of the cells. It then excretes them into the bile canaliculi, this being affected by cholestasis. It is feasible to investigate the functional competence of parenchymal cells by measuring the removal from the plasma of a suitable substance. Bromsulphthalein, an easily measured coloured compound, has been widely used and it is normally more than 80 per cent excreted into the bile after conjugation. Its excretion is therefore similar to that of bilirubin, but is more sensitive to damage of cell function. Indocyanine Green, which is excreted without conjugation, may also be used and is claimed to provide a more sensitive test. It is more expensive but is non-toxic whereas bromsulphthalein occasionally produces reactions. Such tests of liver function are not now used in the United Kingdom for clinical purposes.

Biochemical changes in liver disease

Neonatal jaundice

The two main causes of jaundice in the newborn are excess production of bilirubin as a result of haemolytic disease (usually from blood-group incompatibility), and delayed formation of the enzymatic conjugating capacity of the liver, principally bilirubin-UDP glucuronosyltransferase. Because of the latter, premature infants may have a plasma unconjugated bilirubin up to 250 μmol/l at 5 days, which returns to normal as the glucuronosyltransferase is synthesized. When there is haemolysis, the unconjugated bilirubin may exceed 300 μmol/l. As at this concentration and above the deposition of the lipid-soluble bilirubin in the basal ganglia is likely to lead to the dangerous kernicterus, the level of 300 μmol/l is taken as the indication for exchange transfusion. Kernicterus may occur at a lower level of bilirubin due to the displacement of bilirubin from albumin by drugs such as sulphonamides and salicylates. Phototherapy is generally used to lower bilirubin levels if it exceeds 340 μmol/l in a fullterm neonate; the concentration is lower for premature infants.

Biliary atresia produces a cholestatic jaundice with increased conjugated bilirubin, but the plasma alkaline phosphatase is usually normal in the early stages, as the immature liver cells cannot synthesize excess enzyme. A number of rare genetic defects in the handling of bilirubin result in neonatal jaundice.

Viral hepatitis

Preicteric hepatocellular damage can be detected by raised plasma transaminases, often to very high levels, and by an increased excretion of urobilinogen in the urine. The symptoms during this stage of the disease are of malaise and anorexia. When the disease is established there is moderate jaundice due to the development of intrahepatic cholestasis with an increased plasma total and conjugated bilirubin and bilirubin in the urine without urobilinogen and pale stools. The plasma albumin may be slightly lowered as in many acute illnesses but never falls below 25 g/l. A slight acute-phase response and increase in IgM are commonly seen. The plasma transaminases are often beginning to fall at this stage. The prothrombin time may be prolonged slightly.

During recovery from the acute attack bilirubin disappears from the urine and urobilinogen reappears. The plasma proteins and enzyme values return to normal.

If the hepatitis becomes sub-acute the plasma proteins remain abnormal with a definite fall in albumin and persistently raised γ-globulin; the plasma alkaline phosphatase is raised, but bilirubin and transaminases may be only slightly raised. In nonicteric hepatitis the changes are similar, but less marked, except that the plasma bilirubin remains within normal limits. Alternatively the disease may progress in the early stages to acute hepatic necrosis or in the sub-acute stage to chronic hepatitis.

Special precautions must be observed in handling blood specimens from patients with hepatitis because of the risks of infection to laboratory staff (p. 254) from hepatitis B.

Chronic active hepatitis

This condition is marked by continuing destruction of liver cells, and most tests therefore give abnormal values. There is a low plasma albumin with much increased γ-globulins (IgG), and a marked increase in bilirubin. High values are found for both plasma alkaline phosphatase and for the transaminases. The ALT is usually increased more than the AST. Smooth muscle antibodies and antinuclear factor can usually be detected in serum and reflect the development of autoimmune responses to liver antigens released into the circulation. These may perpetuate the damage which eventually, if unabated, results in cirrhosis.

Cirrhosis

Cirrhosis is the development of fibrous septae within the liver lobules together with disorganized regeneration of liver cells following death. The result is a loss of the normal architectural arrangement of the lobules with increased portal blood pressure due to failure of portal blood to drain through the sinusoids to the hepatic vein in the normal manner. This, together with impaired lymphatic drainage, results in accumulation of ascitic fluid in the peritoneal cavity due to passage of hepatic lymph across the liver capsule. The biochemical changes are very variable and depend on the rate at which the underlying damaging process is continuing and the number of functioning lobules left. There is thus a variable and dissociated damage to the functions of the liver. The plasma total bilirubin level may be normal or slightly raised and there is often excess urobilinogen in the urine but no bilirubin. The plasma albumin level is progressively decreased as healthy liver cells are lost and there is a rise in the γ-globulins due to failure to excrete IgA in the bile and the development of autoimmune antibodies to liver elements released by the damage. A typical electrophoretic pattern is usually found, for the excess IgA which is present has a high mobility and results in β-γ fusion (Fig. 8.1, p. 92). The plasma transaminases may be raised only moderately unless there is a flare-up in the process causing hepatocellular damage. The plasma alkaline phosphatase and γ-glutamyltransferase are usually slightly raised. Plasma cholesterol tends to be low, with diminished esterification. Type I coproporphyrinuria is usually present. There is often impaired glucose tolerance. There is almost always hyponatraemia which is largely dilutional, and a multifactorial potassium deficiency.

The damaged liver fails to metabolize hormones, including ADH. Feminizing changes in men, and the spider naevi often found in this condition, have been ascribed to excess of circulating oestrogens.

Ascites

Local factors contributing to the formation of ascites in cirrhosis include portal hypertension and impaired hepatic lymph drainage. Systemic factors include the low circulatory albumin concentration and the retention of excess sodium and excess water associated with secondary aldosteronism (p. 212).

Ascites may be due to many primary disorders. Ascitic fluid in cirrhosis and in congestive heart failure is usually a transudate, whereas that associated with peritoneal infections or malignancy is usually an exudate (p. 104).

Primary biliary cirrhosis

In this form of cirrhosis autoimmune damage to biliary epithelial cells results in destruction and disordered proliferation of the intrahepatic bile ducts with fibrosis. There is a mild and late cholestatic jaundice with a raised plasma total and conjugated bilirubin, and bilirubin in the urine. The plasma alkaline phosphatase is often great-

ly raised. The plasma transaminases increase when there is active hepatocellular damage, but parenchymal cell function may be only slightly impaired. Albumin levels fall slightly and late in the disease and there is a rise in γ-globulins, due mainly to IgM. Antimitochondrial antibodies can usually be detected in serum. Marked alteration of lipid metabolism develops, plasma cholesterol and phospholipids are increased, electrophoresis shows lipoprotein X and excess β-lipoproteins, and xanthomatosis is common.

Posthepatic (large bile duct) obstruction

This is commonly due to gallstones or carcinoma at the head of the pancreas. There is cholestatic jaundice, with a markedly raised plasma conjugated bilirubin and bilirubin in the urine. Urobilinogen will be found in the urine and faeces only if the obstruction is incomplete or intermittent. The plasma alkaline phosphatase and the total cholesterol level may be increased. Unless the obstruction is longstanding, parenchymal liver cell function is not severely damaged. The plasma transaminases are usually only moderately raised, and the plasma albumin level is normal. However, obstruction may cause hepatocellular damage with 'bile infarcts'.

Prolonged obstruction may cause secondary biliary cirrhosis which is biochemically indistinguishable from primary liver cirrhosis. However mitochondrial antibodies are then absent.

Acute hepatic necrosis

All functions of the liver are profoundly altered. There is usually severe jaundice, with a high plasma total and unconjugated bilirubin, and bilirubin (but no urobilinogen) in the urine. The plasma transaminases are very greatly increased during the active phase and the alkaline phosphatase may be slightly increased. Failure of conversion of amino acids to urea leads to an increase in total plasma amino acids and increased urinary amino acids without specific changes on chromatography. Blood ammonia is usually raised. The plasma urea is usually low, but if there is severe dehydration a normal and even slightly increased level may be found. The concentrations of all plasma proteins, except γ-globulins, are decreased, in particular, the clotting factors. Occasionally, for example in paracetamol poisoning, damage is so severe that death occurs before plasma protein levels fall. Hypoglycaemia may be profound, and the blood pyruvate and lactate concentrations are high, with an acidosis.

Hepatic coma

This is a frequent end-stage of cirrhosis but is occasionally seen following severe hepatitis and usually occurs before death in acute hepatic necrosis. The abnormal laboratory findings are related to the stage of the underlying liver disease and its nature together with secondary factors such as poor renal function, diuretics or vomiting.

The toxins affecting the central nervous system have not been clearly identified though the role of ammonia seems certain. Cerebral metabolism may be disturbed due to the excess ammonia accelerating the conversion of oxoglutarate to glutamate, and thus depriving the tricarboxylic acid cycle of oxoglutarate. There is an increased blood concentration of lactate, and of pyruvate and keto acids, giving a metabolic acidosis often accentuated by renal failure. There may also be respiratory alkalosis due to hyperventilation. The distinctive odour (the *foetor hepaticus*) is due to mercaptans which are thought to arise from excess circulating methionine. Though there is often slight proteinuria the plasma urea is usually only slightly raised; however acute renal failure may develop. Ammonia measurement is only indicated if hepatic coma is suspected but clinically unproven in an unconscious patient, and this particularly applies to young children.

Drug effects

Many drugs can cause jaundice, some by affecting bilirubin metabolism and some producing liver disease by a toxic effect on the cells. Examples of the first mechanism are the sulphonamides which may produce haemolysis, and novobiocin which may inhibit the conjugation of bilirubin. On the other hand, some drugs can induce the microsomal glucuronosyltransferase, and phenobarbitone is thus used for the treatment of unconjugated hyperbilirubinaemia by promoting conjugation and therefore excretion of the excess bilirubin.

There are many types of toxic reaction. Carbon tetrachloride is an example of a directly toxic drug, which produces acute hepatic necrosis; the similar effects of paracetamol are dose-related. Hypersensitivity is blamed for a clinical and biochemical picture resembling mild or severe infective hepatitis due to halothane; sensitivity to some other drugs, such as rifampicin or monoamine oxidase inhibitors, produces only a transient rise in plasma transaminase, and only rarely hepatitis. Susceptibility to methyltestosterone or oral contraceptives produces cholestasis (with an early rise in plasma alkaline phosphatase, and also in transaminases) which is usually transient, but hypersensitivity to chlorpromazine, with cholangiolitis, occasionally progresses to resemble biliary cirrhosis.

Malignant disease

Primary hepatoma is commonly marked by an increase plasma concentration of the oncofetal antigen, α-fetoprotein (p. 233). Jaundice may be late, and is preceded by increased plasma values for alkaline phosphatase and γ-glutamyltransferase.

In the far more common metastatic carcinomatosis, α-fetoprotein is normal, and there is (with the other biochemical changes of primary hepatoma) an increase in serum transaminases. An increase in liver-derived alkaline phosphatase typifies the local obstruction caused by metastatic deposits and is commonly seen without any other changes in the liver tests.

Gallstones

The major component of most gallstones is cholesterol, and they usually also contain variable amounts of calcium carbonate and phosphate and of bile pigments. In the bile, cholesterol is held in solution in micelles with the aid of phospholipids (mainly lecithin) and bile salts: the ratio of the concentrations of phospholipids plus bile salts to that of cholesterol determines its solubility. Amongst the factors that promote stone formation are alterations of this ratio by an abnormality in the secretion of hepatic bile, and stasis or infection in the gallbladder which can provide sites for the initiation of cholesterol precipitation.

Pigment stones may be formed in haemolytic states when there is greatly increased bilirubin excretion in the bile. Their main individual component is bilirubin.

Choice of liver function tests

Biochemical tests of liver function have decreased in importance in the diagnosis of liver disease as a result of the development of isotope scanning and radiological and imaging techniques. These newer techniques provide anatomical evidence for the location and type of lesion in the liver. Thus scanning techniques are valuable in identifying hepatic metastases and percutaneous cholangiography is effective in indicating the site of cholestasis.

Many laboratory tests for liver function have been examined and described over the years but a relatively limited number have stood the test of time and been shown to provide useful information. The tests currently available in most laboratories are total bilirubin, alanine transaminase (or aspartate transaminase), alkaline phosphatase, total protein, albumin and globulin. In addition some laboratories would offer γ-glutamyltransferase, electrophoresis, and immunoglobulin assays in certain defined situations such as the possibility of primary biliary cirrhosis.

Biochemical tests detect cell injury or response to it and impairment of specific aspects of liver function. The clinical questions of importance are: to detect the presence of hepatobiliary damage; to establish diagnosis; to assess severity; to assess prognosis and to evaluate therapy. Such tests depend on either the release of substances from dead or damaged hepatocytes and biliary epithelial cells or failure of the liver to synthesize or metabolize some compound. The changes seen are very nonspecific and are poor at providing diagnostic information about the pathogenesis of hepatic disorders, though they may be quite sensitive to damaging processes in general. Although there are typical patterns of test results found, for example, in extrahepatic cholestasis and hepatocellular damage, each of these processes may give rise to elements of the other, thus rendering the test useless for detecting the underlying cause of the condition. Biochemical tests are however useful for: (a) detecting the presence of liver damage or disturbance in function; (b) following the course of disease and identifying recurrent or continuing chronic disease; (c) identifying the type of jaundice (prehepatic can be distinguished from hepatic and posthepatic, though the last two cannot be distinguished from each other). The tests are however not useful for: (a) distinguishing between intra- and extrahepatic obstruction (hepatic and posthepatic jaundice); (b) assessing the severity of liver damage; (c) assessing the residual functional liver cell mass.

Further reading

Hargreaves T. Which biochemical liver tests should we use? *Health Trends* 1985; **17**: 78–80.

Price CP, Alberti KGMM. Biochemical assessment of liver function. In: Wright R, Alberti KGMM, Karran S, Millward-Sadler GH, eds. *Liver and Biliary Disease*. London: W.B. Saunders, 1979.

Roberton NRC. Neonatal jaundice. *Rec Adv Paediatrics* 1986; **8**: 157–84.

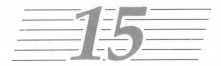

The Alimentary Tract

Objectives

In this chapter the reader is able to

- revise the physiology of secretion, digestion and absorption
- study the biochemical changes in diseases of the stomach and duodenum
- study the metabolic effects of loss of intestinal secretions and of general and specific malabsorption syndromes.

At the conclusion of this chapter the reader is able to

- use the laboratory in the investigation of salivary gland diseases
- investigate gastric acid secretion, and understand the role of the tests
- use the laboratory in the investigation of acute pancreatitis
- use the laboratory in the screening and investigation of pancreatic cystic fibrosis
- use the laboratory in the investigation of chronic pancreatitis
- understand the causes of steatorrhoea and their relation to the metabolic effects and to tests for diagnosis and differential diagnosis
- understand the causes and significance of a positive faecal occult blood.

Salivary glands

The salivary glands secrete about 1500 ml of saliva every 24 h, mainly from the parotid glands. The electrolyte composition of saliva is variable. The average composition is Na^+ 30 mmol/l, K^+ 20 mmol/l, Cl^- 30 mmol/l, HCO_3^- 10 mmol/l. The saliva contains amylase, and if there is acute obstruction to the outflow of the secretions from the parotid glands amylase is retained and regurgitated into the bloodstream. This is a different isoenzyme from that produced by the pancreas. The obstruction may be intraglandular, due to swollen cells as in acute parotitis, and particularly in mumps, or extraglandular, if there is a salivary duct stone. The plasma amylase level may rise during the acute phase of the obstruction to over 1000 U/l (reference range 70–300 U/l).

Stomach and duodenum

Every 24 h the normal stomach produces about 1000 ml of gastric juice when the subject is fasting, whilst the stomach of a subject who is taking a normal diet secretes 2000–3000 ml of juice per 24 h. Gastric juice is a mixture of secretions. Parietal cells secrete hydrochloric acid and intrinsic factor, and zymogen cells (chief cells) secrete the pepsinogens and other enzymes; other cells produce an alkaline mucus. The average pH of mixed gastric juice is about 1.5, and the average concentration of the principal electrolytes is H^+, 70 mmol/l, Na^+, 70 mmol/l, K^+, 10 mmol/l, Cl^-, 140 mmol/l. The principal physiological stimulants to gastric secretion are the vagus nerve impulses and the polypeptide hormone gastrin(s) released from specialized antral cells in response to food, and finally both stimulation and inhibition of this secretion by intestinal hormones stimulated by food in the duodenum.

In diseases of the stomach and duodenum alterations of gastric secretion often occur. Analysis of gastric secretions has a limited but specific value in the diagnosis and assessment of disorders of the upper gastrointestinal tract. In particular, they are useful in the management of patients with recurrent peptic ulceration which has not responded to medical treatment with histamine (H_2) blockers.

Simple examination of the resting juice

The resting juice is obtained by emptying the stomach through a nasogastric tube after the patient has fasted for 12 h overnight.

Appearance

Gastric juice should be clear and colourless, and average about 50 ml in volume. A trace of bile from duodenal reflux has no significance. If there is delay in gastric emptying, food residues may be present and the volume may exceed 150 ml. A trace of fresh blood may be seen in the normal resting juice sample, and this is due to trauma caused by the passage of the tube. A large quantity of digested blood (the 'coffee grounds' appearance) shows that there has been oesophageal or intragastric bleeding; this is abnormal and usually indicates that cancer of the stomach or a bleeding gastric ulcer is present. A small amount of mucus may be present normally mainly from swallowed saliva; excessive quantities of mucus may be found when there is gastritis.

Acidity

The possible measurements of gastric acidity are as hydrogen-ion activity with a pH meter, and as titratable acidity by titration with alkali to within the range of pH 7.0 (physicochemical neutrality) to pH 7.4 (physiological neutrality). The concentration of acid is expressed as millimoles per litre.

Pepsin(s)

Pepsins, produced from pepsinogens by acid, are normally present in gastric juice, and are secreted in parallel with gastric acid.

A small amount of pepsin is secreted into the plasma and excreted into the urine as uropepsinogens. Its excretion very roughly follows the peptic secretory activity of the stomach. Measurements of pepsinogen in gastric juice, plasma and urine are not used routinely.

Tests for gastric acidity

The original stimulus applied to the stomach to test its capacity to secrete acid was a simple meal such as tea and toast: hence the term 'test meal'. Oral stimulants are unsatisfactory as they do not produce maximum secretion of acid, they mix with and dilute the gastric secretions, and give variable results. If gastric secretory response is to be measured, a stimulus must be used which gives maximum stimulation to the gastric secretion of acid by all the parietal cells (parietal cell mass). Histamine was formerly used, especially as the augmented histamine test with its unwanted effects blocked by an antihistamine, or by using an analogue (ametazole: *Histalog*). These have now been replaced by a synthetic gastrin: this is a better stimulant and more pleasant for the patient.

Pentagastrin test

Pentagastrin (*Peptavlon*: ICI) is a synthetic pentapeptide which contains the key C-terminal portion of the gastrin molecule (*cf.* tetracosactrin, p. 213).

Method

(i) The test is preceded by a 12 h overnight fast.
(ii) Pass a wide-bore stomach tube (a Levin or a Ryle's tube, size 12–16 French) into the stomach, and check the positioning of the tube by fluoroscopy.
(iii) Aspirate the resting juice completely.

This may be examined for volume and general appearance.

(iv) Collect the basal, spontaneously-secreted, gastric juice quantitatively by continuous suction for a period of 60 min, at a sub-atmospheric pressure of 30–50 mmHg (4.0–6.5 kPa).

 (v) Inject intramuscularly 6 μg pentagastrin/kg body weight.

(vi) Continuously aspirate the stimulated secretion for the next 60 min dividing this collection into four separate specimens representing 0–15, 15–30, 30–45, and 45–60 min samples.

The five collections of gastric secretion (basal and four stimulated) are sent to the laboratory in separate containers, each clearly labelled with the times of collection.

Interpretation
In normal subjects the total basal acid output (BAO) is less than 5 mmol/h, and the maximum acid output (MAO) in the 60 min after pentagstrin is about 20 mmol in a man and 10 mmol in a woman.

The average outputs of patients with duodenal ulcer are about twice the normal and about one-third of the patients have diagnostic hypersecretion. The peak acid output (PAO) is calculated as twice the secretion in the highest two consecutive 15-min periods, and is normally less than 45 mmol/h in a man and 30 mmol/h in a woman.

A high BAO (more than 5 mmol/h) and/or a high PAO suggest a duodenal ulcer, whereas a PAO less than 15 mmol/h is evidence against a duodenal ulcer. Patients with gastric ulcer generally have a normal acid secretion. Patients with carcinoma of the stomach may have achlorhydria or may secrete normally.

Absolute achlorhydria (anacidity) exists if none of these specimens has a pH less than 7. This occurs regularly in pernicious anaemia, occasionally in gastric carcinoma, and rarely otherwise; absolute achlorhydria excludes any form of peptic ulcer. Hyposecretion, with no 'free acid' (pH 3.5–6.5) and less than 1 unit change in pH

after pentagastrin, is a non-specific finding that is seen in a variety of conditions, e.g. hypochromic anaemia or gastritis.

Insulin test

This is used to investigate the completeness of a vagotomy which has been performed for the treatment of peptic ulcer. Insulin-induced hypoglycaemia causes (via the hypothalamus) vagal stimulation of gastric acid secretion if the vagus nerves are still intact.

Method
Pass a gastric tube and collect a 1-h basal secretion. Inject soluble insulin (0.2 units/kg) intravenously and collect complete samples of gastric juice every 15 min for 2 h, and of blood for glucose estimation every 30 min.

The patient must be closely observed, and intravenous 50 per cent glucose kept available, because of the risk of severe hypoglycaemia.

Interpretation
An increase of acid secretion of less than 20 mmol/l above the basal activity is taken as indicating that vagotomy has been complete, provided that (i) adequate hypoglycaemia (less than 2 mmol/l) has been produced, and (ii) the stomach has been found capable of secreting hydrochloric acid in response to pentagastrin stimulus, which may follow directly after the insulin test. As vagotomy is rarely absolutely complete, the acid response to insulin is a function of residual innervation.

Role of gastric secretion tests

In general all the tests of acidity show the same pattern of responses. Patients with gastric ulcers have the same range of acid secretion as do normal subjects, so there is little point in testing them routinely. The only disease consistently associated with achlorhydria is Addisonian pernicious anaemia, though this finding is rarely needed for diagnosis (p. 144). Achlorhydria is sometimes found in patients with gastric carcinoma or mucosal atrophy (e.g. in severe hypochromic anaemia), though gastric function tests are rarely needed.

Hyperchlorhydria usually accompanies a duodenal ulcer, though there is no consensus relating degree of secretion to choice of treatment.

After partial gastrectomy or vagotomy, tests are necessary to investigate the completeness of the operation or the cause of recurrent ulceration.

Measurement of gastrin

Gastrin is present in the serum and may be measured by radioimmunoassay. The normal biologically active form has 17 amino acids (G17) but big gastrin (the 34 amino acid intracellular precursor) and little gastrin, G14, may be present. The latter has no biological activity. Gastrin production is inhibited by acid in the stomach antrum cell and the level remains constant during most of the day, rising following a meal and falling during sleep. The normal fasting level is less than 40 pmol/l; very high values are found in achlorhydria, particularly in pernicious anaemia.

The main value of gastrin measurement is in the *Zollinger-Ellison syndrome* of severe peptic ulcers and hypersecretion caused by a gastrinoma, usually of the islet cells of the pancreas but sometimes of antral G-cells: the massive basal secretion of acid (more than 200 ml of juice with an HCl content of more than 20 mmol/h) is little increased by pentagastrin. Immunoassay of plasma gastrin in cases of hyperacidity shows a diagnostic high value of greater than 100 pmol/l. About 80 per cent of patients with gastrinoma produce a greater than 50 per cent rise in serum gastrin after secretin stimulation. This may be part of a pluriglandular syndrome of multiple endocrine adenomas (p. 185).

Biochemical effects of disease of the stomach and duodenum

The biochemical assessment of a patient who is suffering from a longstanding disease of the stomach e.g. carcinoma or duodenal ulcer, or after surgery, must be concerned with the effects of malnutrition and of loss of secretions. The extent of malnutrition is best estimated by measurement of the blood haemoglobin and of the plasma albumin concentration which often falls below 24 g/l in cases of carcinoma of the stomach. If the albumin is below 35 g/l restorative measures should, if possible, be undertaken before the patient is submitted to surgery. The protein deficiency is caused both by a low intake and by loss from the surface of the ulcer or cancer (*protein-losing enteropathy*). Vomiting causes loss of secretions. Because of the acidity of gastric juice prolonged vomiting leads to severe hypochloraemic alkalosis (p. 41) and often to ketosis as well as to water and potassium depletion; this alkalosis will not develop if there is vomiting in a patient with achlorhydria. The alkalosis may be accentuated by medication with alkali, or caused by prolonged alkali treatment without vomiting. Bleeding from gastric or duodenal disease gives rise to a high plasma urea (p. 85).

After gastrectomy or gastroenterostomy the patient may develop either the 'dumping syndrome', or postgastrectomy hypoglycaemia, or both. The dumping syndrome is seen shortly after a meal, associated with the osmotic effect of food rapidly entering the duodenum. The cause of all the symptoms is not known, but there is a hypovolaemia and a temporary fall of the plasma potassium level. Postgastrectomy hypoglycaemia occurs about 2 h after a carbohydrate meal: it is due to the reaction that follows temporary hyperglycaemia, which is caused by rapid gastric emptying and consequent over-rapid absorption of carbohydrate. These patients show a 'lag storage' glucose tolerance curve (p. 60).

Pancreas

The pancreas is an organ that is relatively inaccessible to biochemical study. In acute pancreatic disease changes which are relatively diagnostic can be found in the blood and, often, in the urine. In chronic pancreatic disease indirect biochemical evidence of disordered function is difficult to obtain in the early stages, and the analysis of pancreatic secretions, which is the direct test of pancreatic function, is difficult because of the necessity for duodenal intubation.

Acute pancreatitis

Acute inflammation of the pancreas is most commonly associated with gall-stones and excessive alcohol consumption. Other causes are viral infections, hyperparathyroidism (p. 184) and hyperchylomicronaemia (p. 76). Swelling of the acinar cells leads to regurgitation of pancreatic enzymes into the blood stream. Of the main pancreatic enzymes, amylase, lipase (triacylglycerol lipase), and trypsinogen and chymotrypsinogen, amylase is more frequently estimated than is lipase: immunoassay for trypsin concentration in plasma offers no advantages. Pancreatic and salivary amylases are closely related isoenzymes (p. 106); the salivary glands do not secrete a lipase or a proteolytic enzyme.

Amylase

During an attack of acute pancreatitis the plasma amylase level rises rapidly, often to over 2000 U/l. A level of over 1000 U/l, in a clinically suspicious case, is usually diagnostic of acute pancreatitis. It is important to perform the estimation within the first 24 h as the enzyme rise may be transient, and the level usually falls to normal within two or three days as the acute attack resolves.

Other disorders of the upper gastrointestinal tract, particularly perforated duodenal ulcer, intestinal obstruction and peritonitis affecting the exposed surface of the pancreas, may be accompanied by a raised plasma amylase. The probable causes are leakage of pancreatic juice into the peritoneal cavity whence the enzymes can be absorbed into the circulation, or involvement of the ampulla in the inflammatory process associated with a duodenal ulcer

which blocks the secretion of pancreatic juice into the duodenum. Administration of morphine also raises the plasma amylase by contracting the pancreatic duct sphincter. In such cases, however, the plasma amylase level usually does not increase above 1000 U/l, and the slow rise and fall of plasma enzyme concentration may take a week or more. Tubal pregnancy may show a high plasma amylase, arising from the Fallopian tube. Amylase is sometimes measured in fluid from an abdominal fistula to see whether this arises from the pancreas.

As the molecular weight of amylase is only 48 000, it is readily excreted: urine amylase is less than about 3000 U/24 h. In all these cases of raised plasma amylase, unless there is a glomerular failure (which itself causes amylase retention), there is a slow rise and fall of urine amylase. In acute pancreatitis the value may be 10 000 U/l.

Macroamylasaemia

This is a rare harmless congenital condition in which a high plasma amylase is caused by a binding to an abnormal globulin, and urine amylase is normal.

Other biochemical changes

Plasma lipase has a similar but probably slower pattern of rise and fall in pancreatitis than amylase; the peak activity is at about 48 h and the level usually remains high for about a week. Leakage of lipase from the inflamed pancreatic surface in acute pancreatitis causes hydrolysis of fat in the peritoneal cavity. Calcium may be fixed as calcium soaps on these patches of fat necrosis and for this reason the plasma calcium may be low (even low enough to cause tetany) between about 2 and 10 days from the onset of the acute attack. However, hyperparathyroidism and pancreatitis sometimes coexist. Plasma trypsin values increase over the same period.

In acute pancreatitis there is often a transient hyperglycaemia and glycosuria. Methaemalbuminaemia develops in acute haemorrhagic pancreatitis due to absorption of altered haemoglobin (p. 139). Serial C-reactive protein measurements are useful in predicting complications such as sepsis or cyst formation after renal damage before they are clinically evident. Hypoxia and blood-stained peritoneal exudation predict patients who will develop potentially lethal complications.

Chronic pancreatitis

In the investigation of non-acute disease of the pancreas, estimation of plasma or urine enzyme in the resting state rarely yields information of diagnostic value: the very slow cell destruction does not release enzyme at a sufficient rate to raise the plasma activity, and in the long-term both pancreatic isoamylase and trypsin values in plasma are lowered. The only reliable biochemical tests are those based on investigation of duodenal aspirate (pancreatic secretion) after injection of the physiological stimulants which are secretin (acting primarily on the intralobular ducts) or pancreozymin/cholecystokinin (acting on the acinar cells), or after stimulation by a standard 'meal'.

Hormonal stimulation tests

Method
After an overnight fast, a double lumen tube is passed, and its position checked radiologically. Continuous suction (by water-syphon or electric pump) is applied both to the stomach and to the duodenum. All duodenal samples are collected into iced bottles to preserve the enzymes.

There is 10 min of preliminary suction, to ensure complete emptying of the gut. Two successive 10 min samples of pancreatic juice, which are the resting controls, are collected from the duodenal tube. An injection of a pancreatic stimulant is then made. *Secretin* (Boots) (1 unit/kg body weight) is given as an intravenous injection, and this causes an increase in the secretion of bicarbonate and in the volume of juice. Following the injection, samples are collected over three successive 10 min periods.

Interpretation
The volume of a 10 min control sample is normally about 10 ml: the pH is about 7.5 and the bicarbonate content 25 mmol/l. All enzymes are present, but only amylase is usually measured.

The injection of secretin into a normal subject causes an increase in the volume of aspirate to at least 2 ml/kg body weight calculated over 1 h; the secretion rate is usually maximal in the first 10 min. There is a rise in the bicarbonate concentration to a peak of above 20 mmol/l, and in the pH to above 8.

Pancreozymin injection causes little change in the volume or alkalinity of the juice, but there is a doubling of the activity of the enzymes.

Maximal stimulation
These simple procedures give sub-maximal stimulation. Tests have been devised that involve continuous intravenous infusion of high doses of secretin + pancreozymin and these achieve a peak bicarbonate output in normal subjects of 30 mmol/h. Their diagnostic indication is uncertain.

In chronic inflammatory pancreatic disease there may be diminished resting values of volume, alkalinity, and enzymes; the typical effect of secretin stimulation is a failure of the bicarbonate to exceed 60 mmol/l with a normal volume response: loss of enzyme response to pancreozymin is late. When there is destruction of pancreatic tissue with obstruction, e.g. due to malignant disease, then the typical effect is loss of volume and enzymes, with only a late fall of bicarbonate response.

Lundh meal

This tests the trypsin response of the pancreas to a protein stimulant: it is simpler than the hormone stimulation tests, but not so discriminating.

Method
After an overnight fast a single-lumen Levin 12 tube is passed, and positioned fluoroscopically in the duodenum. The

patient is given a standard meal which contains 18 g corn oil, 18 g *Casilan* (casein hydrolysate) and 10 g glucose, in 300 ml water. A complete 2 h duodenal aspirate is collected by continuous suction, and stored on ice. There are many varieties of procedure.

Interpretation

The normal stimulated pancreatic juice has a trypsin activity, in the pooled sample, of 25–80 μmol/ml·min (TAME method). In chronic pancreatic disease or carcinoma the activity is usually below 20 units.

Pancreatic cystic fibrosis (mucoviscidosis)

The disease, which is probably the commonest inborn error of metabolism in Caucasians, is a general hereditary dysfunction of the exocrine glands. Cysts may be found in the lungs (and also the liver) as well as in the pancreas, and these produce viscid secretions rich in glycoprotein. It presents in children as failure to thrive, and there is often steatorrhoea, and bronchitis with obstructive pulmonary disease. The diagnostic feature is a high content of sodium and chloride in the sweat, the concentrations tending towards those found in the plasma, and may be more than twice those found in the resting sweat of control children. In this disease even moderate sweating may cause serious sodium depletion. In healthy children the sweat sodium rarely exceeds 50 mmol/l, and a sweat sodium of more than 65 mmol/l is highly suggestive of pancreatic cystic fibrosis; in adults the sweat sodium is more variable, but a value exceeding 90 mmol/l is suggestive of cystic fibrosis. For the detection of doubtful cases it is necessary to collect sweat with care and assay its sodium concentration.

Owing to obstruction in the early stages, there is often a high plasma trypsin; as secretion of trypsin is generally deficient, this often leads to excess albumin in the meconium of the newborn. Measurement of serum immunoreactive trypsin (IRT) is a useful screen of cystic fibrosis: blood should be collected as soon after birth as possible, and not later than 6 weeks of age.

Biochemical effects of pancreatic disease

Faecal fat

The process of normal digestion of fat, and the excretion of the end-products of fat digestion, have been discussed in Chapter 6. In chronic pancreatic disease, fat digestion is impaired because lipase secretion is deficient. The percentage of fat which is absorbed falls from the normal 90 to 95 per cent of the total output, to within the range 20–70 per cent, and fat globules are seen on microscopical examination of the faeces.

The term 'steatorrhoea' is applied to abnormal ill-formed stools that contain excessive quantities of fat. Both the daily volume and the total wet and dry weight of faeces are increased; they are pale, bulky, greasy, often frothy, and offensive – and may float. Simple diarrhoea usually causes a slight increase in the total faecal fat though the stool does not appear greasy. The effects of the high excretion of fat in chronic pancreatic disease are similar to those which develop in steatorrhoea from any cause, and are discussed below (p. 170).

Faecal nitrogen

The process of normal digestion of protein and the excretion of the end-products of protein digestion have been discussed in Chapter 7. In chronic pancreatic disease, protein digestion is impaired because trypsin secretion is deficient. Undigested muscle fibres are found in microscopical examination of the faeces, and the faecal nitrogen output is greatly raised. When it is important to establish whether there is sufficient digestion of protein (or deficient absorption of amino acids, or excess protein loss in the gut), a nitrogen balance test can be done (p. 83).

Loss of pancreatic secretions

Pancreatic secretions may be lost (with bile and intestinal secretions) through an ileal fistula or in diarrhoea, or by themselves through a pancreatic fistula. About 2000 ml/24 h of an alkaline fluid, with an average electrolyte concentration of Na^+ 130 mmol/l, K^+ 4 mmol/l, HCO_3^- 60 mmol/l, Cl^- 60 mmol/l, may be lost from the body. If this loss of secretions is prolonged there will be sodium and water depletion and a metabolic acidosis (p. 42); there may also be potassium deficiency. Loss of enzymes and of bile salts gives rise to protein maldigestion and malabsorption and to steatorrhoea.

Other effects

Chronic disease of the pancreatic acinar tissue does not initially involve the islet tissue, and carbohydrate metabolism is not affected in the early stages of the disease. However, in patients who have had pancreatic carcinoma or severe chronic pancreatitis for some time, or following total pancreatectomy, impaired glucose tolerance with hyperglycaemia and glycosuria are often seen (p. 53). Deficient digestion of protein leads to a negative nitrogen balance; protein malnutrition and a low plasma albumin result. Sufficient amylase is usually secreted for starch digestion to be unaltered. The plasma calcium, vitamin B_{12}, and iron are usually normal, because mucosal absorptive capacity is little altered.

Intestinal tract

Loss of intestinal secretions

A healthy subject secretes about 3000 ml of intestinal secretions every 24 h. Their electrolyte content depends on the site of secretion, but an average value for ileal secretions is Na^+ 130 mmol/l, K^+ 15 mmol/l, HCO_3^- 35 mmol/l, Cl^- 100 mmol/l. Almost all the water and electrolytes that are secreted are reabsorbed and faecal loss of electrolytes in health is negligible; similarly

about 50 g of mucosal and enzyme protein altogether passes into the gut and is digested and reabsorbed daily. Intestinal secretions may be lost as vomit or diarrhoea (especially from high intestinal obstruction), through a fistula or ileostomy, or by suction. Loss of intestinal secretions may be very severe in diarrhoea. The very alkaline pancreatic juice and bile are usually lost at the same time as are the intestinal secretions.

Such losses lead to gross water and sodium depletion, with metabolic acidosis and potassium deficiency. Nitrogen may also be lost. Diarrhoea has a high potassium content (often 30 mmol/l); it is also particularly dangerous in infants, because they have a low intracellular fluid reserve and more easily become water depleted (p. 20). Acidosis and potassium deficiency tend also to be more marked in infants. Purgation causes potassium depletion and acidosis.

When, as in the blind loop syndrome, there is pooling of intestinal secretions and bacterial colonization of the small bowel, then there is excess indole synthesis from dietary tryptophan with high urinary indican secretion and deficiencies of vitamin B_{12} and of folic acid. Alterations in bile salt metabolism result in the deconjugation of bile salts with steatorrhoea due to a lack of conjugated bile salts and diarrhoea due to the irritant effects of free deconjugated bile salts.

Protein loss

Nitrogen loss can also occur due to protein exudation through the mucosa in a variety of conditions with increased permeability of the gut mucosa when albumin and globulins are lost (protein-losing gastroenteropathies) (p. 83). Faecal nitrogen need not be grossly increased if the disorder is high in the gastrointestinal tract, for much of the protein is digested to amino acids which are absorbed and metabolized. The rate of loss exceeds the reserve capacity of the liver for the synthesis of albumin and a low plasma albumin results. The condition may be diagnosed by intravenous injection of a substance that is treated by the mucosa similarly to albumin but not digested, e.g. ^{131}I-polyvinyl pyrrolidine of molecular weight about 40 000. This is therefore excreted into the gut in the gastroenteropathies, and the radioactivity in the faeces can be detected and measured. The faecal concentration of α_1-antitrypsin, a protein inhibitor resistant to digestion, may also be measured.

Biochemical effects of intestinal malabsorption

The biochemical effects of primary intestinal malabsorption (e.g. in coeliac disease) are due to the multiple absorption deficiencies of the small intestine. The major abnormality is of fat absorption (not fat digestion) and steatorrhoea is a prominent symptom. The amount of absorbed dietary fat is usually within the range 45 to 85 per cent, and the stool can be seen to contain microscopic fat globules, fatty acid crystals and soap plaques. Unsaturated fatty acids are more easily absorbed than are saturated fatty acids.

Steatorrhoea, as part of the malabsorption syndrome, occurs at the preabsorptive stage in chronic pancreatic disease and pancreatic cystic fibrosis due to lipase deficiency; in intrahepatic or posthepatic biliary obstruction, due to bile salt deficiency (with generally well-formed stools); after massive resection of the gut or severe disease of the small intestine; in gastrocolic fistula and sometimes after gastrectomy, partly due to inadequate mixing and rapid passage through the intestines and to secondary deficiency of pancreatic function. In primary malabsorptive disorders (which include tropical sprue, coeliac disease, and Whipple's disease) the pathological alteration of the small intestinal mucosa prevents the absorption of fat. Tropical sprue may be of dietary or infective origin. Coeliac disease in children, and usually also in adults, is caused by sensitivity to the gliadin fraction of dietary wheat gluten, which leads to damage of the mucosa. There is a heavy chain disease (p. 104) of α-chains in which intestinal lymphoid infiltration causes steatorrhoea and diarrhoea.

In all types of steatorrhoea the failure of fat absorption leads to deficient intake of energy. The total plasma cholesterol level is often low. There is also malabsorption of the fat-soluble vitamins A, D and K, which may lead to clinical vitamin deficiencies, particularly in the sprue syndrome. There is a low fasting plasma carotene level. The plasma vitamin A level rises little after oral vitamin A administration (100 000 units) and this finding may be useful as a screening test in the investigation of steatorrhoea: the value would normally double in 6 h. Deficiencies of the B group vitamins develop when the intestinal bacterial flora is altered as in the 'blind loop syndrome'.

Digestion of protein is not affected, and absorption of amino acids is impaired only in severe cases and the plasma protein concentrations may be normal, or there may be a slight fall in the albumin level; the prothrombin time is prolonged, and the immunoglobulin concentrations may be reduced. Absorption of carbohydrates is diminished, and the patient may have attacks of hypoglycaemia, and a flat glucose tolerance curve (p. 61); there may also be secondary disaccharidase deficiencies (p. 47). The deficiency of calcium absorption, which is due to the mucosal defect, and partly to malabsorption of vitamin D and to excessive calcium excretion in the stools as calcium soaps, causes osteomalacia and occasionally hypocalcaemia and tetany. There may also be impaired absorption of phosphate, and hypophosphataemia (p. 182).

There may be deficient absorption of vitamin B_{12}, iron, and folic acid (this particularly in tropical sprue). Tests using radioactive vitamin B_{12}, such as the Schilling test (p. 144) can be used to investigate ileal absorption.

In prolonged steatorrhoea, or if there is also diarrhoea, electrolytes are lost. The patient may have water and sodium depletion, hypokalaemia may be marked, and there is often phosphate loss.

Tests of malabsorption

The symptoms of generalized malabsorption are diverse and usually depend on the consequences of nutritional or vitamin deficiency. Bowel symptoms are usually present but the hallmark is the demonstration of a failure to absorb fat or the presence of steatorrhoea. In its absence, generalized malabsorption is unlikely though specific absorptive defects may be present (p. 171).

The amount of fat present in the stool varies from day to day and a single 24 h collection cannot be considered representative. A minimum 3 day collection is required on a dietary fat intake exceeding 30 g per day. A mean stool fat of greater than 18 mmol/day indicates steatorrhoea; severe steatorrhoea of 50 mmol or more per day suggests defective lipolysis due to pancreatic insufficiency. Fat absorption may be measured by oral administration of ^{14}C-labelled triglyceride followed by measurement of $^{14}CO_2$ in expired air. This test avoids the hazards of handling faeces in the laboratory.

Differential diagnosis of pancreatic and intestinal malabsorption

The commonest causes of steatorrhoea are biliary obstruction, chronic pancreatitis, and coeliac disease; the differential diagnosis of the second and third of these may not always be possible on clinical grounds alone. The results of fat absorption tests or of faecal fat analysis are not diagnostic.

The trypsin deficiency and impairment of protein digestion which is found in pancreatic disease, and the impairment of carbohydrate absorption which is found in coeliac disease (in contrast to the 'diabetic' impaired glucose tolerance of pancreatic disease), are more characteristic if present. If the facilities are available, more definite biochemical diagnosis of pancreatic disease can be obtained by duodenal intubation and examination of pancreatic juice after stimulation.

Xylose absorption test

The best test of carbohydrate absorption uses the poorly metabolized pentose, D-xylose. After an oral dose of 25 g to adults, in the fasting state, a normal subject excretes 4.5–8 g (30–50 mmol) of xylose in the urine in the next 5 h. In the sprue syndrome less than 4 g (28 mmol) is excreted; in pancreatic disease absorption and excretion are usually unaltered. The test is not valid in old persons or when there is impairment of renal function: in the latter case, when urine values are unreliable, a plasma xylose level less than 2.0 mmol/l at 90 min is considered abnormal.

As 25 g of xylose sometimes causes nausea, a dose of 5 g is becoming popular though the test is not so discriminating. The critical level of excretion in 5 h is then about 1.25 g (8 mmol).

Other tests

In the investigation of disease of the gastrointestinal tract (including the pancreas), non-biochemical modes of investigation may be more diagnostic than those described here.

Specific failures of intestinal function

The above disorders generally affect all aspects of intestinal function. There are a variety of specific alterations of the brush-border membrane, which may primarily affect digestion (e.g. alactasia, p. 47) or absorption (e.g. Hartnup disease, p. 90).

Gastrointestinal hormones

The APUD concept

A variety of similar cells throughout the body, of presumed common embryological origin, are capable of producing peptides, of storing amines, and of *a*mine *p*recursor *u*ptake and *d*ecarboxylation, and are therefore called APUD cells, and their tumours sometimes generically called apudomas. These cells produce the various hormones of the gastrointestinal tract, and also comprise the anterior pituitary, the parathyroid, and the thyroid C cells. The APUD cells exist in nervous tissue, and are thought to be present in the bronchi.

Knowledge of the physiology of the growing number of identified peptide hormones from diffuse endocrine cells in the gastrointestinal tract is advancing rapidly. Gastrin, and secretin and pancreozymin, have long been used as stimulants in tests of gastrointestinal function, and immunoassay is enabling certain plasma assays to become valuable in diagnosis. Glucagon and insulin are discussed in Chapter 5.

Vasoactive intestinal peptide

This hormone (VIP), produced in excess by a pancreatic tumour (VIPoma), gives rise to the Werner-Morrison syndrome of very severe spasmodic watery diarrhoea, with water and salt loss, hypokalaemia, and achlorhydria. This can be diagnosed by finding a very high plasma VIP.

Argentaffin system

The argentaffin cells, which are scattered diffusely throughout the mucosa of the alimentary canal, produce as an internal secretion 5-hydroxytryptamine (serotonin, 5-HT) via 5-hydroxytryptophan (5-HTP) – this is not a polypeptide. Serotonin is present in blood platelets, and]lso in the nervous system. Its full physiological and psychological significance is at present not known, but it can cause capillary constriction and affect gastrointestinal motility.

The rare metastasizing malignant *carcinoid tumour* produces excess serotonin, which leads to a syndrome characterized by flushing attacks, diarrhoea, and right heart valvular disease and heart failure. Pellagra, and even protein deficiency, may be caused by deviation of tryptophan to the excess hormone (p. 111). The plasma serotonin level is increased, and the condition is usually diagnosed by the excessive urinary excretion of a serotonin metabolite, 5-hydroxyindolylacetic acid – ingestion of bananas gives a false positive result. A simple urinary screening test is available. Occasionally the precursor, 5-HT, is produced in tumours and excreted in excess.

Faecal occult blood

The nature of blood in the faeces depends on the quantity, and on whether it has been digested. Significant quantities of unaltered blood are bright red, and of altered blood produce a dark 'tarry' stool or melaena.

Occult blood is not identifiable by direct visual examination. It can be detected in faeces by similar methods to those used for detecting blood in urine. The usual methods are sensitive and will respond to a haemorrhage of 5–10 ml. For maximum sensitivity the patient must be taken off all meat for three days before collection of the specimen for analysis, as haemoglobin derivatives from ingested meat give a positive reaction to the test in the same way as haemoglobin derivatives which have originated from the patient's blood. Most iron preparations that are given by mouth, although they may colour the faeces black, do not interefere with the chemical tests. However, iron(II) (ferrous) sulphate tablets may cause gastrointestinal bleeding, or iron(II) carbonate and iron(II) fumarate can give false positive reactions with the sensitive tests. Simple commercial sideroom tests are available (p. 260).

The occult blood test detects blood which may have come from any site in the gastrointestinal tract. The test is valuable in the investigation of obscure anaemias, and in the search for pathological lesions, such as malignant disease or peptic ulcer. If a sensitive technique gives a negative result on three consecutive daily samples of stool then bleeding from the alimentary tract may be excluded.

For accurate quantitative determination of gastrointestinal bleeding it is necessary to measure haemoglobin in the faeces derived from radioactively labelled erythrocytes which have been injected intravenously.

Further reading

Davenport HW. *Physiology of the Digestive Tract.* 5th edn. Chicago: Year Book Medical Publishers, 1982.

Moosa AR. Diagnostic tests and procedures in acute pancreatitis. *New Engl J Med* 1984; **311**: 639–43.

Theodossi A, Gazzard BG. Have chemical tests a role in diagnosing malabsorption? *Ann Clin Biochem* 1984; **21**: 153–65.

16

Calcium, Phosphate, and the Bones

Objectives

In this chapter the reader is able to

- revise the physiology of bone
- revise the physiology of calcium and phosphate distribution, and their control by vitamin D, parathyroid hormone, and other hormones
- study the metabolic changes in hyperparathyroidism and hypoparathyroidism.

At the conclusion of this chapter the reader is able to

- understand the factors which may alter calcium, phosphate, and magnesium distribution
- use the laboratory to investigate hypercalcaemia and hypocalcaemia
- understand the causes of metabolic bone disease and their relation to tests for differential diagnosis.

General metabolism

Calcium and phosphorus intake and absorption

The usual daily dietary intake of calcium in adults is about 25 mmol (1.0 g), with a wide variation, and calcium balance can be maintained on a minimum intake of about 10 mmol (0.4 g). During late pregnancy and lactation a higher intake (30 mmol (1.2 g) has been recommended) is required to provide calcium for the fetus and for the milk – which contains about 7.5 mmol (0.3 g) of calcium per litre. More calcium is also needed during periods of active growth.

The absorption of calcium ions, which takes place principally in the upper small intestine, is promoted by vitamin D. To stimulate calcium absorption, by promoting the synthesis of calcium-binding protein in the enterocyte, it must be present in the general circulation, not within the lumen of the intestine.

The normal daily intake of phosphorus (in all forms) in adults is 1.5–3.0 g, and 1.0–1.5 g is the minimum recommended. A diet which is otherwise satisfactory is never deficient in phosphorus. Inorganic phosphate is absorbed as the phosphate ion, whereas phospholipid or nucleic acid phosphate has to be liberated by hydrolysis before it can be absorbed. When there is defective absorption of calcium then defective absorption of phosphate usually results, as the excess calcium in the gut causes precipitation of calcium phosphate. Vitamin D has an independent direct stimulatory action on the net absorption of phosphate.

Calcium and phosphorus in the blood

The reference range of plasma/serum calcium in adults is 2.1–2.6 mmol/l. About 50 per cent of the plasma calcium is ultrafiltrable calcium, and most of this is present as free calcium ions (Ca^{2+}), reference range 1.0–1.2 mmol/l; the remainder is non-ionized and bound to citrate and other small ions. The other 50 per cent of the plasma calcium is bound to plasma proteins, particularly albumin: alkalosis encourages calcium-binding and reduces ion activity. It is the free calcium ions that are physiologically active and are responsible for the effects of calcium on the parathyroid glands, bones, and neuromuscular tissue. The concentration of the non-ultrafiltrable or protein-bound fractions in plasma varies with the pH and with the plasma protein concentration, and blood for calcium estimation must therefore be collected without stasis because venous constriction raises the plasma protein concentration (p. 94). Total plasma calcium is usually measured. Some laboratories correct all values for plasma albumin or total protein concentrations; a frequently used formula is to assume that each 1 g/l increase in albumin concentration above 40 g/l binds 0.02 mmol/l of calcium, and vice versa. This is controversial, but plasma albumin should always be measured at the same time as calcium so that a qualitative assessment can be made. Measurement of ionized calcium, which is pH-dependent, requires a special electrode (p. 10).

The reference range of plasma inorganic phosphate in adults is 0.8–1.4 mmol/l, and about 10 per cent of this is protein-bound. Plasma also contains organic phosphorus, most of which is as phospholipids (p. 72). The phosphorus content of erythrocytes is high, and phosphate estimations should always be performed fasting (there is a daily variation of ±0.3 mmol/l because of meals), and on unhaemolysed plasma or serum, either freshly separated or preserved with fluoride because erythrocyte organic phosphates are easily hydrolysed.

In infants the normal plasma calcium and plasma phosphate levels are higher than in adults (p. 266).

Calcium–phosphate product

There is in general a reciprocal relation between the plasma calcium and phosphate, maintained homoeostatically by solution of bone salt. This can be expressed that the product of the concentrations in the plasma of 'ionized calcium' and of 'phosphate' is about 1.2, and of 'total calcium' × 'phosphate' is about 2.8. Plasma is not quite saturated with calcium and phosphate: metastatic calcification becomes a hazard when the total calcium–phosphate product exceeds about 5.5.

The excretion of calcium and phosphorus

The calcium and phosphorus in the faeces consist both of unabsorbed calcium and phosphorus from the diet, and also of calcium and phosphorus which have passed from the plasma into the intestine. Of a daily intake of 25 mmol (1 g) of calcium, 2.5–7.5 mmol (0.1–0.3 g) is excreted in the urine, normally only traces in the sweat and skin, and the remainder in the faeces. Normally about one-third of the intake of phosphorus is excreted in the faeces and two-thirds in the urine.

Normally almost all of the filtered calcium is reabsorbed: calcium behaves as a threshold substance, and when the plasma calcium level falls below about 1.8 mmol/l its excretion in the urine normally ceases. When renal function is normal, the amount of calcium excreted in the urine increases as the plasma calcium level increases; however in 'idiopathic' hypercalciuria (p. 188) the plasma calcium is often normal. Except in the investigation of calculi (p. 123) the value of urine calcium measurements is doubtful unless the intake is known.

The clearance of phosphate is altered both by disorders of the glomeruli and of the tubules, phosphate excretion falling when there is glomerular damage (p. 118) and increasing in renal tubular disorders (p. 121). Excess parathyroid hormone decreases phosphate reabsorption: this measurement, calculated as Tm_P (the tubular maximum for phosphate reabsorption) is sometimes useful in investigating parathyroid disease.

Bone

In biochemical studies a bone may be considered principally as a metabolic pool of calcium and phosphate: its mineral fraction (65 per cent) consists largely of a hydroxyapatite type of crystal, $3Ca_3(PO_4)_2.Ca(OH)_2$. About 99 per cent of the body calcium (about 25 mol: 1 kg) and more than 75 per cent of the phosphate (about 20 mol: 620 g) is in the bones, and about 150 mmol (6 g) of calcium is readily exchangeable. Only about 25 mmol of calcium (1 g) is present in extracellular fluid. Bone contains a considerable store of sodium (amounting to at least one-third of the total body sodium), of magnesium and potassium, and of carbonate, fluoride and citrate. These ions are absorbed on the hydroxyapatite crystals. Bones are not static structures, for calcium, phosphate, and other ions are continuously being laid down and reabsorbed, and there is normally dynamic equilibrium in a steady state.

Figure 16.1 shows an idealized bone, and the general processes of calcium transport.

Bone formation is governed by osteoblasts. These

(i)   manufacture the protein of the bone matrix (osteoid) which is composed mainly of collagen and are then converted to osteocytes. Matrix formation may be deficient when there is protein malnutrition, or other causes of severe negative nitrogen balance;

(ii)   secrete alkaline phosphatase, both spontaneously, and in response to local strain. This acts partly by hydrolysis of pyrophosphate, which is an inhibitor of hydroxyapatite formation, and is also associated with matrix production;

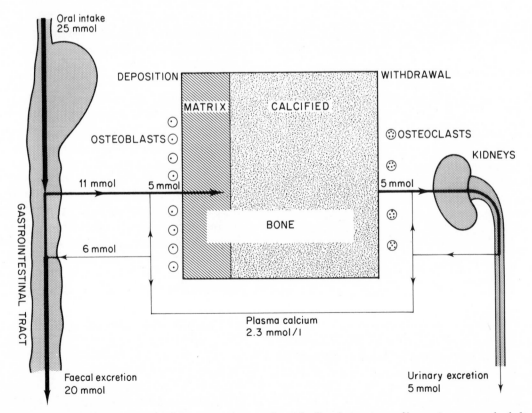

Fig. 16.1   The general processes of calcium transport, and an idealized structure of bone, in a normal adult. Values are for calcium, mmol/24 h.

(iii)   secrete osteocalcin (bone GLA protein), which is stimulated by vitamin D; this has an important but unclassified role in bone mineralization. Plasma osteocalcin concentration (a research assay) can serve like 'bone' alkaline phosphatase (p. 180) as an index of osteoblast activity.

Bone resorption is governed by osteoclasts, which are a type of macrophage. They act to demolish matrix and release its mineral content. The action of osteoclasts is influenced by osteoblast activity, and bone resorption is also encouraged by a low plasma concentration of calcium, phosphate, or bicarbonate. The eventual net effect of parathyroid hormone is to cause release of calcium and phosphate ions from bone salt – and hydroxyproline (p. 89) is released from bone matrix.

Other sites of metabolism

Although the largest part of the calcium and much of the phosphate of the body is concerned with the metabolism of bone, these elements have many other essential functions. Calcium ions are essential for the conversion of prothrombin to thrombin. Calcium ions act at the plasma membrane, for example affecting neuromuscular conduction; within cells their functions are manifold. Phosphate ions are involved in very many ways in cell metabolism as a constituent of nucleic acids, and of ATP, metabolic intermediates, and phospholipids. Phosphate plays an important part in the buffering mechanisms of plasma and urine.

Control of calcium balance
Parathyroid hormone

Only a single active polypeptide is produced by the chief cells of the parathyroid glands. The secretion of parathyroid hormone (PTH) is not governed by a trophic hormone of the pituitary gland, but is stimulated by a low plasma calcium ion activity and inhibited by a high activity. A low magnesium ion also inhibits release of PTH.

The effects of PTH are to raise the plasma calcium and lower the plasma phosphate: chemical solubility of bone salt would alone maintain the plasma calcium at about 1.7 mmol/l, and it is raised above that level by the influence of PTH. The accepted actions of PTH are

(i)   on the bone, via the osteoclasts, to promote dissolution of matrix, breakdown of bone salt, and liberation of calcium, phosphate, hydroxyproline, and some hydroxyl ions: adequate vitamin D must be present. This is an indirect action, as the PTH receptors in bone are osteoblastic;

(ii)   on the kidney, (a) to promote the 1α-hydroxylation of 25-hydroxycholecalciferol to calcitriol, thus indirectly promoting intestinal absorption of calcium, (b) to diminish tubular reabsorption of phosphate and thus promote phosphate excretion, (c) to increase tubular reabsorption of calcium, and (d) to a lesser extent (if in excess), to diminish reabsorption of bicarbonate leading to a hypercholoraemic acidosis: there may also be an aminociduria.

Urinary cAMP increases, derived from both bone and kidney.

Assay
Measurement of plasma PTH (by radioimmunoassay) may be valuable in combination with assay of plasma calcium and phosphate in the investigation of problems of hypercalcaemia or hypocalcaemia. However, assays involving different sites on the molecule (carboxy-, midregion, amino-terminal) may give different results. A cytochemical assay (p. 191) has been developed.

Calcitonin

This polypeptide hormone is primarily of thyroidal origin (p. 199) from the parafollicular cells. It plays an unclarified role in the maintenance of a steady plasma calcium level, and its secretion is modified by the plasma calcium ion activity. It diminishes bone resorption by inhibition of osteoclast activity and is therefore used in the treatment of Paget's disease. When in high concentration, it increases the renal excretion of calcium and phosphate, and lowers the plasma calcium and phosphate.

An immunoassay is available and is useful for diagnosis of the rare calcitonin-secreting medullary cell carcinoma of the thyroid, in which the plasma calcium and phosphate are usually normal.

Other hormones

Thyroxine stimulates bone turnover, particularly the activity of osteoclasts. In hyperthyroidism there may be increased bone resorption with an increase in urinary calcium excretion, and sometimes mild hypercalcaemia.

The oestrogens and androgens influence bone metabolism mainly by their effects on the production of the bone matrix. When there is oestrogen and androgen deficiency (postmenopausal, or in old age) matrix production is diminished, and this can sometimes be reversed by appropriate replacement therapy.

The glucocorticoids also influence bone metabolism mainly by their actions on protein catabolism affecting the production of bone matrix. When excess glucocorticoids are present, as in iatrogenic or idiopathic Cushing's syndrome (p. 209), matrix production is diminished, bone breakdown stimulated, and skeletal mass reduced (leading to an increased urinary calcium). Growth hormone stimulates growth of cartilage: excess activity in acromegaly (p. 194) often raises the plasma phosphate by an action on the renal tubules.

Vitamin D – the calciferols

There are a number of related substances that have vitamin D activity (Fig. 16.2). Ergocalciferol (vitamin D_2) is produced by artificial irradiation of ergosterol (from plants) with ultraviolet light. Cholecalciferol (vitamin D_3) is produced by irradiation of 7-dehydrocholesterol in human skin by the ultraviolet component of sunlight (which opens the B ring, p. 78), and also occurs naturally in some animal food sources. Cholecalciferol is converted in the liver to 25-hydroxycholecalciferol (calcifediol). This is further activated in the kidney, under the influence of parathyroid hormone and with some stimulation by a low plasma phosphate, to 1,25-dihydroxycholecalciferol (calcitriol), and to 24,25-dihydroxycholecalciferol and other hydroxylated metabolites. When plasma calcium, and also phosphate, are not low, instead of formation of the highly active calcitriol, the much less active 24,25 derivative is preferentially synthesized (compare the control of rT_3 synthesis, p. 197). Ergocalciferol is metabolized similarly. The increased synthesis of vitamin D in the skin during the summer in Britain causes a seasonal variation in the reference ranges for all related compounds.

Because cholecalciferol is produced naturally in the skin, and the body's requirements are only supplemented from the diet, calcitriol can be considered to be a hormone.

The actions of calcitriol (and related compounds) raise the levels of both the plasma calcium and the plasma phosphate. The principal site of action is on the intestine, where the absorption of both calcium and phosphate is promoted. Vitamin D acts directly on bone to promote normal growth and development mainly by promoting resorption and utilization of calcium via production of calcium-binding proteins by osteoblasts.

Assay
25-Hydroxycholecalciferol is by far the most abundant metabolite in plasma. Its assay can be useful in determining whether hypocalcaemia, and bone disease, is caused by vitamin D deficiency. Assay of other derivatives is a research procedure.

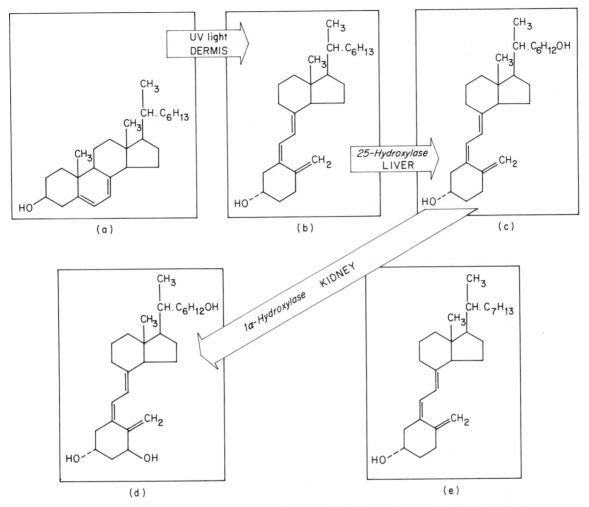

Fig. 16.2 Structures of compounds related to vitamin D: (a) 7-dehydrocholesterol; (b) cholecalciferol (vitamin D_3); (c) 25-hydroxycholecalciferol (calcifediol); (d) 1,25-dihydroxycholecalciferol (calcitriol); (e) ergocalciferol (vitamin D_2)

Hypervitaminosis D

The primary effect of therapeutic overdosage with vitamin D is excessive absorption of calcium, some excessive absorption of phosphate, and eventually increased bone resorption. There is progressive hypercalcaemia with usually a raised plasma phosphate, and secondary depression of parathyroid activity. Symptoms of hypercalcaemia, including calcium deposition in the tissues and secondary renal damage, will develop if treatment is not stopped when the plasma calcium level exceeds about 3 mmol/l.

Hypovitaminosis D

This leads to rickets or osteomalacia (p. 187).

Enzymes – the phosphatases

The phosphatases are a group of enzymes that promote the hydrolysis of organic phosphates with liberation of phosphate ions. They can be divided into two main groups, the classification depending on whether the enzyme has maximum activity in an alkaline or an acid medium. Alkaline phosphatase is considered here because of its major concern with bone metabolism. Acid phosphatase has significance in chemical pathology as a cancer marker (p. 234).

Alkaline phosphatases

These enzymes are produced in many cells of the body, and the diagnostically important sites of secretion are the osteoblasts and the hepatocytes. Isoenzymes from intestinal mucosa (after a fatty meal; but only in subjects of blood group A who are non-secretors of ABH) and from placenta (after midpregnancy) may also be detected in plasma. Alkaline phosphatase is found both in urine and in bile, in both cases arising from local cells.

The usual reference range in adult plasma (though this is method-dependent) is 35–130 U/l in men; 30–110 U/l in women, the enzyme being derived about equally from the liver and bone. The plasma activity varies with age (p. 266), tends to be higher in males, and is higher (up to 200 U/l) during late pregnancy and periods of active bone growth, from excess placental and osteoblastic isoenzyme respectively.

A raised plasma alkaline phosphatase is found either when there is excess production or release of the enzyme from relevant cells. When there is increased osteoblastic activity excess alkaline phosphatase is secreted. In hyperparathyroidism with bone disease (p. 184), malignant disease with an osteoblastic response (osteosarcoma or certain secondary carcinomas), rickets and the other forms of osteomalacia, and the healing phase of major fractures, the plasma activity is usually 150–350 U/l, and in Paget's disease the value may be over 500 U/l. Normal plasma values are almost always found in osteolytic bone disease (for example in multiple myeloma and some types of malignant deposits in bone), and in osteoporosis.

There is a rare benign transient hyperphosphatasia of infancy.

Isoenzymes
Liver alkaline phosphatase is increased in various types of hepatobiliary disease (p. 155). In cases where both osteoblastic and liver isoenzymes may be present it is necessary to perform electrophoresis to identify and measure the isoenzymes. Other abnormal alkaline phosphatases, usually of placental type, may be produced by malignant tissue (p. 234).

Alterations of plasma calcium and phosphate
Hypocalcaemia (Scheme 16.1)

A low ionized calcium activity causes hyperexcitability of the nervous system, which may present clinically as convulsions, and as tingling and numbness leading to tetany. Other effects of long-standing hypocalcaemia are cataracts, calcification of the basal ganglion, a prolonged coagulation time, and mental depression.

Hypocalcaemia associated with hypoproteinaemia alone, when there is a normal ionized calcium, yields no metabolic abnormalities.

A reduction in both total plasma calcium concentration and ionized calcium activity may be due to

(a) deficient dietary intake related to physiological need;
(b) deficient intestinal absorption: vitamin D deficiency, the malabsorption syndrome, phytate excess, or improper high-phosphate infant feeding;
(c) deficient withdrawal from bone: particularly hypoparathyroidism;
(d) increased loss: via the intestines (usually combined with (b)); via the kidneys, tubular disorders;
(e) acute pancreatitis, anticonvulsant therapy, and hypomagnesaemia.

A reduction only in ionized calcium may be due to

(a) alkalaemia;
(b) binding of calcium to other ions, particularly intravenous EDTA or citrate. Such citrate toxicity may develop from massive blood transfusions as in cardiac surgery or liver transplants,

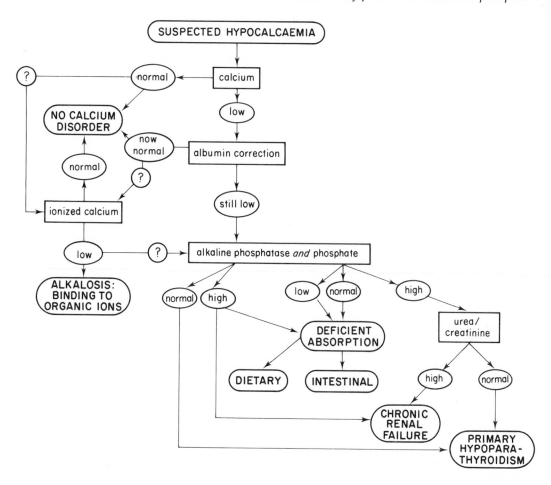

Scheme 16.1   Typical findings shown by plasma biochemical analysis, supplementing clinical evidence, in the investigation of suspected hypocalcaemia in an adult. The further tests are described in the text. Tests marked ⊘ are to be considered if evidence is contradictory

or during plasmapheresis: assay of ionized calcium (p. 175) is essential for management.

Hypercalcaemia (Scheme 16.2)

An increased ionized calcium activity causes muscular weakness, gastrointestinal symptoms, giddiness, extreme thirst, and marked lassitude. There may be deposition of calcium phosphate at various sites as metastatic calcification, and hypercalcaemia leads to hypercalciuria and often to renal damage (with polyuria) and then to renal calculi, especially when there is also hyperphosphataemia. Severe acute hypercalcaemia carries the risk of a cardiac arrest.

Hypercalcaemia associated with hyperproteinaemia alone, when there is a normal ionized calcium, yields no metabolic abnormalities.

An increase in both total and ionized calcium may be due to

(a) increased intestinal absorption: hypervitaminosis D, and formerly in the milk-alkali syndrome;
(b) increased withdrawal from bone; malignancy whether local or general (the commonest cause in hospital patients), hyperparathyroidism (the commonest cause when found on screening), immobilization, thyrotoxicosis, or chronic acidosis;

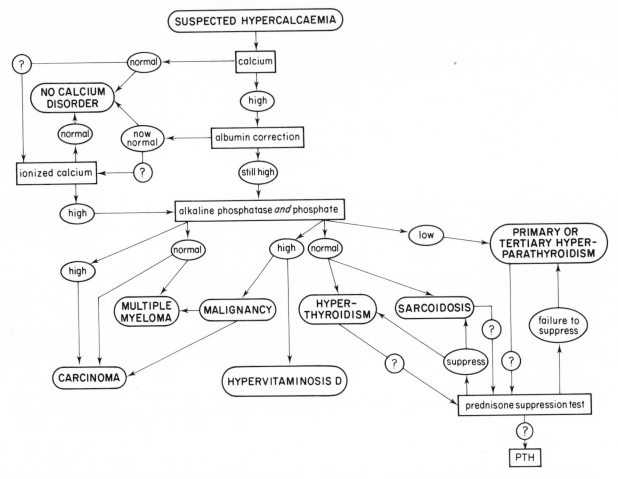

Scheme 16.2 Typical findings shown by plasma biochemical analysis, supplementing clinical evidence, in the investigation of suspected hypercalcaemia in an adult. The further tests are described in the text. Tests marked ⓘ are to be considered if evidence is contradictory

(c) decreased renal excretion: from thiazide diuretics;

(d) sarcoidosis.

Excessive dietary intake alone will not cause hypercalcaemia.

Hypophosphataemia

This causes, through depletion of ATP, central and peripheral neurological disorders, and cardiac and skeletal muscular weakness; a direct effect on bone can lead to osteomalacia and rickets.

A decrease in plasma phosphate concentration may be due to

(a) deficient intake: in general malabsorp-

tion; or from imperfect intravenous fluid replacement or dialysis;

(b) deficient intestinal absorption: from phosphate-binding agents such as aluminium hydroxide;

(c) redistribution from ECF to cells: into bone, during healing of rickets, after parathyroidectomy, or from (rare) osteoblastic metastases; into somatic cells, principally from any acceleration of carbohydrate metabolism as in acute treatment of diabetes mellitus;

(d) increased loss: via the intestines, in severe diarrhoea; via the renal tubules, in hyperparathyroidism or in specific disorders with failure of reabsorption.

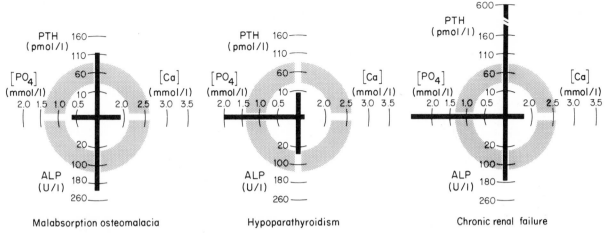

Fig. 16.3   The use of radial diagrams in understanding the biochemical differential diagnosis of hypocalcaemia. Four measurements, plasma calcium (Ca), phosphate (PO$_4$), alkaline phosphatase (ALP), and parathyroid hormone (PTH) are made and the results plotted on the diagram. The reference ranges form the shaded circle. The thick black line shows a finding for each measurement which is typical for the condition

Hyperphosphataemia

This has no direct metabolic effects, and affects bone through alteration of calcium distribution.

An increase in plasma phosphate may be due to

(a)   excessive intake: from dietary laxatives or enemas;

(b)   increased intestinal absorption: in hypervitaminosis D;

(c)   redistribution from cells to ECF: from bone destr   tion (see hypercalcaemia), or in acromegaly; from somatic cell breakdown e.g. chemotherapy of lymphoma;

(d)   decreased renal excretion; in hypoparathyroidism or in glomerular failure.

Diseases affecting the metabolism of bone

Hypoparathroidism

Idiopathic (autoimmune) atrophy of the parathyroid glands is sometimes seen, but hypoparathyroidism is usually caused by accidental vascular damage to the glands, or their complete removal, during thyroidectomy, or sometimes by irradiation or iron overload.

The biochemical findings (Fig. 16.3) are due to deficiency of PTH (plasma PTH may be unmeasurable) affecting bones and renal tubules, and to secondary effects from diminished renal formation of calcitriol. There is a low plasma calcium level which may be below 1.5 mmol/l, and a high plasma phosphate which may exceed 2 mmol/l. There is decreased withdrawal of calcium from bone, and osteoblast activity and bone formation may also be reduced. The plasma alkaline phosphatase level is normal or low. A low plasma calcium may lead to absence of detectable calcium in the urine.

The clinical features are caused by the low plasma ionized calcium concentration (p. 180), and are predominantly neurological (including tetany) though cataracts are common. Treatment by calcium and vitamin D must be controlled by serial estimations of the plasma calcium concentrations. There are risks of overdosage with vitamin D causing a high plasma calcium, and then of nephrocalcinosis with renal failure.

Neonatal hypocalcaemia

This may present in the first 48 h with tetany and convulsions, and is usually due to delayed development of PTH secretion secondary to maternal hypercalcaemia.

Pseudohypoparathyroidism

In this group of rare familial disorders, the syndrome of hypoparathyroidism is often associated with abnormal body build. It is caused by diminished tissue (bone and kidney) receptor-system sensitivity to PTH. Plasma PTH values are normal, or raised due to secondary hyperparathyroidism. Urinary cAMP excretion (p. 177) does not increase after PTH injection, in contrast to the response in normal subjects and in patients with hypoparathyroidism. The condition responds to calcium and vitamin D.

Primary hyperparathyroidism

Primary hyperparathyroidism may be caused either by benign or malignant tumours of one or more parathyroid glands, or by hyperplasia of all the glands: a single adenoma is the most common finding. Certain tumours elsewhere may produce an ectopic PTH-like substance (p. 233). The autonomous adenoma that follows stimulation by prolonged hypocalcaemia and secondary hyperparathyroidism is called tertiary hyperparathyroidism (p. 187).

The biochemical findings (Fig. 16.4) are

due to an excess of PTH activity. There is a raised plasma calcium concentration which may exceed 4 mmol/l but which may only manifest itself when provoked by a low phosphate or high calcium diet; less regularly the plasma phosphate is low, sometimes below 0.5 mmol/l. The urinary phosphate excretion is high and the urinary calcium excretion is high: cAMP excretion is increased. If there is secondary renal damage the plasma phosphate level may be above normal, with a raised plasma urea. In about half of the cases, usually those of longer duration, and depending on bone involvement, there is a high plasma alkaline phosphatase and increased urinary hydroxyproline excretion. There is a tendency to an alkaline urine, and to a hyperchloraemic metabolic acidosis.

If the plasma calcium rises above about 3 mmol/l signs of hypercalcaemia may appear (p. 181), of which the earliest are loss of appetite and muscular hypotonicity. There is increased bone turnover with a drain of calcium from the bones from increased osteoclastic activity; the increase of calcium deposition in the bones is associated with increased osteoblastic activity. When the bones are effected they show a generalized rarefaction with pain, and in advanced cases the cyst formation, deformities, and fractures, of osteitis fibrosa cystica (von

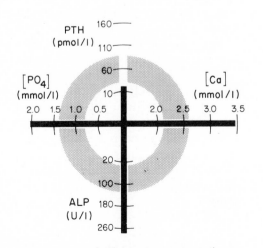

Metastases

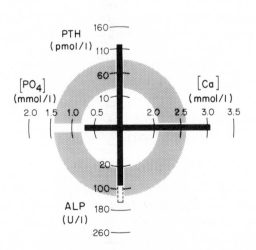

Primary hyperparathyroidism

Fig. 16.4 The use of radial diagrams in understanding the biochemical differential diagnosis of hypercalcaemia. Symbols are the same as in Fig. 16.3

Recklinghausen's disease). A marked degree of hyperparathyroidism may be present without any demonstrable clinical or radiological changes in the bones. The high urinary calcium and phosphate lead to tubular damage, polyuria, and polydipsia. Formation of calcium phosphate and calcium oxalate stones (or deposition in joints) is a common presenting symptom, though in such cases there is very often no obvious bony disease especially when there is a high calcium intake. In all cases of renal calculi (p. 123) the plasma calcium and phosphate should be estimated on more than one occasion, as perhaps about 5 per cent of cases are due to primary hyperparathyroidism. In long-standing cases renal damage may raise the plasma phosphate level.

After removal of the enlarged parathyroid(s) by surgery, there may be a dangerous fall in the plasma calcium, which needs to be monitored for a week, and occasionally in the plasma magnesium and phosphate (p. 189).

Investigations
The diagnosis can usually be made on the clinical and biochemical signs. When hyperparathyroidism is suspected, repeated estimation of plasma calcium (with plasma proteins) is usually as valuable a method of diagnosis as are more complex investigations – when hypercalcaemia is marginal, correction for possible hypoproteinaemia may be necessary (p. 175). Plasma phosphate and urea/creatinine analyses should always be done at the same time, and finding an increased plasma alkaline phosphatase and urinary hydroxyproline indicates bone involvement.

Though plasma PTH is almost always high, this assay is rarely needed, for most cases are diagnosable by simpler means. Measurement of PTH in blood obtained by selective venous catheterization of the neck veins may help in locating an adenoma.

The mechanism of the useful *glucocorticoid suppression* test is unknown. When a patient with hypercalcaemia due to primary or tertiary hyperparathyroidism (or familial

hypocalciuric hypercalcaemia) is placed on a high dose of prednisone (60 mg daily for 10 days), the plasma calcium remains unaltered, whilst hypercalcaemia due to sarcoidosis, and usually to metastases or thyrotoxicosis, is significantly reduced.

Multiple endocrine adenomas (or neoplasia, MEN)
Hyperparathyroidism may be a part of two distinct familial syndromes. In type I it is associated with the Zollinger-Ellison syndrome (p. 165; pancreatic gastrinomas) and pituitary chromophobe adenomas. In type II it is associated with medullary carcinoma of the thyroid and phaeochromocytoma; the rare related type III also has multiple neuromas. These may be related to the distribution of different APUD cells (p. 171).

Familial hypocalciuric hypercalcaemia
This is an important differential diagnosis as parathyroidectomy is contraindicated. The biochemical features resemble primary hyperparathyroidism except for low renal clearance of calcium. The cause may be lowered sensitivity of the parathyroid glands to feedback from the plasma calcium.

Osteoporosis

In osteoporosis there is reduction of bone mass, both matrix and mineral, without alteration of their ratio, to an extent greater than expected for the patient's age and sex. This is probably never primarily a disorder of mineral balance though it may coexist with osteomalacia. Osteoporosis develops when bone mass is lost, or when matrix formation is imperfect with adequate calcium and phosphate available for calcification. It may present with pain, deformities, and fractures.

Primary osteoporosis

The classification is unsatisfactory, the causes obscure, and the categories overlap. It is common. It mainly develops either postmenopausally, or generally with ageing. In the first group bone loss predominates and oestrogen deficiency plays an important but unclarified role: other hormone deficiencies, particularly calcitonin and adrenal androgens, have been implicated. Disuse plays a part in senile osteoporosis, and deficient bone formation predominates.

Undetermined (and possibly genetic) factors contribute both to postmenopausal and to senile osteoporosis, as only a proportion of possible subjects develop these conditions. In chronic osteoporosis the plasma levels of calcium, phosphate, and alkaline phosphatase (unless there are fractures) are generally within the reference range, though there may be a slight postmenopausal increase in plasma calcium.

Treatment is unsatisfactory; a high intake of oestrogens is considered to be helpful in prevention in susceptible subjects.

Secondary osteoporosis

This term is used when a specific known cause can be implicated. It includes the following disorders.

Disuse osteoporosis
This may develop after prolonged decubitus or immobilization of a limb. When of rapid onset, there can be hypercalcaemia, and hypercalciuria with calculi is frequent.

Cushing's syndrome
In iatrogenic or spontaneous Cushing's syndrome (p. 209) the primary pathogenesis is the effect of excess glucocorticoid activity on the synthesis of bone matrix.

Other endocrine disorders
Osteroporosis is a feature of non-menopausal gonadal deficiency in males or females, with deficient synthesis of bone matrix. It is also an occasional feature of thyrotoxicosis.

Osteomalacia and rickets

In osteomalacia there is deficient calcification of a normal mass of bone matrix. It is a disorder of mineral balance. Defective calcification of the matrix develops when there is deficiency of calcium (the more important) or phosphate at the bone-forming surface (the plasma calcium-phosphate product is usually less than 1.6), and also directly due to deficiency of vitamin D. Acidosis promotes osteomalacia by increasing urinary calcium loss, and also by a direct effect on dissolution of bone salt. The result of the deficient formation of calcified bone, with relatively normal bone destruction, is rarefaction.

The mineral deficiency may result from decreased absorption or increased excretion.

Decreased absorption
This occurs

(i) when dietary intake of calcium is low – this can occur with a 'normal' intake, when needs are greater particularly during lactation;

(ii) (of phosphate) when there is prolonged hypophosphataemia from use of phosphate binders such as aluminium hydroxide, or from improper intravenous feeding;

(iii) from vitamin D deficiency, leading to calcium and phosphate malabsorption – this can result from dietary deficiency; deficient skin synthesis; decreased absorption (in the malabsorption syndrome from any cause); deficient hydroxylation in chronic renal disease and possibly in advanced liver disease; anticonvulsant therapy (e.g. treatment with phenytoin), perhaps by enzyme induction increasing the catabolism of calciferol;

(iv) from other intestinal causes.

Calcium absorption is decreased by a high concentration in the intestine of any anion which forms an insoluble calcium salt. If there is excess of phosphate (as in uraemia; p. 120), then insoluble calcium phosphate will be precipitated. Fatty acids, present in excess in steatorrhoea, likewise form insoluble calcium soaps within the intestine.

Phytic acid (inositol hexaphosphoric acid), which is present in many cereals, gives rise to insoluble calcium salts. A high dietary phytic acid contributes to the calcium deficiency of some Asians, especially vegans, in Britain. In coeliac disease absorption of calcium is deficient also because of the flattened mucosa, and absorption of phosphate may be impaired. In other chronic gastrointestinal diseases, after gastrectomy, and occasionally in patients who are receiving ion-exchange resin therapy, calcium absorption may be impaired.

In Britain osteomalacia is often due to a combined effect of malnutrition (generally from poverty) leading to deficient intake of calcium and vitamin D, and of the low-sunshine climate leading to deficient synthesis of cholecalciferol in the skin. In dark-skinned immigrants this skin synthesis may be particularly deficient, and dietary phytic acid plays a part. Poor children who live in a sunny climate are less likely to develop vitamin D deficiency.

Rickets is the special name given to vitamin D-deficient osteomalacia in children; in addition to rarefaction there is disordered growth of cartilage and bone with characteristic pathological changes at the epiphyseal lines and bone deformities.

Increased excretion
This results from

(i) proximal renal tubular disorders, including the Fanconi syndrome – from a combination of phosphate loss and acidosis;
(ii) renal tubular acidosis, which leads to loss of bone calcium;
(iii) familial hypophosphataemic ('tubular') rickets, with phosphate loss alone – leading to a vitamin D-resistant rickets-like disorder. There is also an adult-onset form.

Secondary effects

Deficiency of calcium initially causes a low plasma calcium concentration: the plasma phosphate is normal, and the alkaline phosphatase usually raised, because stresses applied to the weakened bones stimulate osteoblastic activity. In renal tubular disorders, a low plasma phosphate may predominate. In osteomalacia the low plasma calcium usually appropriately causes some *secondary hyperparathyroidism*, which may restore the plasma calcium level to normal (but not above) and lower the plasma phosphate: the calcium × phosphate product remains low. In rickets, because of this effect and particularly because of defective absorption of phosphate, the plasma phosphate level is always low, and the plasma calcium low or normal. In severe steatorrhoea the plasma calcium usually remains low, with a low or low/normal plasma phosphate (Fig. 16.3).

The parathyroid hyperactivity associated with osteomalacia is insufficient to cause hypercalcaemia unless an autonomous parathyroid adenoma develops (*tertiary hyperparathyroidism*) and in these patients osteitis fibrosa cystica does not develop.

Treatment of osteomalacia is treatment of its cause. Extra vitamin D and calcium should be given in all cases, and if necessary parenterally.

Some other disorders of calcium and phosphate balance

Renal osteodystrophy

Chronic renal failure with uraemia is associated with this syndrome: the bone disorder usually combines, in variable proportions, features of osteomalacia, osteoporosis, and hyperparathyroidism. The main biochemical causes are phosphate retention (due to glomerular damage) leading to an increased plasma phosphate, and impaired renal hydroxylation of 25-hydroxycholecalciferol to calcitriol. Calcium absorption is diminished. The resultant low plasma calcium (and probably other factors) causes secondary parathyroid hypertrophy with a high plasma PTH (and there is some peripheral resistance to the hormone), and this will return the plasma calcium towards normal; alkaline phosphatase values are usually raised (Fig. 16.3). Acidaemia contributes to the loss of calcium from bone. There is a high calcium–phosphate product and soft-tissue calcification.

After long-term dialysis, phosphate depletion and aluminium toxicity (p. 122) contribute to the bone disease.

Renal rickets (or 'glomerular' rickets) is the bone disorder in children with chonric renal failure, due both to impaired vitamin D metabolism and to phosphate retention causing intestinal loss of calcium: the bone changes are associated with epiphyseal changes as in rickets.

Hepatic osteodystrophy

When there is cholestasis, and particularly in biliary cirrhosis, osteomalacia often develops, though some osteoporosis may be seen. There is lack of absorption of vitamin D (due to the steatorrhoea), and defective hydroxylation may be present. Plasma calcium and phosphate are low/normal, bone and liver alkaline phosphatase raised, and secondary hyperparathyroidism sometimes develops.

Paget's disease (osteitis deformans)

There is disseminated irregular bone destruction and a marked tendency to new bone formation. The plasma calcium and phosphate levels are normal, but the alkaline phosphatase level is extremely high, often over 500 U/l. The plasma acid phosphatase activity may also be slightly increased. Urinary hydroxyproline, from collagen turnover, is also high.

Hypophosphatasia

This is a rare hereditary disorder, which presents as a skeletal condition resembling rickets. There is deficient tissue synthesis of alkaline phosphatase, a very low plasma alkaline phosphatase, and high urinary excretion of phosphorylethanolamine (a natural substrate for the enzyme) resulting from the failure of hydrolysis of organic phosphates.

Idiopathic hypercalcaemia of infants

In this rare disorder there is a raised plasma calcium level, secondary renal damage with a raised plasma urea, and a normal plasma phosphate, alkaline phosphatase, and bicarbonate. The cause is probably excessive calcium absorption from the gut due to hypersensitivity to vitamin D – though many cases are caused by overdose (p. 181). Clinically there is failure to thrive and often mental retardation.

Absorption hypercalcaemia and hypercalciuria

Hypercalcaemia due to excessive absorption of dietary calcium is occasionally seen, associated with alkalaemia and secondary renal damage. This *milk–alkali syndrome*, now rare, occurred in patients who took, for long periods, excessive absorbable alkalis and milk for the treatment of peptic ulcer.

A common cause of hypercalcaemia, leading to renal calculi (p. 124), is increased absorption of calcium, and possibly fluctuating hypercalcaemia and PTH suppression. The cause is unknown. There may be an initial renal phosphate leak, with a variable and fluctuating increase in plasma vitamin D; alternatively a general defect in calcium transport has been suggested. Some cases of renal calculi are thought to be due to hypercalciuria caused by specific defective tubular reabsorption of calcium.

Sarcoidosis

The cause of this hypercalcaemia syndrome is probably increased absorption of calcium, due to increased formation of calcitriol in the granulomatous tissue which contains a 1α-hydroxylase. The hypercalcaemia and hypercalciuria of sarcoidosis returns to normal after high doses of prednisone, which does not affect the hypercalcaemia of hyperparathyroidism (p. 185).

The differential diagnosis of sarcoidosis,

and its subsequent monitoring, is helped by the finding of a raised serum angiotensin-converting enzyme (p. 208) in more than half the cases.

Malignant disease

This is the commonest cause of hypercalcaemia, and is usually associated with hyperphosphataemia and may lead to urinary calculi (Fig. 16.4). Overt osteolytic malignant disease in bone, whether primary or metastatic (including myelomatosis), destroys bone with the release of calcium, phosphate, and bicarbonate. The malignant tissues directly produce a bone-resorbing substance, and also act indirectly by secreting an osteoclast-activating factor (humoral hypercalcaemic protein). In most such cases, but not in myelomatosis, there is an osteoblast response and an increase in plasma alkaline phosphatase.

However, hypercalcaemia can develop in malignant disease even without detectable macroscopic or microscopic metastases in bone. Various mediators produced by the primary tumour (p. 235) have been implicated, including osteoclast-activating factor, prostaglandins, and ectopic PTH-like substances.

Magnesium

Magnesium balance in health and disease has been studied less extensively than has calcium balance.

The minimum daily intake to maintain long-term balance is about 10 mmol, though the average mixed diet contains ample magnesium. About one-third is absorbed in the upper small intestine, and this is not dependent on vitamin D; balance is maintained by the equivalent quantity being excreted in the urine. Almost all of the 750 mmol of body magnesium is in the cells (about half in the bone) at a concentration about 10 times that in the plasma. About 80 per cent of plasma magnesium is diffusible, and the remainder is bound to protein in the same way as is plasma calcium.

Although changes in the activity of magnesium ions affect neuromuscular conductivity in the same way as do changes in calcium ions, alterations of clinical significance are less common.

Hypermagnesaemia

This leads to weakness due to impairment of neuromuscular transmission, and to nausea and mental confusion. Hypermagnesaemia is not common, but can be found when there is severe acute or chronic renal failure, and is caused by failure of filtration. It is accentuated if there is treatment with magnesium salts.

Hypomagnesaemia

This leads to twitches, tremor, and mental confusion. Hypomagnesaemia usually develops slowly, and may be caused by

(a) failure of intestinal absorption. This occurs in severe malnutrition, the malabsorption syndrome, chronic diarrhoea, and after major gastrointestinal surgery with suction and imperfect fluid replacement;

(b) renal tubular loss in hyperaldosteronism, and from many diuretics, or in drug nephropathy (e.g. aminoglycosides, cisplatin);

(c) diversion from plasma in acute pancreatitis (compare calcium, p. 180), after parathyroidectomy, or in recovery from ketoacidosis – this may develop rapidly;

(d) chronic alcoholism: this is multifactorial.

Further reading

Editorial. Measuring the PTH level. *Lancet* 1988; i: 94–5.

Elin RJ. Assessment of magnesium status. *Clin Chem* 1987; **33**: 1965–70.

Heath D, Marx SJ. Calcium disorders. *BIMR Clinical Endocrinology no 2*. London: Butterworth, 1982.

Insogna KL, Broadus AE. Hypercalcaemia of malignancy. *Annu Rev Med* 1987; **38**: 241–56.

Jamieson MJ. Hypercalcaemia. *Br Med J* 1985; **290**: 378–82.

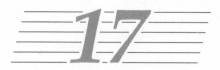

General Diagnostic Endocrinology: The Hypothalamus and Pituitary Gland

Objectives

In this chapter the reader is able to

- study the principles of hormone assay and of endocrine investigation
- revise the physiology and biochemistry of the hypothalamic regulating hormones, the anterior pituitary hormones, the posterior pituitary hormones, and of their neural and feedback control
- study the biochemical changes in primary hypothalamic disorders
- study the biochemical changes produced by deficiencies of, and tumours of, the anterior pituitary
- study the biochemical changes in, and investigate syndromes of, primary and secondary antidiuretic hormone excess and deficiency.

At the conclusion of this chapter the reader is able to

- understand the application of stimulation and suppression tests especially in differentiating trophic and target components of endocrine disease
- use the laboratory in the investigation of hypothalamic–pituitary disease
- use the laboratory in the investigation of diabetes insipidus.

Diagnostic procedures

Hormone assay

Blood/plasma analysis gives a measure of hormone concentration, whether total or free (unbound), only at a point in time, whilst many hormone concentrations vary both episodically and in a circadian rhythm: because of the pulsatile secretion of many pituitary hormones, taking three blood samples at 20-min intervals is sometimes recommended. Results of urine analysis can represent integrated secretion over a longer period but are influenced by variations in metabolism (mainly in the liver) and in renal excretion. Salivary hormone analysis is being introduced as offering the same results as for urine free hormones. The relative merits, and problems, of measuring total hormone, free (unbound) hormone, and hormonal metabolites, are discussed under the individual endocrine glands. Carefully selected stimulation and suppression (dynamic) tests may be essential. Measurement of actual secretion rate is always difficult and expensive. The local laboratory should be consulted for details of tests that are not described here.

The anterior pituitary hormones can be estimated biologically, although the techniques are generally difficult and tedious: new in vitro cytochemical procedures can measure biological effects of a hormone on target cells. Radioimmunoassay and other immunoassays (which may give different results from those of bioassay) for all these hormones in plasma have been developed and are generally used in endocrine investigation. Radioreceptor assay is being developed, using isolated hormone receptors as the initial binding site: this resembles bioassay in its specificity for effective hormone activity. If not available locally, the assays can be done (in Britain), if essential for diagnosis, at special centres (p. 253): reference ranges should be obtained locally.

An increased excretion in urine of the placental hormone chorionic gonadotrophin is easily measured semiquantitatively immunologically as a pregnancy diagnosis test; a similar rapid test for luteinizing hormone is now available.

In assays of the various peripheral hormones, competitive protein binding and related methods, as well as the above procedures, have largely replaced chemical methods, and gas chromatography may be necessary for quantitation of individual hormones.

Dynamic tests

Stimulation and suppression tests of endogenous hormone secretion are valuable both for investigating mild degrees of alteration of endocrine gland function, and for determining the level of a lesion. Details of appropriate tests are given under the individual glands: different institutions may use different procedures with variation in responses.

Stimulation tests

These are used when, with slight hypofunc-tion, resting values of hormones may be low–normal; the reserve capacity will be low and does not respond fully to an appropriate stimulant. Stimulation tests may also be necessary to distinguish between central and target gland deficiency.

Primary deficiency of target glands (such as primary hypothyroidism) typically shows low resting plasma (and urinary) values of the appropriate peripheral hormone (such as free thyroxine), and these values are not raised by stimulation with the specific pituitary trophic or hypothalamic releasing-hormone (such as TSH, or TRH). The plasma concentration of the trophic hormone (TSH) will be high due to withdrawal of negative feedback.

When primary pituitary deficiency is causing deficiency of target gland function, the low resting values for peripheral hormone will respond to stimulation by the appropriate trophic hormone. The plasma values for the pituitary trophic hormone will be low, and these (and the peripheral hormone values) will not respond to stimulation by the hypothalamic releasing-hormone.

To test hypothalamic function it is possible to modify feedback controls (e.g. insulin-hypoglycaemia (p. 214), metyr-apone (p. 214), clomiphene (p. 221)) and then to measure changes in trophic hormones or in peripheral hormones. Releasing-hormones cannot be measured in plasma.

Suppression tests

These are used when, with slight hyper-function, resting values of hormones may be high–normal; this is sufficient to act on negative feedback which cannot therefore be further fully suppressed. Suppression tests may also help in distinguishing between central and target gland overactivity, though this is usually less of a problem than for deficiency.

Autonomous primary overactivity of target glands (such as Cushing's syndrome due to adrenal tumour) typically shows high resting plasma or urinary values for peripheral hormones (such as cortisol): these are not lowered by suppressing the stimulant system (e.g. by dexamethasone). The plasma value for the trophic hormone (ACTH) will be low due to excess negative feedback.

When primary hypothalamic–pituitary excess is causing target gland overaction, the resting plasma values for the trophic hormone will be high as feedback is ineffective; the high values for peripheral hormone will respond to appropriate suppression – except for pituitary *tumours* which do not so respond, being autonomous.

The hypothalamus and anterior pituitary

Hormones of the anterior pituitary gland

Six separate hormones or hormone complexes which are probably secreted independently by different cells (somatotrophs etc.), have so far been isolated from the human anterior pituitary gland and their individual actions are relatively well understood. They are

growth hormone (GH, or somatotrophic hormone, STH)
thyrotrophic hormone (TSH, thyroid-stimulating hormone)
adrenocorticotrophic hormone (ACTH and the related β-lipotrophin)
prolactin (PRL)
follicle-stimulating hormone (FSH)
luteinizing hormone (LH).

The term 'gonadotrophins' combines FSH and LH (from common gonadotrophs), and also placental 'human' chorionic gonadotrophin (hCG). TSH and the gonadotrophins are structurally similar glycoproteins.

There is no human melanotrophin (MSH) independent of ACTH, and no separate MSH-regulating factors. The function of the related lipotrophins and endorphins is unclarified.

The hormones of the anterior pituitary

gland (except GH and PRL) mainly act on other, target, endocrine glands to stimulate the production or release of peripheral hormones. An increase in the plasma concentration of peripheral hormone, whether secreted by the target gland or administered therapeutically, will depress the secretion by the anterior pituitary of the appropriate trophic hormone both directly and by acting on the hypothalamus. Removal of the target gland, or cessation of its secretions, withdraws this negative feedback control of the anterior pituitary and an increased secretion of the trophic hormones results. The secretion of the hormones of the anterior pituitary gland is influenced via its hypothalamic regulating hormones directly and indirectly by the central nervous system, by such factors as stress and trauma, by circadian rhythms

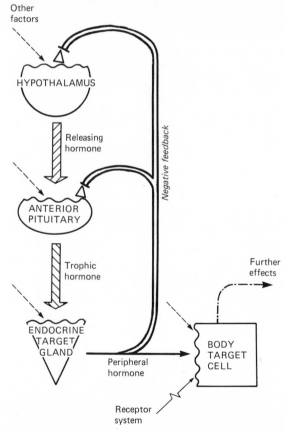

Fig. 17.1 The control of general peripheral hormone secretion by the anterior pituitary gland and the hypothalamus, and the pathways of negative feedback

(p. 15), as well as by the feedback mechanisms of circulating peripheral hormones, and by many drugs (Fig. 17.1). The anterior pituitary hormones themselves also have a direct negative feedback effect on the hypothalamus.

Hypothalamic regulating hormones

A number of peptide hormones secreted by the hypothalamus have been identified and chemically characterized, their actions on the anterior pituitary elucidated, and assay methods are being developed. At present these are

growth hormone-releasing factor (GHRH, specific for GH)
growth hormone-inhibiting hormone (GHRIH or somatostatin, with multiple other inhibitory actions on gastrointestinal hormones, and also on TSH)
thyrotrophin-releasing hormone (TRH, acts on TSH and PRL)
corticotrophin-releasing hormone (CRH, specific for ACTH)
prolactin-inhibiting factors (PIF/mainly dopamine)
gonadotrophin-releasing hormone (GnRH or LHRH, acts on FSH and LH).

In pharmacy these are sometimes called '-relins', e.g. GnRH is gonadorelin.

Endocrine disorders due to direct hypothalamic abnormality

Overactivity

Precocious puberty, in either sex, may be caused by premature hypothalamic stimulation of the pituitary, which causes release of gonadotrophins to give plasma values within the adult reference range. This may sometimes be due to pressure on the hypothalamus by a pineal tumour, or to its independent effects.

One cause of Cushing's syndrome is a block of feedback in the hypothalamus and pituitary with consequent excess CRH and ACTH secretion (p. 209).

Underactivity

There may be selective failure of GHRH, TRH, CRH or GnRH, with consequent deficiency of the appropriate pituitary secretion, and of the activity of the target organ.

General disorders of the anterior pituitary gland

Overactivity of the anterior pituitary need not involve all its hormones; a tumour usually causes excessive secretion of only one hormone and may depress secretion of other hormones. Underactivity of the anterior pituitary may involve all hormones, or be partial as an isolated hormone deficiency. Although it is possible to perform a combined pituitary function test, for example combining the effects of insulin (p. 214), TRH (p. 200), and GnRH (p. 221), individual tests are usually indicated.

Panhypopituitarism

When anterior pituitary activity is diminished the secretion of GH, PRL, and gonadotrophins are lost first, and the patient presents with symptoms of failure of lactation, amenorrhoea, and loss of sexual hair before any other symptoms of hypopituitarism develop. The typical initial biochemical abnormality is the low gonadotrophins, with an impaired response to GnRH and a low plasma oestradiol or testerosterone. Later TSH secretion, and then ACTH secretion, are impaired. This pattern, when seen after postpartum haemorrhage, is often called Sheehan's syndrome; it may also be due to local non-endocrine lesions or injury. Carbohydrate metabolism is usually unaltered and the patient is relatively well.

Anorexia nervosa endocrinologically resembles Sheehan's syndrome. It is a psychogenic disorder and the patient suffers from depressed hypothalamic function and from malnutrition with associated biochemical changes – a rise in LDL-cholesterol may be marked, and hypokalaemia is common. Secretion of gonadotrophins is depressed early, leading to amenorrhoea.

Changes in thyroid and adrenocortical hormones are variable: there can be hypoglycaemia which leads to increased GH secretion.

Single hormone deficiencies

Growth hormone deficiency leads to dwarfism.

Pituitary myxoedema, pituitary Addison's disease, or pituitary amenorrhoea/eunuchoidism, may also occur. These terms imply that there is defective pituitary secretion specifically of TSH, or of ACTH, or of gonadotrophins, but that there is no general pituitary deficiency or primary disease of the thyroid, adrenal cortex, or gonads. These diseases are rare, and must be distinguished from mild general hypopituitarism in which perhaps the particular target organ (thyroid, adrenal cortex, or gonads) responds less readily to stimulation by its trophic hormone.

Growth hormone

Secretion of GH is controlled by its releasing hormone, and also by a non-specific inhibiting hormone, somatostatin. GH acts mainly via GH-induced circulating polypeptides from the liver, somatomedin (insulin-like growth factors), which affect tissues to promote nitrogen retention and growth. It has diabetogenic and anti-insulin actions. Normally the fasting plasma GH level (reference range <10 mIU/l) falls to less than 5 mIU/l after glucose, and rises (due to hypoglycaemia) after insulin.

Pituitary dwarfism

This rare condition is due to decreased activity of somatotroph cells, from many causes. There is usually a destructive lesion, and other manifestations of hypopituitarism are present, though there may be pure GH deficiency. The plasma GH may be low, and does not rise after insulin-induced hypoglycaemia used as a provocative test. Tests for other pituitary hormone deficiencies should also be made. The

biochemical effects are increased tolerance to glucose and increased sensitivity to insulin.

Acromegaly

This results from excessive secretion of GH, caused by a somatotroph adenoma, or less usually by carcinoma or hyperplasia. It is rare in children, before the epiphyses have closed, and then leads to gigantism.

For diagnosis the fasting plasma GH level is usually raised, and this is not suppressed by an oral glucose load. The most marked effect is a stimulation of growth of bone and cartilage, but internal organs may also be enlarged. There is demineralization of the skeleton; the plasma calcium is normal with a high urinary calcium, but the plasma phosphate is usually raised. During the active phase there may be a goitre but not necessarily hyperthyroidism. Occasionally lactation is present, with a high serum PRL. Patients with acromegaly may develop diabetes.

Late destruction of gonadotrophs by the tumour diminishes gonadotrophin secretion and causes loss of sexual functions; if the disease stabilizes there is generalized hypopituitarism but GH remains high. Tests for other pituitary hormones should then be made.

Prolactin

In the control of PRL secretion its inhbitory factors (PIF) are more important than stimulation by releasing hormone. PRL initiates and maintains lactation in breasts prepared by oestrogens and progestogens. Its secretion, stimulated by suckling, also inhibits ovulation.

Prolactinoma is the commonest form of pituitary tumour. The resulting hyperprolactinaemia, which can be measured, is associated with diminished secretion of FSH and LH if amenorrhoea and infertility are presenting symptoms (p. 219), and there may be galactorrhoea.

Other causes of hyperprolactinaemia include hypothalamic disease, and drugs (e.g. methyldopa) that inhibit the secretion or action or dopamine. These produce galactorrhoea and amenorrhoea.

The neurohypophysis

The two principal hormones secreted by the hypothalamus, and stored in the posterior pituitary, are the related peptides antidiuretic hormone and oxytocin.

Antidiuretic hormone (ADH; arginine vasopressin)

This acts on the kidneys to promote distal tubular reabsorption of water and a concentrated urine: in pharmacological doses it causes peripheral vasoconstriction. The vasopressive actions of ADH on smooth muscle will not be considered further. The posterior lobe of the pituitary acts as a store for ADH, whence it is released in response to water deprivation. This is principally due to the effects of the increased plasma osmolality on hypothalamic receptors, but thirst and a fall in blood volume play a part.

Antidiuretic hormone deficiencies and related syndromes

Cranial (neurogenic) diabetes insipidus
This results from deficient secretion of ADH, of many pathological causes, and the patient suffers from polyuria (4–20 l/24 h) of low osmolality (<150 mmol/kg), and polydipsia in response to increased thirst. This polyuria of diabetes insipidus causes only slightly increased plasma osmolality unless drinking is restricted, when it may be dangerous. A diagnostic test combines first water restriction for 8 h under close supervision (which does not increase urine osmolality to more than 50 per cent above plasma osmolality, in contrast to the change in healthy subjects); then ADH (or analogue) administration (which raises urine osmolality by more than 750 mmol/kg). Although plasma ADH is low, this assay is a research procedure and is rarely required.

Nephrogenic diabetes insipidus
This results from severe chronic renal disease, secondary tubular damage (e.g. from myelomatosis), and specific ADH receptor defect which may be familial or due to drugs (e.g. lithium). The polyuria and low urine osmolality do not respond to ADH.

Solute-induced diuresis must be excluded in differential diagnosis.

Psychogenic polydipsia
This relatively common condition produces a fall in plasma and urine osmolality. The polyuria may exceed 20 l/24 h, and responds to water deprivation. Urinary concentrating ability may be temporarily impaired.

Essential hypernatraemia
This rare condition is due to failure of ADH response to osmotic stress, usually caused by intracranial tumour or head injury affecting the hypothalamus. Thirst is impaired.

Inappropriate secretion
'Non-endocrine' tumours, particularly those of the bronchus, may 'ectopically' synthesize, and produce a *S*yndrome of *I*nappropriate secretion of *ADH*. A 'non-ectopic' SIADH may also be seen after brain damage and in lung disease. There is high urine osmolality, water retention (and gain of weight) with a low plasma osmolality, and low concentrations of all plasma components from haemodilution with slowly developing hyponatraemia symptoms (p. 27). Although plasma sodium concentration may be very low, total body sodium content is normal.

The differential diagnosis is from hyponatraemia of sodium loss, often caused by diuretics; in this, other plasma concentrations are normal, ECF volume may be low, and prerenal uraemia may develop: urinary osmolality may be less than that of plasma.

Oxytocin

This causes contraction of uterine muscle

when this is under the influence of oestrogens, and produces ejection of milk during suckling. It also has some antidiuretic activity. Oxytocin abnormalities are not measured.

Further reading

Hockaday TDR. Assessment of pituitary function. *Br Med J* 1983; **287**: 1738–9.

Ney L, ed. Investigation of endocrine disorders. *Clin Endocrinol Metab* 1985; **14**: (no. 1).

18

The Thyroid Gland

Objectives

In this chapter the reader is able to

- revise the pathways of thyroid hormone metabolism, and their control
- revise the actions of the thyroid hormones
- study the biochemical changes in the principal abnormalities of the thyroid gland.

At the conclusion of this chapter the reader is able to

- understand the principles of thyroid function tests
- use the laboratory in the investigation of suspected disorders of thyroid function.

Control by higher centres

Secretion of TSH is controlled by TRH (p. 193). TSH acts on the thyroid gland to promote the release and synthesis of the thyroid hormones, whilst anatomically it causes hypertrophy and hyperplasia of the thyroid cells. There are thyroid-stimulating IgG immunoglobulins (thyroid plasma membrane receptor antibodies), whose production and relation to hyperthyroidism, exophthalmos, and the mucopolysaccharide deposition of pretibial myxoedema are not fully elucidated, and will not be discussed further here.

Free thyroxine and tri-iodothyronine (the thyroid hormones), by acting on the anterior pituitary, partly control the secretion of TSH as a negative feedback control by opposing the action of TRH. Dopamine (p. 193) also inhibits TSH secretion.

Iodine

The minimum daily requirement of iodine in adults is about 100 µg, the normal intake in Britain being about 200 µg. Iodine circulates as iodide, and is concentrated in certain secretions (e.g. saliva, milk, gastrointestinal) as well as in the thyroid, and is excreted in the urine. A small amount of organic iodine is lost in the bile. A deficiency of iodine in the diet or drinking water, which occurs in certain inland mountainous areas, causes a simple goitre: the mild deficiency of thyroxine synthesis leads to increased TSH secretion and anatomical as well as physiological stimulation of the thyroid. Cretinism results when there is gross iodine deficiency in infancy, because of inadequate thyroid hormone production for brain development. Iodine-deficiency goitre can be prevented by the addition of sodium iodide to table salt (sodium chloride) in the proportion of 1/10 000.

When iodine is given for the treatment of thyrotoxicosis it acts principally by inhibiting the action of TSH, possibly by reducing the sensitivity of the thyroid cells to this hormone, and also inhibits hormone release. Reduced secretion of thyroxine results, and this inhibition reaches its maximum in 10 to 14 days but is short-lived.

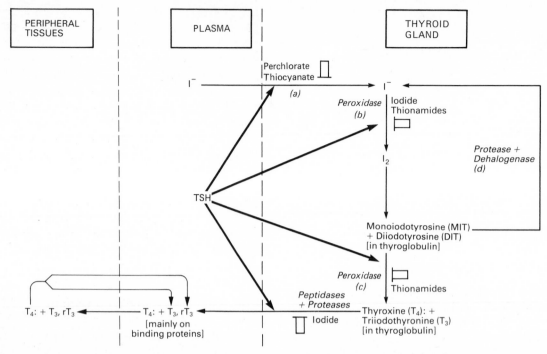

Fig. 18.1   The main pathways of thyroid hormone biosynthesis and control. The probable sites of action of antithyroid drugs are indicated (inhibition shown as □), and the locations of the commoner genetic enzyme defects shown as (a), (b), (c), (d)

Hormone synthesis in the thyroid gland

This may be summarized and simplified (Fig. 18.1).

1 The acinar cells remove iodide from the plasma at a rate which is controlled by the plasma/gland iodide gradient (normally about 1:20), and by TSH activity.
2 Iodide is oxidized to iodine.
3 The iodine is immediately taken up by a tyrosine residue of an intracellular protein (thyroglobulin) to produce mono- and di-iodotyrosine globulin – this forms the colloid.
4 Two iodinated tyrosine molecules condense to form thyroxine (T_4) and tri-iodothyronine (T_3), which remain part of the peptide chain of thyroglobulin: those which are not condensed are dehalogenated, and almost all the iodine is recycled.
5 Thyroglobulin is hydrolysed by lysosomes, and thyroid hormones (mainly thyroxine) are released into the circulation. Traces of thyroglobulin are also released into the plasma.

Antithyroid drugs

The thionamides (e.g. carbimazole) act principally by restricting the oxidation and coupling of iodide to tyrosine in the thyroid gland, and diminish the synthesis of thyroid hormones. The secretion of TSH then increases because of diminution of circulating thyroxine, and hypertrophy and hyperplasia of the thyroid results. Thiocyanates and perchlorates, on the other hand, act competitively to diminish iodide uptake by the thyroid.

Propranolol and related drugs act on peripheral receptors, not on the thyroid gland, but inhibit the peripheral effects of thyroid hormones by blocking conversion of T_4 to T_3.

Thyroid hormones

Figure 18.2 shows the structures of the compounds that are important in thyroid metabolism, and there are other derivatives.

3,5,3'-Tri-iodothyronine (T_3) is more po-

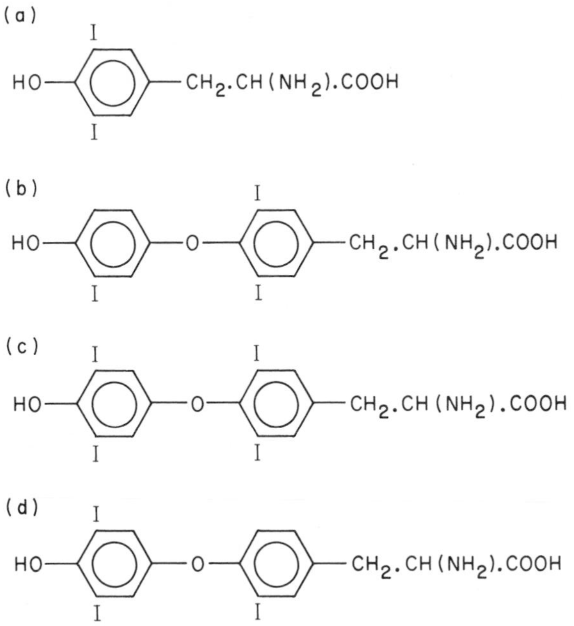

(a)

(b)

(c)

(d)

Fig. 18.2 Structures of the thyroid compounds: (a) diiodotyrosine, (b) 3,5,3′-tri-iodothyronine (T_3); (c) thyroxine (T_4); (d) reverse-T_3 (rT_3)

tent than thyroxine (T_4) in effects on peripheral cell metabolism, though probably less effective in its feedback effect on TSH secretion: it has a shorter half-life. The relative importance of these two hormones in affecting cell metabolism, and to what extent T_4 is a prohormone only active after peripheral conversion to T_3, are uncertain. About 0.02 per cent of the thyroxine in plasma is active and in the free state; the remainder is bound to a T_4- and T_3-binding α-globulin (TBG), to prealbumin, and also to albumin; tri-iodothyronine, also bound to plasma proteins, is about 0.3 per cent free.

T_3 and its inactive alternative reverse-T_3 (rT_3) are normally produced about equally from peripheral (mainly hepatic) deiodination of T_4; in malnutrition, after trauma, or in chronic disease there is a shift from T_3 to rT_3 production, possibly to reduce overall catabolism. Drugs that induce hepatic enzyme synthesis, such as phenytoin, cause increased conversion to T_4 to T_3, and plasma T_4 concentration therefore falls.

The principal biochemical action of the thyroid hormones is calorigenesis with acceleration of tissue oxidation, and there is general stimulation of all metabolic processes. In physiological concentrations they are protein anabolic, but in excess they are inhibitors of protein synthesis and protein-catabolic, causing a negative nitrogen balance, and stimulating breakdown of muscle creatinine to creatine. T_4 and T_3 are to a certain extent anti-insulin and diabetogenic for they stimulate gluconeogenesis, but the abnormal glucose tolerance test curve (lag storage or diabetic) found in thyrotoxicosis is principally due to rapid absorption of carbohydrate from the intestine. The thyroid hormones lower the plasma concentration of cholesterol and to a lesser extent the lipoproteins. They directly stimulate the breakdown of bone leading to decalcification and loss of matrix. The cardiovascular system, and some aspects of the autonomic nervous system, are sensitized to the action of catecholamines.

Calcitonin, from the parafollicular (C) cells, is unrelated to the other thyroid activities (p. 177).

The assessment of thyroid function

There are three complementary approaches: measurement of circulating thyroid or pituitary hormones, of thyroidal metabolism of iodine, and of secondary effects of thyroid hormones. No tests are universally reliable or applicable.

Thyroid hormones in plasma

Total plasma hormone
Protein-bound iodine (PBI), no longer used, includes all thyroid hormones and metabolites, and also contaminating organic iodine such as intravenous X-ray contrast media.

The most widely used investigation is total plasma thyroxine (reference range 60–130 nmol/l). Assay of total T_3 is less precise (reference range 2–3 nmol/l). In hyperthyroidism total T_4 is usually above 160 nmol/l and in hypothyroidism is less than 50 nmol/l.

Free thyroid hormones

Assay of *true* free T_4 or T_3 is possible for research by a dialysis method.

Clinical (analogue) free T_4 analyses are done by a radioimmunoassay method (usual reference range 9–23 pmol/l); true results are not found in certain disorders of binding proteins or in the presence of antibodies to thyroid hormones, but these analogue values are otherwise useful. Typical values in hyperthyroidism are above 30 pmol/l, and in hypothyroidism below 5 pmol/l.

Free thyroxine index

This is a widely used but indirect procedure for determining the unsaturated binding capacity of TBG for thyroid hormones. It involves mixing serum (or plasma), a resin, and $[^{125}I]$ T_3. If plasma thyroxine is high (with a normal thyroxine-binding globulin, as in thyrotoxicosis), then the $[^{125}I]$ T_3 cannot be taken up by the plasma because the binding sites on TBG are saturated. It therefore is absorbed on to the resin where the high uptake can be measured. Conversely, the resin uptake is low in hypothyroidism because binding sites are unoccupied.

Changes in thyroxine binding

With normal thyroid function and free T_4 concentration, the nephrotic syndrome lowers thyroxine-binding globulin by urinary loss, and cirrhosis by reducing protein synthesis, and produce a low plasma thyroxine and a high resin uptake; protein malnutrition may also reduce thyroxine-binding globulin. Excess oestrogens (particularly in pregnancy and from the contraceptive pill) increase thyroxine-binding globulin and produce a high plasma total T_4 and T_3 and a low resin uptake. Salicylates displace thyroxine from binding-globulin, usually leading to increased resin uptake and initially to increased free hormone concentrations, though equilibrium is soon restored.

Using resin uptake, it is possible to express plasma thyroxine corrected for changes in protein-binding – i.e. 'free'. The usual measure is free thyroxine index (FTI) (reference range 50–140). If it is suspected that there is a change in total T_4, but not in free T_4, then free thyroxine index is a useful measurement if free T_4 is not available.

Thyroxine-binding globulin

This can be measured directly. Its assay is useful for suspected disorders of binding-proteins, or in combination with total plasma thyroxine as an alternative to the indirect (resin) procedures for unsaturated binding capacity.

Thyroglobulin

An increase in plasma thyroglobulin is not related to increased hormone production, but reflects leakage from benign or malignant tumours, or radiation thyroiditis. The assay is occasionally used to test for recurrence of malignancy after surgery.

Pituitary hormone

Alteration of thyroid function is always associated with alteration of TSH secretion, either primary or by feedback.

The usual, less sensitive, assay for TSH is most valuable in the diagnosis of hypothyroidism, where a raised level is the most reliable early indication. This is particularly important in neonatal hypothyroidism (p. 202).

Recently-introduced *sensitive* methods are able to distinguish between low and normal values (reference range 0.5–5.0 mU/l). In hyperthyroidism, plasma 'sensitive' TSH is <0.2 mU/l. The assay of plasma TSH can distinguish between pituitary hypothyroidism, in which plasma TSH is low (0.2–0.5 mU/l), and primary hypothyroidism, in which it is high at an early stage and may exceed 25 mU/l. The assay is also useful in monitoring replacement therapy with thyroxine.

TRH-stimulation test

A useful test for depression of pituitary thyrotrophic function, when clinical and plasma hormone assessment are borderline, is to measure the response of plasma TSH to intravenous TRH: the procedure, and reference ranges for the responses, vary locally but the following is acceptable.

Method
09:00   Collect 10 ml blood for TSH assay.
Inject i.v. 400 μg TRH.
09:30, 10:00   Collect further blood samples for TSH assay.

Interpretation
In a normal subject the basal value is less than 5 mU/l, the 30-min value 5–30 mU/l, and the 60-min value 2–10 mU/l.

An impaired response is found even in early hyperthyroidism due to the excess circulating thyroxine causing pituitary suppression; a normal response excludes hyperthyroidism. A low response is also found in pituitary (but not hypothalamic) hypothyroidism and in successfully treated hypothyroid patients: primary hypothyroidism usually gives an enhanced response.

Tests based on iodine metabolism

All tests of thyroid function which are based on investigation of iodine metabolism in the gland are disturbed by the presence of circulating exogenous iodine. In states of iodine deficiency, radioactive iodine uptake is increased.

Tests using radioactive iodine usually employ ^{131}I: however isotopes with a shorter half-life have great advantages in safety. Technetium, which is also taken up by the thyroid, may also be used as [^{99}Tc^m] pertechnate.

Of the dynamic tests of thyroid function only radioactive iodine uptake (RAIU), usually 24 h after an oral dose, was regularly used before the development of sensitive hormone assays for plasma.

Indirect tests – basal metabolic rate

The basal metabolic rate (BMR) of a patient is the basal energy output, measured as oxygen uptake, compared with that of equivalent healthy subjects. Accurate measurement of the BMR is difficult, and the test, which is non-specific, is now obsolete except for metabolic research.

A raised BMR is typically found in thyrotoxicosis and is proportional to the degree of toxicity. However, anxiety states, and various systemic disorders, also raise the BMR. A low BMR is typically found in hypothyroidism. However, other endocrine deficiencies also lower the BMR.

Unlike the hormone assays and in vivo iodine tests, the BMR takes account of possible altered tissue sensitivity to thyroid hormones.

Other biochemical abnormalities in thyroid disease

The plasma cholesterol concentration is occasionally lowered in thyrotoxicosis, but this is of no value in diagnosis. A raised plasma cholesterol is usually found in hypothyroidism, and the value is proportional to the severity of the disease in an individual patient: this has been used in following the effects of therapy. Phospholipids are similarly altered, and in hypothyroidism there is also carotinaemia. Effects of thyroxine on muscle can be shown by an increase of urinary creatine in thyrotoxicosis; however plasma creatine kinase does not increase. Occasionally increased bone breakdown leads to hypercalcaemia.

Summary of biochemical changes in thyroid disease

Thyrotoxicosis

This term is used for the syndrome produced by an excess of circulating free thyroid hormones, and the clinical features, which include anxiety, tremor, weight loss, sweating and tachycardia, result from an increase both in oxidative metabolism and in sensitivity to catecholamines, though the characteristic exophthalmos is not fully explained. Thyrotoxic crisis is a life-threatening exacerbation with severe hypermetabolism and hyperpyrexia, from a variety of causes but particularly arising after surgery. Most causes of thyrotoxicosis are caused by primary overactivity of the thyroid gland (*hyperthyroidism*), associated with goitre (Graves's disease). Otherwise there may be hyperactive thyroid nodules, or *secondary hyperthyroidism* due to excess secretion of TSH ectopically (p. 233) or from a pituitary tumour. Non-thyroidal thyrotoxicosis, without goitre, is caused by excess intake of thyroid hormone – usually as an aid to slimming (*thyrotoxicosis factitia*).

In typical thyrotoxicosis plasma free and total T_3, and to a lesser degree free and total T_4, are increased. Plasma TSH is decreased, and RAIU increased. Two unusual variants are *T_3-toxicosis*, where an altered pattern of thyroidal hypersecretion leads to excess production only of T_3 so plasma T_4 is unaltered, and *T_4-toxicosis*, where in the presence of severe intercurrent illness hypersecreted T_4 is not converted to excess T_3 but to the inactive rT_3 (p. 199).

In secondary hyperthyroidism there will be an increase in plasma TSH, T_3 and T_4, and in RAIU. In thyrotoxicosis factitia the exogenous thyroid hormone depresses both TSH secretion and RAIU.

A lag storage or diabetic type of glucose tolerance curve, and a low plasma cholesterol may be present, but these findings are insufficiently consistent to be of more than secondary interest. Demineralization of the skeleton, with increased urinary calcium and sometimes hypercalcaemia, is found in severe cases.

Hypothyroidism

This term is used for the syndrome produced by a deficiency of circulating free thyroid hormone; and the clinical features (usually of insidious onset), which include tiredness, apathy, dry skin, weight gain and hypothermia, result from depression of tissue oxidation and sensitivity to catecholamines, though the characteristic myxoedema tissue is not fully explained. Most cases in adults (*primary hypothyroidism*) are caused by a deficiency of active thyroid tissue from many causes – when fully developed called myxoedema. *Secondary hypothyroidism* ('trophoprivic') can result

from deficiency of hypothalamic or pituitary secretion (p. 194). Hypothyroidism may be associated with goitre.

In typical primary hypothyroidism plasma free and total T_4, and to a lesser degree free and total T_3, are decreased. Plasma TSH is increased with an excessive response to TRH stimulation (p. 201), and RAIU decreased. In secondary hypothyroidism however plasma TSH is decreased and the response to TRH is variable depending on the status of the pituitary.

Neonatal hypothyroidism is common and may be difficult to diagnose clinically. When not associated with goitre it is usually due to an anatomical failure of development.

There are also various rare *genetic defects* causing goitre and hypothyroidism which are thought to be due to the enzyme deficiencies shown at (*a*), (*b*), (*c*), or (*d*), in Fig. 18.1. In neonates measurement of serum TSH on the blood sample taken for the Guthrie test for phenylketonuria (p. 89) is probably the best screening test, and a value above 80 mU/l is diagnostic; there is disagreement as to whether thyroxine should also be measured. More detailed hormone studies are needed for the elucidation of enzyme defects, and biochemical analysis of a biopsy may be required.

Endemic goitre is due to dietary iodine deficiency; compensatory hypersecretion of TSH often maintains the euthyroid state by enlarging the gland.

Abnormal findings of secondary interest in hypothyroidism are a high plasma cholesterol and β-lipoproteins. A flat glucose tolerance curve is sometimes found. The urinary corticosteroid excretion is often low: plasma creatine kinase may be high, though the cause is not decided.

Euthyroid syndromes

Sick euthyroid syndrome

In chronic illness, and in malnutrition, there is often impaired synthesis of thyroxine-binding globulin and impaired conversion of T_4 to T_3 with rT_3 being produced instead; plasma free T_4 and TSH are normal, but total T_4 may be low due to a decreased level of binding protein. These are abnormalities of peripheral thyroid hormone metabolism, and thyroid function is normal.

Euthyroid hypothyroxinaemia

In these conditions total plasma T_4 is decreased due to diminished binding to available thyroxine-binding globulin. This is usually either from overall protein depletion, a genetic abnormality of TBG, or if drugs interfere with binding. Plasma free T_4 remains unaltered.

Euthyroid hyperthyroxinaemia

In these conditions total plasma T_4 is increased (with a normal free T_4) due to increased binding to available thyroxine-binding proteins. This is usually from increased thyroxine-binding globulins in hyperoestrogenaemia (p. 217). A high total T_4 can be caused by alteration of thyroid-hormone metabolism by propranolol or amiodarone. There are also rare disorders of binding protein such as familial dysalbuminaemic hyperthyroxinaemia, where clinical free T_4 is raised but true free T_4 is normal (p. 200) with a normal TSH.

Choice and order of tests in suspected thyrotoxicosis or hypothyroidism

For efficiency and economy a large number

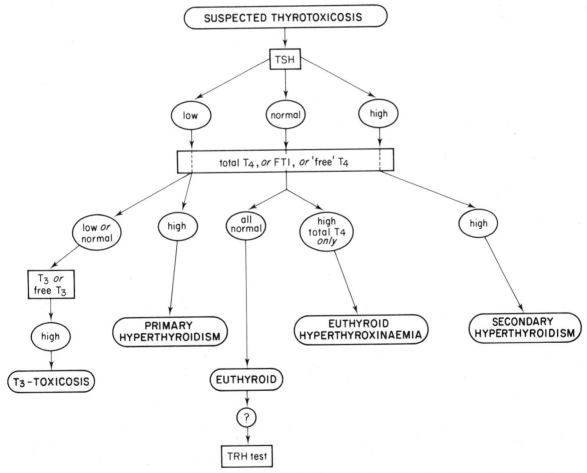

Scheme 18.1 Typical findings shown by plasma hormone analysis, supplementing clinical evidence, in the investigation of suspected thyrotoxicosis in an adult, and using 'sensitive' TSH as the initial test. The further tests are described in the text. Tests marked ⑦ are to be considered if evidence is contradictory

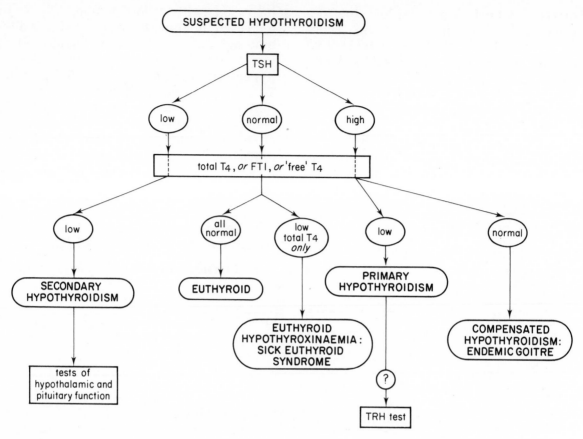

Scheme 18.2   Typical findings shown by plasma hormone analysis, supplementing clinical evidence in the investigation of suspected hypothyroidism in an adult, and using 'sensitive' TSH as the initial test. The further tests are described in the text. Tests marked ⑦ are to be considered if evidence is contradictory

of complex tests should not be carried out if a few simple ones will suffice, but the choice also depends on the facilities of the laboratory.

For thyrotoxicosis (Scheme 18.1)

(a) Plasma sensitive TSH if available;
(b) plasma total T_4 if test (a) is abnormal or doubtful, and in all cases if test (a) is not done. If TSH is raised with an increased T_4, this suggests secondary hyperthyroidism;
(c) free T_4 or equivalent (e.g. FTI) in doubtful cases, especially when protein-binding may be altered: some laboratories do this as an alternative to total T_4;
(d) if T_3-toxicosis is suspected, then plasma total T_3;
(e) in assessment of therapy no laboratory test is ideal, though plasma T_4 and T_3 may be helpful.

For hypothyroidism (Scheme 18.2)

(a) Plasma TSH;
(b) plasma total T_4 as in thyrotoxicosis;
(c) free T_4 or FTI as in thyrotoxicosis;
(d) a TRH-stimulation test may be useful for suspected secondary hypothyroidism;
(e) in assessment of therapy plasma TSH is generally useful.

Further reading

John R. Screening for congenital hypothyroid-ism. *Ann Clin Biochem* 1987; **24**: 1–12.

Khir ASM. Suspected thyrotoxicosis. *Br Med J* 1985; **290**: 916–21.

Mardell RJ, Gamlen TR. *Thyroid function tests in clinical practice*. Bristol: John Wright and Sons, 1983.

Pearce CJ, Byfield PGH. Free thyroid hormone assays and thyroid function. *Ann Clin Biochem* 1986; **23**: 230–7.

19

The Adrenal Glands

Objectives

In this chapter the reader is able to

- revise the pathways of adrenocortical hormone metabolism and their control
- revise the physiology of glucocorticoid and mineralocorticoid hormone activity
- study the biochemical changes in the principal abnormalities of adrenocortical function
- study catecholamine metabolism.

At the conclusion of the chapter the reader is able to

- understand the principles of adrenal function tests
- use the laboratory in the investigation of suspected disorders of adrenocortical function
- use the laboratory in the investigation of phaeochromocytoma.

Control by higher centres

The chemistry of the corticotrophin group of hormones is complex; the related lipotrophins, endorphins, and enkephalins will not be discussed further in this book. Secretion of ACTH is controlled by CRH, with feedback from the level of circulating plasma cortisol. ACTH acts on the adrenal cortex to produce hyperplasia, and to promote the uptake of cholesterol (probably from LDL) and its conversion to pregnenolone and progesterone, and thus stimulates the formation of the glucocorticoids and adrenal androgens. There is a combined circadian and pulsatile (episodic) rhythm of ACTH secretion. ACTH also has a slight melanophore-expanding activity because the ACTH polypeptide contains the active amino acid sequence of melanophore-stimulating hormone activity. Extra-adrenal actions of ACTH are unimportant physiologically.

As a result of various stimuli, such as injury, infections, or operations (mediated neurologically and by interleukin 1, p. 232); or exercise; or acute mental stress or attacks of depression, the secretion of ACTH by the anterior pituitary gland is increased due to excess production of CRH which overrides the negative feedback control. This ACTH secretion promotes an increased output of adrenal glucocorticoids: if the external stimulus is long continued, exhaustion of the adrenal cortex occurs and resistance to further noxious stimuli is lowered.

Hormones of the adrenal cortex

Two main types of hormone, corticosteroids and androgens, are synthesized in and secreted by the adrenal cortex (Fig. 19.1); it also normally secretes a small quantity of oestrogens and progestogens.

Corticosteroids

The principal corticosteroids secreted by the human adrenal cortex are aldosterone (from the zona glomerulosa), cortisol (in pharmacy often called hydrocortisone, from the zona fasciculata), and corticosterone (from both layers). Cortisol is synthesized from progesterone by the action of successive hydroxylases (steroid mono-

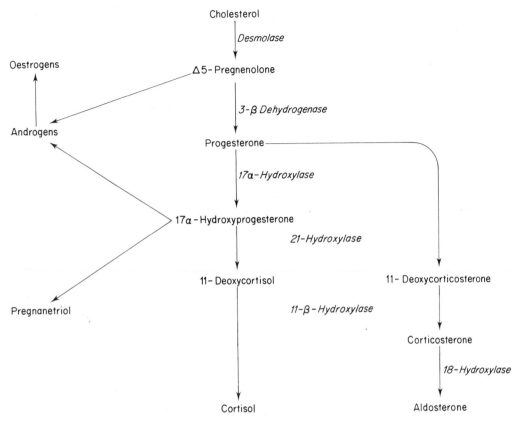

Fig. 19.1 The principal steps in the synthesis of the hormones of the adrenal cortex

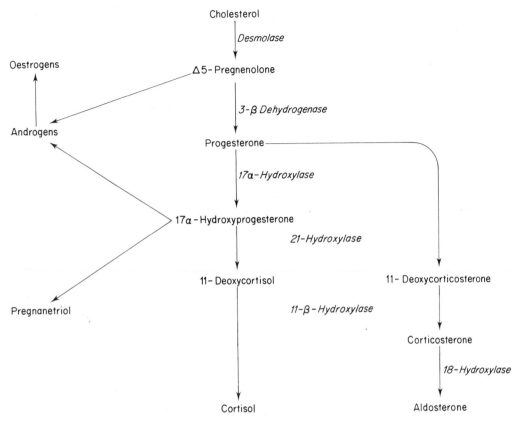

Fig. 19.2 Structures of the corticosteroids: (a) corticosterone; (b) cortisone; (c) cortisol (hydrocortisone); (d) aldosterone

oxygenases), and aldosterone by a different pathway via corticosterone: cortisone is a synthetic product. Their structures are shown in Fig. 19.2.

Aldosterone is very potent, and is secreted in small amounts, about 0.5 μmol/24 h: the normal secretion of cortisol is about 70 μmol/24 h.

Mineralocorticoid activity

The major mineralocorticoid functions of the adrenal are performed by aldosterone: particularly by an action on the distal renal tubules (and to a lesser extent on the small intestine, and salivary and sweat glands) which promotes sodium reabsorption and potassium exchange. The result is retention of sodium, chloride, and secondarily of water; and loss of potassium.

The final stages of the secretion of aldosterone are not under primary ACTH control. Renin is produced in the juxta-glomerular cells of the kidney (p. 117) by a feedback mechanism principally responding to volume changes of the extracellular fluid that affect renal perfusion pressure.

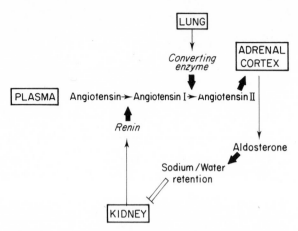

Fig. 19.3   The renin–angiotensin–aldosterone system

Renin, which is a proteolytic enzyme, produces the decapeptide angiotensin I from a circulating α_2-glycoprotein angiotensinogen, and the peptidase angiotensin converting enzyme, principally in the lung, transforms it to the active octapeptide angiotensin II, which stimulates synthesis and release of aldosterone (Fig. 19.3). Angiotensin II is also vasopressive, whilst the minor angiotensin III only promotes aldosterone synthesis. Sodium or water depletion promotes aldosterone secretion, and vice versa, by affecting the production of renin. In addition a high plasma potassium directly increases aldosterone synthesis, and vice versa.

Cortisol and corticosterone have some mineralocorticoid activity.

Natriuretic hormones

The group of related peptides known as atrial natriuretic factor (ANF) has potent diuretic, natriuretic, and vasorelaxing properties. It blocks renin and angiotensin secretion, and also opposes the sodium-retaining action of aldosterone. ANF is released into the plasma from specific granules in response to expansion of blood volume; it may function as a natriuretic hormone in man under physiological conditions. At present assays of ANF are not used in the investigation of patients.

Glucocorticoid activity

The main glucocorticoid functions of the adrenal are performed by cortisol, supplemented by corticosterone. They stimulate gluconeogenesis from protein by mobilizing amino acids, and decrease carbohydrate utilization, but promote glycogen deposition in the liver: insulin sensitivity is decreased. In excess they cause fat deposition and are protein catabolizers, breaking down protein to carbohydrate, and causing a negative nitrogen balance, though physiological amounts may be protein anabolic. They help in the maintenance of the glomerular filtration rate and of the normal blood pressure.

Cortisol, but not corticosterone, is anti-inflammatory and immunosuppressive, and depresses the number of circulating eosinophils, basophils, and lymphocytes.

The secretion of the glucocorticoids is stimulated by ACTH. The very slight glucocorticoid activity of aldosterone has no significance at physiological concentrations.

Androgens

Their secretion in the zona reticularis of the adrenal glands is stimulated by ACTH, possibly with PRL synergism: the principal compound is dehydro*epi*androsterone. Adrenal secretion is normally only weakly androgenic and protein anabolic.

The adrenal androgens and oestrogens act as promoters of growth of hormone-dependent carcinoma of the prostate and breast respectively, the latter having a high content of oestrogen and progesterone receptors (p. 217) – for prostatic carcinoma the receptor situation is uncertain. The rationale of adrenalectomy, when performed (in combination with gonadectomy) as palliative treatment of these tumours, is the removal of the 'controlling' hormonal background. Hypophysectomy is performed for the same purpose, and the rationale here is principally the removal of ACTH, the gonadotrophins, and GH.

Adrenocortical hormones in plasma and urine

Cortisol is the principal glucocorticoid in the plasma. About 5 per cent of it is active and circulates in the free state, the remainder being bound to a relatively specific cortisol-binding β-globulin (CBG, transcortin), and also to albumin. The plasma concentration of CBG, therefore of bound and of total cortisol, is increased by endogenous and exogenous oestrogens – particularly in pregnancy and from hormonal contraceptives. Plasma cortisol is usually estimated specifically by competitive protein binding. There is a marked circadian variation which masks irregular fluctuations due to secretory pulses of ACTH – reference ranges for plasma cortisol at midnight are 50–280 nmol/l, and at 09:00 are 200–700 nmol/l.

The glucocorticoids are excreted in the urine principally in reduced forms, conjugated with glucuronic acid. Methods can measure urinary cortisol and its metabolites ('corticosteroids', but including pregnanetriol) as 17-oxogenic steroids; the alternative measurement of Porter–Silber reacting 17-hydroxycorticosteroids gives similar results except in cases of biochemical disorders of adrenal hormone synthesis. More specific methods for urinary free cortisol, whose excretion follows the plasma free cortisol, have largely replaced these assays – reference range <250 nmol/24 h.

Estimation of plasma aldosterone is by radioimmunoassay (the patient should be on a normal Na/K diet), and urinary assay is possible.

The plasma cortisol level reflects mainly adrenocortical secretion of cortisol at the time of venepuncture, or recent exogenous cortisol administration. The 24 h urinary excretion represents integration of the circadian variation, but is affected by renal failure or altered hepatic metabolism. Misleading results are sometimes found in metabolic disorders of the adrenal cortex when unusual derivatives are excreted and measured as hydroxycorticosteroids. These values are therefore in general increased when there is increased ACTH secretion, or hyperplasia or tumour of the adrenal cortex, and decreased when there is decreased ACTH secretion, or damage to the adrenal cortex.

Plasma ACTH may be measured by radioimmunoassay, and a cytochemical method of bioassay is being developed as a research procedure. This is a direct measure of pituitary or ectopic hormone production in diagnostically difficult cases, and may distinguish between primary and secondary adrenocortical deficiency or excess.

Adrenocortical hyperactivity

Oversecretion of adrenal cortical hormones may arise from hyperplasia or tumour of the adrenal cortex, and may be secondary to increased ACTH secretion. The symptomatology depends on the nature of the cortical hormones which are secreted in excess.

Cushing's syndrome

This is characterized by an increased circulating free cortisol concentration.

High ACTH
This is usually caused by excess secretion of ACTH by an overactive anterior pituitary, with abolition of the circadian rhythm. The relative responsibility of a primary corticotroph adenoma, or of primary impairment of the feedback cycle at the hypothalamus with consequent continual excessive secretion of CRH and ACTH, is controversial. The syndrome is sometimes present in chronic alcoholics, probably due to 'stress' stimulation of hypothalamic CRH. There may also be extrapituitary ectopic secretion of an adrenocorticotrophic hormone by a 'non-endocrine' tumour, such as carcinoma of the bronchus (p. 233). Prolonged therapeutic use of ACTH may also be responsible.

Low ACTH
The syndrome may less commonly be caused by an adrenal tumour that secretes excess cortisol, with consequent suppres-

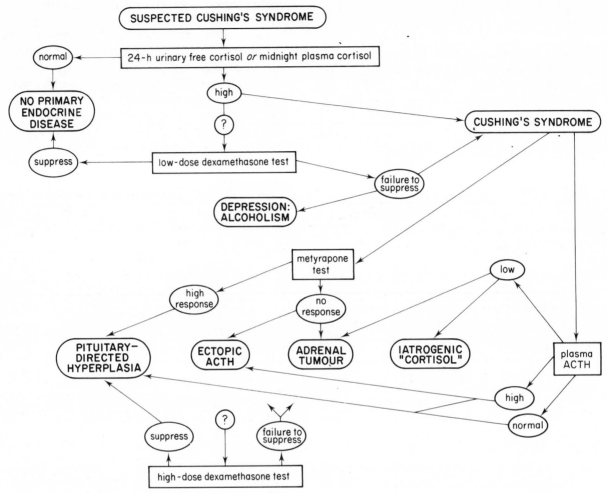

Scheme 19.1   Typical findings shown by biochemical hormone analysis, supplementing clinical and imaging evidence, in the investigation of suspected Cushing's syndrome. Tests marked ⑦ are to be considered if evidence is contradictory

sion of ACTH secretion: there may be autonomous adenoma, or carcinoma. Excessive and prolonged treatment with cortisol or a synthetic analogue is a common cause of Cushing's syndrome.

Insulin-resistant diabetes and glycosuria result from effects on carbohydrate metabolism; cessation of growth, muscular wasting, osteoporosis (with loss of skeletal calcium and hypercalciuria) and atrophy of collagen leading to the characteristic striae, from effects on protein metabolism; increased body fat, with a moon-face and buffalo-hump and hypertriglyceridaemia from effects on lipid metabolism. A mild hypokalaemic alkalosis, and sodium and water retention, from effects on electrolyte metabolism, are found. Hypertension, polycythaemia, lymphopenia, and eosinopenia, usually occur: there is a tendency to infection. Adrenal androgen secretion is usually little altered (except in adrenocortical carcinoma); hence in women virilism is rare though hirsutism may be seen. Psychotic symptoms are common.

The plasma cortisol is high, with early abolition of the circadian rhythm which first raises the midnight level even with a normal morning level. Urine free cortisol, representing integrated plasma free cortisol values, is typically above 300 nmol/24 h. There is failure to suppress on low-dose dexamethasone (p. 211).

Should biochemical tests be required for differential diagnosis, it is often necessary to use more than one investigation (Scheme 19.1). The plasma ACTH value (best taken at 09:00) depends on the aetiology of the syndrome, being low when the syndrome is due to primary adrenocortical disease or to iatrogenic corticosteroids, and is otherwise high–normal or raised. The metyrapone test (p. 214) is probably more reliable than the high-dose dexamethasone test (p. 213) in differentiating between hyperplasia and tumour. Tests have been developed that involve measuring the response to CRH infusion, but their place is undecided.

An important differential diagnosis is from the common *pseudo-Cushing's disease* of obesity, with depression, hypertension, and often diabetes. It is likely that increased disposal of cortisol leads to excess secretion, maintaining a normal plasma cortisol but with increased urinary corticosteroids which are not suppressed by dexamethasone.

Congenital adrenal hyperplasia (adrenogenital syndrome)

These inborn errors of metabolism are due to excess secretion of androgens and present usually as virilism. They are caused by a metabolic block (Fig. 19.1) in the synthesis of adrenocortical steroids from cholesterol, and the deficiency of circulating cortisol or corticosterone (generally low–normal) results in excess ACTH secretion by removal of feedback inhibition. The excess ACTH stimulates adrenal hyperplasia and the production of androgens along other pathways. Diagnosis depends on demonstration of high amounts in plasma of the steroid immediately before the block and of its metabolites, and sometimes also in urine. In borderline cases stimulation with ACTH may be needed to demonstrate an abnormality.

The commonest variety is 21-hydroxylase deficiency. The accumulation behind the block of progesterone and 17-hydroxyprogesterone (diagnostically raised in plasma) leads to excess androgen production, and to a high urinary excretion of pregnanediol and pregnanetriol. There is sodium loss, and the cortisol deficiency may lead to neonatal hypoglycaemia. Assay of 17-hydroxyprogesterone on the Guthrie test blood spot (p. 89) has been proposed for neonatal screening; the assay on second trimester amniotic fluid has been suggested for screening at-risk families.

The second commonest variety of the syndrome has a block at 11-hydroxylation, and also shows hypertension, possibly due to the mineralocorticoid effect of the excess 11-deoxycortisol and 11-deoxycorticosterone produced.

There are many other varieties. When aldosterone deficiency predominates, particularly in 18-hydroxylase deficiency, the patients are primarily salt-losers with pseudo-Addison's disease.

Tumours

Benign or malignant tumours of the adrenal cortex usually give rise to a syndrome with mixed metabolic and virilizing (or feminizing) aspects, either of which may predominate: ACTH secretion is depressed. In general, benign tumours produce one hormone (but are often non-secreting), and malignant tumours can produce multiple hormones. Adrenal tumours often give rise to excess 3β-compounds such as dehydro*epi*androsterone.

Primary aldosteronism (Conn's syndrome)

These are rare tumours of the adrenal cortex (or sometimes bilateral hyperplasia) which produce only excess aldosterone and cause primary aldosteronism – *inappropriate secretion*. This is characterized by hypokalaemia and a urine potassium above 30 mmol/24-h (and muscular weakness), alkalosis, hypertension, polyuria, and usually sodium retention. There is often a diabetic glucose tolerance curve associated with the potassium deficiency. Renin secretion is suppressed. The diagnosis can be confirmed biochemically, when the patient is on a standard Na/K intake, by showing a high plasma and urinary aldosterone concentration, or a high aldosterone secretion rate, with a low plasma renin activity.

Complex tests may be helpful in the differential diagnosis of borderline cases of hypertension with hypokalaemia. For example, sodium loading by intravenous infusion of saline suppresses plasma aldosterone in patients without primary endocrine disturbance, but not in primary aldosteronism.

Secondary aldosteronism

This common condition will be found in conditions where there is loss of sodium from the extracellular fluid with a fall in plasma volume, such as nephrotic syndrome, cirrhosis and ascites, congestive heart failure, and due to many diuretics. In these conditions hypokalaemia and alkalosis are rare, and plasma renin and aldosterone are increased – this is *appropriate secretion*, and hormone assay is not required.

Adrenocortical hypoactivity

Chronic secondary hyposecretion of adrenal cortical hormones may result from hypopituitarism; other features of hypopituitarism are then usually present, but aldosterone secretion is retained so sodium and potassium balance are then little altered. Specific ACTH deficiency often follows prolonged or excessive treatment with corticosteroids.

Addison's disease

This is a primary lesion of the adrenal gland due to destructive or atrophic disease (and also affecting the medulla), in former times commonly tuberculous, but now usually autoimmune in origin when plasma antibodies against adrenocortical cells can usually be demonstrated, or due to metastatic deposits. The symptoms that develop are due to deficiency of all adrenocortical hormones. There is salt depletion due to excess urinary sodium and chloride loss

with water depletion, and potassium retention. Plasma electrolyte changes are a sign of the loss of adrenal functional reserve. A low renal plasma flow and reduced perfusion are caused by the sodium deficiency and hypotension, and this leads to an early increase in plasma urea. Mild hypercalcaemia, with a normal ionized fraction, is common. Loss of weight, weakness, hypotension, and gastrointestinal disturbances, regularly occur. Increased glucose utilization and decreased gluconeogenesis lead to hypoglycaemia (p. 58) in severe cases: there is a flat glucose tolerance curve, and hypersensitivity to insulin. There is secretion of excess ACTH: this stimulates the adrenal remnant, and causes the characteristic pigmentation because of the associated melanocyte-stimulating action.

Though in severe cases adrenocortical hormones will be undetectable, whilst adrenal hyperplasia (p. 211). It may be a and urinary corticosteroids may only be low–normal, and a tetracosactrin stimulation test may be needed.

Hypoaldosteronism

The commonest causes are Addison's disease and certain varieties of congenital adrenal hyperplasia (p. 211). It may be a feature of chronic renal disease, perhaps due to failure of renin production.

Acute adrenal insufficiency

This may develop in Addison's disease or after adrenal haemorrhage, and sometimes in meningococcal or similar septicaemia. In an Addisonian crisis the metabolic features of Addison's disease are severe, in particular hyponatraemia and hypotension with a high plasma urea, dehydration and metabolic acidosis, hyperkalaemia and total body potassium deficiency, and hypoglycaemia.

It is not uncommon for long-term corticosteroid therapy markedly to suppress the secretion of ACTH. These patients, who show mild adrenocortical deficiency after cessation of treatment, may develop acute adrenal insufficiency when cortisol requirements are increased by stress e.g. by severe infection, trauma and surgery, or parturition.

Stimulation and suppression tests for adrenocorticoid function

Although measurement of baseline plasma or urinary cortisol will often be diagnostic in cases of overt disease of the anterior pituitary–adrenocortical axis, further information can be obtained from appropriate stimulation or suppression tests in doubtful cases.

Short tetracosactrin tests

The standard rapid procedure is to measure the plasma cortisol response to synthetic corticotrophin polypeptide, tetracosactrin.

Method
A midnight sample may be collected for studies of the circadian rhythm.

09:00   Collect 10 ml heparinized blood for cortisol assay (baseline). Inject intramuscularly 250 μg tetracosactrin.
09:30   Collect blood for cortisol assay.

Interpretation
In a normal subject, the baseline value is more than 200 nmol/l, and there is an increase of at least 300 nmol/l over the baseline, usually at 30 min. In Addison's disease there is a low baseline and a response to tetracosactrin of less than 150 nmol/l, and in hypopituitarism (including from exogenous suppression) there may be a subnormal rise at 30 min. In Cushing's syndrome (hyperplasia) there may be an exaggerated response; an autonomous adrenal tumour generally gives no response.

Prolonged tetracosactrin test

This gives a greater stimulus than does the short test, and is useful in doubtful cases and especially in checking function after long-term steroid therapy. All hormonal treatment must be discontinued from at least three days before the control period until the end of the test.

Method
First test day:
09:00   Collect 10 ml heparinized blood for cortisol assay (baseline).
        Inject intramuscularly 1 mg depot tetracosactrin (an alternative protocol gives 0.25 mg of tetracosactrin intravenously over 6 h).

Second and third test days:
        Repeat the blood collections and the stimulant injections.

Interpretation
In a normal adult there is a rise in plasma cortisol on the first day to above 1400 nmol/l. In Addison's disease there is no rise even after three days, whereas in adrenocortical hypofunction secondary to pituitary deficiency the value may exceed 700 nmol/l after the third injection.

Dexamethasone suppression tests

Dexamethasone is a synthetic steroid that inhibits ACTH secretion, and suppresses the plasma and urinary corticosteroids in normal subjects. The test can be used to differentiate hyperadrenocorticism from dubious normals (p. 211), and may be used to differentiate adrenal hyperplasia from tumour.

Method

(i)   Collect 24 h urine samples for baseline corticosteroid estimation for 2 days (days 1 and 2)
(ii)   collect blood samples for baseline cortisol estimation at 09:00 on days 1 and 2
(iii)   dexamethasone is given 6-hourly in 0.5 mg oral doses for 8 doses (low dose test: days 3 and 4) followed by 2.0 mg oral doses 6-hourly for 8 doses (high dose test: days 5 and 6)
(iv)   24-h urine samples are collected for corticosteroid estimation while on dexamethasone (days 3, 4, 5, and 6)
(v)   blood samples for cortisol are collected preceding the dexamethasone dose on days 4, 5, 6, and 7.

Interpretation

In a normal subject the urine and plasma corticosteroids are suppressed on the lower dosage below 50 per cent of the baseline values. On the lower doses of dexamethasone, patients with Cushing's syndrome will show no suppression irrespective of cause. On the higher dose, those with hyperplasia (of hypothalamic–pituitary origin) have suppression of 50 per cent or more, while those with either adenoma or carcinoma, or ectopic ACTH production, are unaffected; however, there is considerable overlap in the responses of the different categories. Patients with hypercortisolism associated with endogenous depression may also fail to suppress.

A useful screening test is to give 1 mg of dexamethasone at 23:00, and measure plasma cortisol at 08:00. A normal subject will suppress below 150 nmol/l, whilst this remains above 600 nmol/l in Cushing's syndrome.

Metyrapone test

Metyrapone inhibits the action of the enzyme 11β-hydroxylase in the adrenal cortex (Fig. 19.1), thus reducing cortisol (and corticosterone) synthesis. This triggers the feedback mechanism, causing CRF and ACTH secretion. The result is excess adrenocortical secretion of the precursor 11-deoxycortisol, which is measured in plasma, or as a urinary corticosteroid. The test is used for investigating hypothalamic or anterior pituitary deficiency if plasma ACTH assays are not available, or to supplement them, or to differentiate between adrenal hyperplasia and tumour. It is essential to know that the adrenals are competent to respond to ACTH.

Method

(i)   Collect 24h urine samples for baseline corticosteroid estimation for 2 days (days 1 and 2)
(ii) metyrapone is given 4-hourly in 750 mg oral doses for 6 doses (day 3)
(iii) collect 24 h urine samples for corticosteroid estimation on day of, and after metyrapone administration (days 3 and 4). A plasma sample may be collected 4 h after the last dose.

Interpretation

A normal subject shows an increase in urine corticosteroid values of at least 35 μmol/24 h, or at least a twofold increase above the resting level. Plasma 11-deoxycortisol normally increases to above 250 nmol/l. A sub-normal response, in the presence of known normal adrenocortical function, shows deficiency at the level of the hypothalamus or anterior pituitary.

In addition, in pituitary Cushing's syndrome, there is often an exaggerated rise in corticosteroids, whilst patients with autonomous adrenocortical or ectopic tumours fail to show a response.

Other tests

These are used mainly in special circumstances to test for hypothalamic–pituitary responsiveness. They involve the use of either insulin-induced hypoglycaemia or pyrogen as stress agents to the hypothalamus via higher centres, or of lysine–vasopressin or other synthetic corticotrophin-releasing factor to stimulate the anterior pituitary.

Adrenal medulla

This secretes, from chromaffin cells, adrenaline and also some noradrenaline. The manifold pharmacological properties of these hormones and their secretion in the nervous system will not be discussed further here.

Catecholamine-producing tumours

An endocrine tumour of the adrenal medulla (phaeochromocytoma, usually benign), or rarely of chromaffin tissue elsewhere (paraganglioma), produces noradrenaline and adrenaline in excess. This leads to progressive sustained or

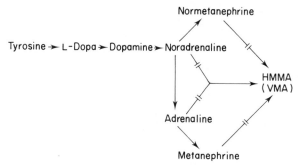

Fig. 19.4   The metabolism of the catecholamines

paroxysmal hypertension, and paroxysms of headache and sweating. There is often increased glycogenolysis with mild impairment of glucose tolerance with hyperglycaemia and glycosuria, and a low plasma insulin. Similar tumours arising mainly in the sympathetic nervous system (neuroblastoma) produce primarily excess dopamine and noradrenaline.

A major end-product of catecholamine metabolism (Fig. 19.4) is vanilmandelic acid (VMA: preferably called HMMA, 4-hydroxy-3-methoxymandelic acid) which is excreted in the urine, and this is measured, if necessary on several occasions, in the investigation of paroxysmal hypertension. Urinary HMMA is normally less than 35 μmol/24 h, whereas in phaeochromocytoma values above 550 μmol/24 h are found in at least one specimen on repeated testing. The patients must be off treatment with drugs, especially monoamine oxidase inhibitors (and vanilla, e.g. in bananas and coffee) for 48 h beforehand. Similar measurement of total urinary metadrenalines (i.e. the metabolic intermediates metanephrine and normetanephrine, normally less than 5 μmol/24 h) is of diagnostic value in doubtful cases. Estimation of the plasma concentrations of adrenaline and noradrenaline or urinary excretion of free catecholamines is difficult. This may be necessary for differential diagnosis of tumours, preferably during a paroxysmal crisis, or for localization of tumours by selective venous sampling.

Further reading

Besser GM, ed. The pituitary-adrenal axis. *Clin Endocrinol Metab* 1985; **14** (no. 4).

Bravo EL, Gifford RE. Phaeochromocytoma: diagnosis, localization and management. *N Engl J Med* 1984; **311**: 1298–1303.

Drury PL. Disorders of mineralocorticoids in investigations of endocrine disorders. *Clin Endocrinol Metab* 1985; **14**: 175–202.

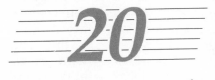

The Gonads

Objectives

In this chapter the reader is able to

- revise the pathways of the metabolism of the sex hormones (ovarian, placental, and testicular) and their control
- revise the biochemical changes related to menstruation, pregnancy, and drugs – especially the contraceptive pill.

At the conclusion of this chapter the reader is able to

- use laboratory tests for the diagnosis of pregnancy
- investigate the integrity of the feto-placental unit in suspected abnormal pregnancy
- use biochemical tests for prenatal diagnosis of fetal disorders
- understand the causes of hirsutism and virilism and investigate a suspected case
- understand the causes of, and be able to investigate, amenorrhoea and infertility of likely hormonal origin.

Control by higher centres

Hypothalamic control of secretion of the pituitary gonadotrophins, FSH and LH, by their specific releasing-hormone is influenced by higher centres and by feedback from circulating oestrogens and androgens.

The specific effects of FSH and LH are on the gonads, and secondarily due to the actions of the sex hormones whose production they stimulate.

Female sex hormones

Oestrogens

The three principal oestrogens are oestradiol, oestrone, and oestriol – oestradiol being the most potent. A steroid ring is not necessary for oestrogenic activity, as shown by the original synthetic oestrogen, stilboestrol. Their structures are shown in Fig. 20.1. Apart from their actions on the sexual organs and activities, the oestrogens are protein anabolizers and have been recommended for the secondary prevention of postmenopausal oesteoporosis (p. 186): they also increase the plasma concentrations of hormone- and metal-binding proteins. They also have a slight sodium and water-retaining activity. By increasing plasma VLDL they act to increase total triglycerides.

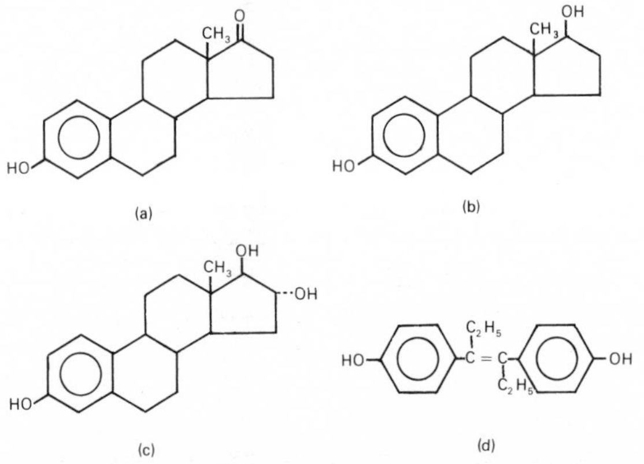

Fig. 20.1 Structures of the oestrogens: (a) oestrone, (b) oestradiol, (c) oestriol, (d) stilboestrol

There is a plasma sex hormone-binding globulin (SHBG), with limited affinity for oestradiol. Oestradiol also binds to albumin, and 2 per cent remains unbound in plasma.

Oestrogens are used for the treatment of carcinoma of the prostate: prostatic growth is maintained by androgens, and oestrogens depress the pituitary production of gonadotrophins, thus reducing in males the secretion of androgens. Oestrogens in large doses have a limited value in the treatment of postmenopausal carcinoma of the breast with metastases, but about half the cases of premenopausal carcinoma of the breast are clinically hormone-dependent, i.e. their growth is stimulated by oestrogens. The continued presence in malignant breast tissue of oestrogen-receptors, and also of progesterone-receptors (as are present in normal breast tissue) is a valuable indication of likely respond to removal of hormone stimulation by surgery or antioestrogen drugs. This may also indicate general freedom from recurrence, and likely response to chemotherapy. Their assay is still a research procedure. About two-thirds of breast carcinoma patients have positive oestrogen-receptors, and two-thirds of these respond – whereas few negatives respond.

Excess oestrogen production takes place in occasional tumours of the ovary, testis, or adrenal cortex.

Oestrogen assays
In plasma it is now usual to assay total oestradiol, or oestriol. Oestrogens are excreted in the urine principally after conjugation with glucuronic acid in the liver, and in cirrhosis there is therefore increased excretion of free oestrogens, with diminished conjugation. Total urinary oestrogen excretion is being replaced by separate estimation of the individual oestrogens, usually oestriol, as required.

Progesterone

The estimation of progesterone in plasma has replaced laboratory assay of the

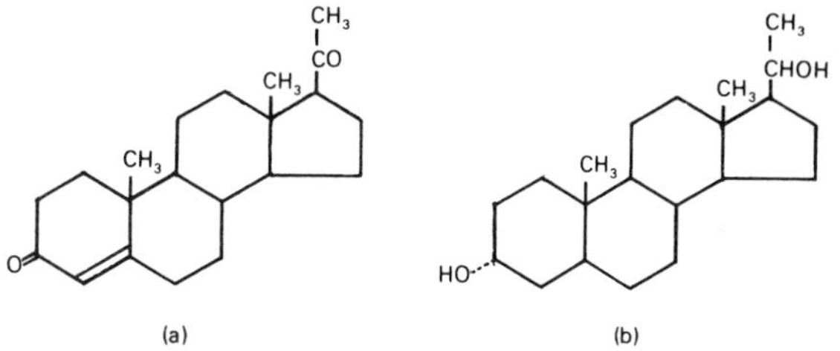

Fig. 20.2 Structures of the progestogens: (a) progesterone, (b) pregnanediol

inactive urinary excretion product, pregnanediol (glucuronide). Their structures are shown in Fig. 20.2. About 5 per cent of plasma progesterone is free, the remainder being bound to cortisol-binding globulin.

Hormonal contraceptives

The most frequently administered sex hormones are the oral hormonal contraceptives (the Pill), which may be a mixture of an oestrogen and a progestogen, or the latter alone, and have a complex mode of action. Effects in some healthy women on normal biochemical patterns are rarely found with contraceptives made up from progestogen alone, or low in oestrogen. By increasing the specific binding proteins, oestrogens cause raised plasma levels of thyroxine (p. 200), cortisol (p. 209), iron, and copper (p. 146); the free fractions are unaltered. There may be diminished glucose tolerance ('steroid diabetes') due to progestogen, and also an increase in plasma free fatty acids. An increase in plasma triglycerides, and to a lesser extent in cholesterol, may be clinically significant where there is pre-existing hyperlipidaemia.

Menstrual cycle (Fig. 20.3)

Just before the beginning of the menstrual cycle hypothalamic stimulation of the anterior pituitary causes release of FSH, and the ovum matures. Just before midcycle there is a peak of ovarian oestrogen secretion (*follicular phase*) with depression of FSH secretion: a surge of GnRH secretion stimulates the midcycle peak of LH, combined with a second shorter FSH peak,

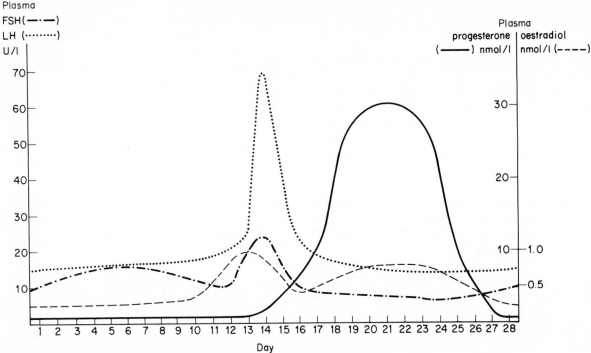

Fig. 20.3   Plasma hormones during an average normal menstrual cycle

and ovulation occurs. Serial measurement of plasma or urine LH can be used to assess the timing of this ovulatory phase, particularly in the management of infertility, though some workers prefer plasma oestradiol. Kits are now available for home-testing of daily urine samples to detect the LH surge.

The follicle ripens to form the corpus luteum. This secretes progesterone, there is a second oestrogen surge, and these peak about 8 days after ovulation. Serial measurement of plasma (or salivary) progesterone may be used to check on the adequacy of this *luteal phase*: a home-testing kit is now available for this purpose that detects the increase in urinary pregnanediol glucuronide.

The progesterone secretion depresses LH production, the corpus luteum ceases to function, the oestrogen and progesterone fall, and there is menstrual bleeding. The final fall in oestrogen is responsible for triggering the hypothalamus to restart the cycle by initiating the release of FSH.

Pregnancy

If fertilization occurs the regular alternation of hormone secretion is altered, and the placenta becomes the principal endocrine organ. It secretes a 'human' chorionic gonadotrophin (hCG) which has similar properties to LH, other hypothalamic and pituitary–trophin-like hormones, and pregnancy-specific proteins. The amounts produced (except for hCG) are proportional to the mass of healthy trophoblasts: the reference ranges, after allowing for gestational age, are very broad. The pituitary itself secretes excess PRL.

Progesterone secretion by the corpus luteum initially increases, but after the third month of gestation this is taken over by the placenta. Cholesterol is converted in the fetal adrenal to dehydro*epi*androsterone, which the placenta converts to oestradiol and other oestrogens: in pregnancy many steroids are produced by such two-organ metabolic processes. In the last month urinary oestrogen excretion, mainly oestriol, rises to 30–50 μmol/24 h.

Biochemical changes

Other changes in normal pregnancy are often secondary to the hormonal changes. The increased plasma concentrations of metals and hormones are caused by binding to transport globulin synthesized in excess, as for the Pill (p. 217). Plasma triglycerides and cholesterol increase significantly. Changes in fluid distribution increase the glomerular filtration rate, and lower the plasma urea and creatinine. Plasma albumin and total protein often fall. Placental synthesis of a specific isoenzyme may double the total plasma alkaline phosphatase activity. Glycosuria may be from a temporary hormonal impairment of glucose tolerance or a lowered renal threshold, and lactosuria (p. 62) is often present.

In *pre-eclampsia*, hypertension is always associated with proteinuria. The plasma urate is usually raised, to a greater extent than urea and creatinine, and the level may be an indication for induction of labour; plasma (hepatic) transaminases are often increased. The mechanisms are uncertain.

Pregnancy diagnosis tests

All present methods for the laboratory diagnosis of pregnancy depend on detection of the increased production and urinary excretion (or plasma concentration) of hCG that occurs in early pregnancy. The classical biological tests depended on the stimulation of the sex glands of a test animal by hCG, and have now been replaced by immunological tests; however, new bioassays using receptors or cytochemistry are being developed.

Widely used commercial immunoassays, with easily visible endpoints based on agglutination, have variable sensitivity, but most give a positive reaction with about 1500 iu of hCG/litre of urine, and are not quantitative. The increased production of hCG in pregnancy may be detectable by such tests on an early morning urine at about 10 days after the first missed period. It rises to a peak from about the 50th to 70th days of gestation, has fallen off by the 120th day, and changes little until delivery. It is always negative one week after delivery, and negative results may be found even in the third trimester. Of the placental products, hCG is unique in peaking in early pregnancy. If the urine of a patient who is thought to be in early pregnancy gives a negative result the test should be repeated one week later. Occasional false positives, due to cross-reaction with LH, are found at the menopause or in amenorrhoea due to ovarian failure. Contamination of urine with blood cells or bacteria may also give a false positive reaction.

Sensitive tests using monoclonal antibodies, which detect 50 iu per litre, are now available: these can give a positive reaction within 10 days of gestation. They are used for suspected ectopic pregnancy which may produce insufficient hCG for a positive result with the standard test, or for early detection of normal pregnancy, and are available in modified form (with a colour endpoint) for self-testing at home. Tests of higher sensitivity will detect pregnancy even earlier, but false positives may then be found, as may positive tests before 'occult abortion'.

Hydatidiform mole, choriocarcinoma, or testicular teratoma contain chorionic tissue, produce hCG, and give strongly positive results with standard 'pregnancy diagnosis tests'; if this is due to the placental tumours there is a rising titre after delivery. The important monitoring of patients for progress and response to treatment (p. 233) is done by a quantitative immunoassay using antibodies to β-hCG: the test may detect 1 mg of residual tumour, more than a year after initial treatment.

Tests for other placental products, e.g. the non-hormonal trophoblastic SP_1 (pregnancy-specific β_1-glycoprotein), have been developed: they can be useful for the diagnosis of pregnancy if the patient is being treated with hCG.

Assessment of fetal and placental integrity

Failure of oestrogen secretion to increase in

late pregnancy (32 to 38 weeks) reflects the integrity of the fetoplacental unit, and may indicate retardation of fetal growth and possibly imminent fetal death, or placental insufficiency e.g. pre-eclamptic toxaemia. The results of isolated assays of plasma oestriol (preferred to urinary oestriol) are of little value because of the wide reference range; a falling titre over a week is serious. Another similar test for placental insufficiency that has been popular involves plasma assays of human placental lactogen (hPL).

However a normal result of a biochemical test does not guarantee a healthy pregnancy, and vice versa. Many workers now consider that these tests add nothing to clinical and imaging assessments such as ultrasound.

Prenatal diagnosis
Further biochemical tests that may be useful in prenatal diagnosis of neonatal disease are the measurement in amniotic fluid of bilirubin for the assessment of erythroblastosis (p. 151), of the lecithin/sphingomyelin ratio or similar index for the assessment of the respiratory distress syndrome (hyaline membrane disease) (p. 72), and of (maternal) plasma and amniotic fluid α-fetoprotein (and amniotic fluid acetylcholinesterase: p. 229), for the diagnosis of spina bifida and other neural tube defects (p. 225). A low plasma and amniotic fluid α-fetoprotein are found in Down's syndrome: the best positive screening test may be a combination of low α-fetoprotein, low unbound oestriol, and high hCG in second trimester maternal plasma, related to age. Specialist laboratories can assay enzymes in cultured fibroblasts from amniotic fluid taken at 14 to 16 weeks, and thereby diagnose a number of inborn errors of metabolism, mainly of lysosomal enzymes.

The increasing use of cytogenetic investigations is outside the scope of this book.

Primary ovarian hyperactivity

Various tumours of the ovary of mixed histological and endocrine pattern may be seen; the majority are not endocrinologically active and are often destructive. Tumours producing exclusively, or mainly, oestrogens or androgens are not uncommon. Germ cell tumours may produce hCG or other hormones.

In the *polycystic ovary syndrome* a high production of androgens (which are converted to oestrogens) is associated with secondary amenorrhoea and hirsutism. LH secretion is increased, but FSH is usually normal.

Hirsutism (excess hair in women) may be associated with a slightly raised plasma androgen (testosterone or dehydro*epi* androsterone), possibly of ovarian or occasionally of adrenal origin; with a decreased plasma sex hormone-binding globulin as a secondary and exacerbating effect raising further the plasma free testosterone. However, in many cases of hirsutism, often familial, no abnormality of androgen metabolism can be demonstrated, and alteration of target organ sensitivity has been proposed.

Virilism implies additional other evidence of masculinization, and is associated with androgen-producing ovarian or adrenal tumours, or with congenital adrenal hyperplasia (p. 211).

If a tumour or congenital adrenal hyperplasia has not been revealed, further biochemical investigation of hirsutism or virilism, including hormonal stimulation tests, is usually unhelpful.

Primary ovarian hypoactivity

At menopause and for some time after oestrogen secretion falls, and there is a feedback increased secretion of FSH and LH. Osteoporosis may appear (p. 186).

Turner's syndrome (45,X gonadal dysgenesis) is a combination of primary ovarian agenesis and other congenital abnormalities. Plasma oestrogens are very low, whilst FSH (and also LH) are increased.

There are many other rare chromosomal disorders, and other forms of deficient ovarian development, with similar hormonal patterns.

Investigation of amenorrhoea and infertility

Primary amenorrhoea implies failure or delay in starting menstruation. Biochemical investigation of infertility is relevant to the presence of primary or secondary amenorrhoea, anovulation, or luteal phase dysfunction.

Biochemical causes, with low plasma oestrogens, may occasionally be centred in the hypothalamus or anterior pituitary (p. 194), where in the former FSH and LH are low-normal, and in the latter both secretions are low. More commonly this is of ovarian origin (including Turner's syndrome and similar disorders), and plasma FSH and LH are increased.

Secondary amenorrhoea implies that menstruation has begun, and later ceased. The main classification is as for primary amenorrhoea, but prolactinoma (p. 194) is now realized to be an important pituitary cause, and polycystic ovaries (p. 220: which sometimes lead to primary amenorrhoea) are an important ovarian cause.

Stimulation tests are available in the investigation of amenorrhoea: both to the pituitary with GnRH and measuring changes in FSH and LH, or to the hypothalamus with clomiphene and measuring LH. However, it is doubtful, once primary non-endocrine disorders are eliminated, such as athleticism or malnutrition, whether these add significantly to the information from the clinical pattern or from the static hormone assays of FSH, LH and PRL.

In the investigation and management of infertility where menstruation is taking place, plasma/salivary progesterone is used to check on the luteal phase of the cycle, and plasma LH or oestradiol on the ovulatory phase (p. 218). In the treatment of infertility of presumed hypothalamic origin (e.g. by clomiphene) or of pituitary origin (e.g. by hCG), the ovarian response may then be monitored by daily plasma or urinary oestradiol measurements. LH assays are essential to determine the timing of ovulation for *in vitro* fertilization programmes.

Male sex hormones

FSH promotes spermatogenesis.

LH stimulates the secretion of the androgens from the interstitial cells of the testes. The principal androgen is testosterone, which is converted in target tissues to the more active dihydrotestosterone, and both circulate bound to sex hormone binding globulin and albumin – about 3 per cent is free. Oestradiol is a major metabolic product of testosterone. The androgens have a feedback action at hypothalamic and anterior pituitary levels on the secretion of LH. The actions of the male sex hormones on the sexual organs and activities will not be further described here. Testosterone is a protein anabolizer and when given therapeutically in large doses raises the plasma calcium level. The protein anabolic action of less virilizing analogues may be utilized to promote a positive nitrogen balance and increase muscle mass, as in athletes.

Testosterone and its analogues are sometimes used for the treatment of carcinoma of the breast with bony metastases. Recession of the metastases with diminution of

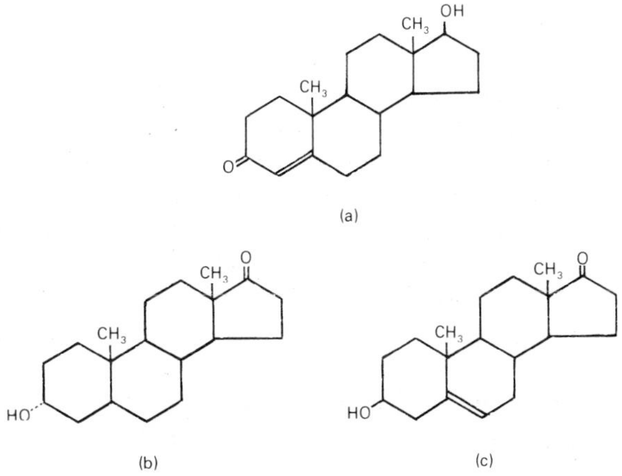

Fig. 20.4 Structures of the androgens:
(a) testosterone, (b) androsterone,
(c) dehydro*epi*androsterone

pain often occurs, but the treatment may have to be stopped because of hypercalcaemia and consequent renal damage.

In the treatment of carcinoma of the prostate the stimulant background of testosterone (p. 217) may be removed by using an analogue, Buserelin, of LH-RH (GnRH, p. 193) which blocks its synthesis.

Testosterone is almost fully metabolized in the body. The urinary excretion products are 17-oxosteroids (the majority of which are derived from adrenal androgens, p. 208) the most important of which is the weakly androgenic androsterone, and oestrogens. The structures of the principal androgens are shown in Fig. 20.4.

Tests of function

About 98 per cent of plasma testosterone is bound to SHBG and to albumin. Plasma testosterone estimation has now largely replaced that of total urinary 17-oxosteroids as a measure of testicular function, whereas dehydro*epi*androsterone (sulphate) represents adrenal androgen secretion. The plasma testosterone response to hCG injection as a stimulation test can be used as an index of Leydig cell reserve. The resting plasma LH is also a marker for testicular function as its secretion is increased by withdrawal of androgen feedback, whilst the LH response to GnRH stimulation can be used to test for relevant pituitary function.

Testicular hyperactivity

Tumours of the testis vary in their histological and endocrine pattern but are usually from the germ cells. Teratoma and chorionepithelioma of the testis produce hCG (and often α-fetoprotein), and the urine of patients suffering from these tumours gives a positive 'pregnancy diagnosis test' at a dilution which may be more than 1/100. For quantitative assay, in the control of treatment, β-hCG assay (p. 219) is used. In these conditions the urinary 17-oxosteroid excretion is generally normal, but interstitial cell tumours give an increased excretion. Seminoma of the testis may produce hCG, or occasionally FSH. There are also rare oestrogen-producing tumours.

Testicular hypoactivity

Delayed puberty is common. Many cases are constitutional, and normal sexual development occurs late. Those with primary gonadotrophin deficiency may not however always show diagnostically low plasma values of FSH and LH even with a low plasma testerostone; primary gonadal failure regularly shows a high plasma FSH and LH.

The full eunuchoid syndrome of impotence, obesity, and muscular wasting (due to loss of the protein anabolizing power of testosterone), may also be due to absence or disease of the testes, or be secondary to pituitary or hypothalamic disease (p. 194). There is a low plasma testosterone, whilst 17-oxosteroid excretion is within normal limits because of continuing adrenal androgen secretion. Measurement of plasma LH, if necessary with stimulation tests, may be used to distinguish between primary and secondary eunuchism. Rarer causes are cellular deficiencies at the receptor or synthesizing stages.

Sub-fertile males with primary testicular deficiency also have a high plasma FSH.

Klinefelter's syndrome (small testes and other abnormalities) corresponds to Turner's syndrome in that an endocrine disorder is due to a chromosome defect (usually XXY).

Gynaecomastia

Pathological gynaecomastia of endocrine origin may be due to deficient testosterone production, increased oestrogens, or both (sometimes secondary to an hCG-producing tumour). The gynaecomastia of liver disease is due to oestrogen excess from non-cleared androgens and other factors, as well as directly to impaired hepatic conjugation and clearance of oestrogens. Oestrogen residues in meat is a known cause. The gynaecomastia of prolactinoma (p. 194) is not due to a direct effect of PRL on the breast, but is probably secondary to suppression of LH secretion leading to low testosterone secretion. Many drugs that produce gynaecomastia act through an endocrine mechanism.

In the investigation of severe gynaeco-mastia of uncertain origin, assay of plasma oestradiol, testosterone (and DHEA), and LH may be helpful.

Further reading

Burger HG, ed. Reproductive endocrinology. In: *Baillière's Clinical Endocrinology and Metabolism*, vol. 1 no. 1. London: Baillière Tindall, 1987.

Chard T. What is happening to placental function tests? *Ann Clin Biochem* 1988; **24**: 435–7.

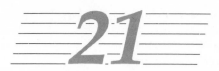

The Nervous System and Muscles

Objectives

In this chapter the reader is able to

- consider the present status of biochemical knowledge of psychiatric disorders
- study the metabolic causes of coma
- study the metabolic causes of secondary mental retardation
- study the biochemical causes of polyneuropathy.

At the conclusion of this chapter the reader is able to

- use biochemical analysis of cerebrospinal fluid in investigation of neurological disease
- investigate biochemically the major neuromuscular and primary skeletal muscle disorders.

Role of laboratory tests

Biochemical changes in the brain, spinal cord, or peripheral nerves have been found in many organic neurological disorders but at present their study is rarely of immediate diagnostic value, though they add greatly to our knowledge of the pathological processes. Nor have biochemical studies in primary psychiatric disorders yet yielded sufficient conclusive information to be an accepted guide to aetiology or diagnosis.

The psychoses

Although certain abnormal biochemical findings are often present in some psychotic disorders, their relation to the aetiology or to the symptoms remains uncertain. With the exception of measurement of plasma drug concentration (e.g. lithium, p. 239) for control of therapy, analysis of blood or other body fluids is at present of no value for diagnosis or management.

Affective disorders

There are indications that changes in the metabolism of the biogenic amines (5-HT, dopamine, noradrenaline) are associated with the affective disorders. Some patients with depression show, as a secondary phenomenon, increased cortisol secretion and diminished suppression with dexamethasone (p. 210): the retention of intracellular sodium that is sometimes found in the depressed phase may be associated with this or directly with altered cell membrane permeability.

Schizophrenia

No unequivocal biochemical changes in brain tissue or body fluids have been demonstrated in schizophrenia. Suggestions of consistent abnormalities of the catecholamine systems, indoleamine systems, or monoamine oxidase activity have not been confirmed.

Secondary psychoses

Psychological symptoms may be present in

a large number of somatic diseases in which there are biochemical changes, although the relation between the specific abnormal chemistry and the symptoms is usually unknown. However, appropriate biochemical investigations in suspected secondary psychoses may reveal such metabolic disorders as severe sodium or potassium depletion (p. 25), magnesium deficiency (p. 189), hypercapnia (p. 41), beri-beri (p. 110), chronic alcoholism (p. 77), pellagra (p. 110), acute porphyria (p. 142), Wilson's disease (p. 147), thyrotoxicosis or hypothyroidism (pp. 201, 202), toxaemia of pregnancy (p. 219), liver failure (p. 160), uraemia (p. 120). Cushing's syndrome (p. 209).

Organic diseases of the central nervous system

The results of analysis of cerebrospinal fluid can often be correlated with certain primary disorders of the central nervous system, but biochemical analyses of blood or urine are, in most such diseases, of little diagnostic or prognostic value.

Specific abnormal findings in different disorders which secondarily affect the nervous system, and where chemical pathology investigation may be helpful, are described under appropriate headings elsewhere in this book. Some of these neurological end-results of biochemical disorders are summarized below.

Coma

This is an end-result of many severe metabolic disturbances such as water depletion (p. 24), hypercapnia (p. 41), uncontrolled diabetes mellitus (p. 55), hypoglycaemia (p. 57), panhypopituitarism (p. 193), myxoedema (p. 202), acute hypercalcaemia (p. 181), liver failure (p. 160), uraemia (p. 120). It is not known whether these very different biochemical abnormalities act through any final common pathway.

Drug coma

This is a separate problem, and is discussed in Chapter 24.

Mental retardation

In some cases this is due to specific biochemical abnormalities, especially inborn errors of metabolism, such as leucine sensitivity (p. 58), galactose or fructose intolerance (p. 58), and other chronic hypoglycaemias (p. 57), many mucopolysaccharidoses and lipidoses (p. 77) phenylketonuria and certain other disorders of amino acid metabolism and organic acidurias (p. 89), lead poisoning (p. 143), hypothyroidism (p. 202), pseudohypoparathyroidism (p. 184), infantile hypercalcaemia (p. 188), kernicterus (p. 157).

Open neural tube defects

These abnormalities result in high concentrations of α-fetoprotein in amniotic fluid, hence in maternal plasma, and of acetylcholinesterase in amniotic fluid: this is important for prenatal diagnosis (p. 220).

Cerebrospinal fluid

Formation and composition

Cerebrospinal fluid (CSF) is secreted into the subarachnoid space, principally through the choroid plexuses, by processes involving active transport: it is not just a plasma ultrafiltrate and the 'blood–brain barrier' is a physiological rather than an anatomical structure. In healthy adults, the rate of production is 100 to 250 ml per 24 h and the total volume of CSF is 100 to 200 ml. CSF is reabsorbed into plasma mainly through the arachnoid villae, and also around the roots of the spinal nerves.

The only chemical components of CSF that are commonly measured are proteins and glucose. Reference ranges in adult lumbar CSF are: total protein 0.15–0.40 g/l, glucose 2.5–4.5 mmol/l; ventricular CSF protein is 0.05–0.10 g/l. As the CSF passes down the spinal cord it tends to equilibrate

Table 21.1

Disease	Protein (g/l)	Glucose (mmol/l)	Cells	Other points
Reference range	0.15–0.40	2.5–4.5	Scanty L (0–4×10^6/l)	Clear
Acute meningitis				
Pyogenic	1.0–10	0–1.5	P+++	Turbid with clot
Tuberculous	0.5–4.0	1.0–2.5	L+P±	Clear with fine clot
Cryptococcal	0.5–3.0	1.0–2.5	L+P±	P± in acute phase
Viral	0.3–1.0	Normal	L++	
Meningism in acute fevers	0.15–0.5	Normal	L+	
Neurosyphilis	0.3–1.0	Normal	L+P±	
Epidemic encephalitis	0.15–1.0	2.5–7.0	L+	
Poliomyelitis				
Pre-paralytic phase	0.15–0.4	Normal	L+P+	
Early paralytic phase	0.4–1.0	Normal	L+	
Multiple sclerosis	0.3–0.8	Normal	L+	Oligoclonal γ-globulin bands
Cerebral tumour	0.15–1.0	1.0–4.0	Normal/L+	Malignant cells sometimes detectable High protein in acoustic neuroma
Spinal block (Froin's syndrome)	0.5–20	Normal	Normal	Opalescent with massive clot: yellow

Cells: L = lymphocytes; P = polymorphonuclears.

to some degree with plasma through the meningeal capillaries. The protein concentration in lumbar CSF is therefore substantially higher than that in ventricular CSF.

A sample of CSF submitted for chemical analysis should, if possible, be fresh and free from blood derived from the tap: after subarachnoid haemorrhage a blood-stained CSF is inevitable. It may be difficult to obtain an absolutely blood-free sample, but if only a small amount of blood is present which is merely sufficient to cause just visible turbidity the analytical findings will not be significantly altered. If the fluid cannot be analysed for glucose within half an hour of withdrawal, then to prevent glycolysis by any cells or bacteria present, the CSF should be put into a bottle which contains sodium fluoride, as for blood glucose. Usually conditions requiring chemical analysis of CSF also require examination of cells, and often microbiological analysis. Local procedures must determine the way such specimens are sent to different laboratories.

Alterations in the chemical content of CSF may not necessarily be caused by disease within the central nervous system, but can be a reflection of changes in the chemistry of the plasma from which the CSF is produced, e.g. in diabetes mellitus hyperglycaemia over the previous 6 h leads to a high CSF glucose concentration, and the converse is seen in hypoglycaemia.

Table 21.1 shows the more important measured changes in the composition of lumbar CSF in disease.

Appearance

Normal CSF is clear, and any colour is usually due to oxyhaemoglobin or to bilirubin. Turbidity in fresh CSF may be due to erythrocytes, leucocytes (usually polymorphonuclear), or bacteria; or occasionally malignant cells. Colour can be seen when the erythrocyte concentrations in the CSF samples exceeds about 50×10^6 cells/l, and opalescence can be seen when the leucocyte concentration exceeds about 200×10^6 cells/l.

If there is blood in the CSF sample that was caused by the lumbar puncture it will disappear from the fluid after a few millilitres have been collected (using three consecutive bottles), and the supernatant fluid will be clear after centrifugation. If there is blood in the CSF that was caused by past haemorrhage, then it will be distributed uniformly throughout the fluid, and the supernatant fluid will usually be pale yellow. The erythrocytes of haemorrhage caused by the puncture have a normal shape; the erythrocytes of a pathological haemorrhage are usually crenated.

Xanthochromia, a yellow coloration in the CSF, can be due either to haemoglobin or to other pigments, usually bilirubin. After haemorrhage the xanthochromia is initially due to oxyhaemoglobin, which is then converted into bilirubin: the oxyhaemoglobin lasts for about 10 days. Bilirubin can be detected in CSF about 6 h after the haemorrhage, and reaches a maximum concentration 3 to 7 days later (by which time the erythrocytes have usually disappeared) and is no longer detectable after three weeks.

Both (unconjugated) bilirubin and conjugated bilirubin pass across into the CSF when the permeability of the blood–brain barrier is altered, or when there is a high plasma bilirubin. A high CSF bilirubin is found for example in chronic cholestatic jaundice and in neonatal jaundice. In premature infants there is increased permeability of the blood–brain barrier.

Carotenoids pass from the plasma into the CSF when the permeability of the blood–brain barrier is altered. The term *'Froin's syndrome'* is given to the yellow fluid of high protein concentration which coagulates spontaneously, and that can be withdrawn from below a spinal block; the xanthochromia results from capillary haemorrhage.

Protein

The total concentration of protein in CSF is usually measured by turbidimetry or colorimetry. Electrophoretic analysis shows that albumin is the main protein, that prealbumin is present in higher concentration than in plasma, and transferrin is present. About 10 per cent of the protein is γ-globulin, whilst higher molecular weight proteins such as lipoproteins and IgM are present in very low concentration. During the first month of life the total CSF protein concentration may be as high as 0.8 g/l, and there is a higher proportion of γ-globulin.

About 80 per cent of protein in normal CSF is derived from plasma, and the rest is from cells in the CNS.

Changes in disease

An increase in CSF protein may be to

(a) increased permeability of the blood–brain barrier

Generally increased permeability is usually caused by meningitis, most commonly acute bacterial meningitis, with a cellular response; by other causes of non-infective meningeal inflammation, including connective tissue disorders, and by metabolic disorders such as uraemia, with no cellular response. Locally increased permeability is responsible in the Guillain-Barré syndrome and other inflammatory conditions of spinal nerve roots. A cerebral tumour may be responsible, depending on its site in relation to the subarachnoid space – acoustic neuroma regularly gives high values. A spinal block is a special case where localized increased permeability and stasis allow equilibration so that the protein concentration may approach plasma values (Froin's syndrome).

(b) increased intrathecal synthesis

Excess B lymphocytes in nervous tissue, and possibly in the CSF itself, secrete excess immune globulins, usually IgG, in a number of local infective and immunologically mediated disorders.

Because CSF is derived from plasma, the CSF proteins will also alter following marked changes in the plasma proteins, as in myelomatosis.

Globulins

Simple qualitative chemical tests for excess CSF globulin (e.g. Pandy reaction using phenol) are mainly sensitive to γ-globulins;

normal CSF gives negative reactions. The Lange test, which involves mixing serial dilutions of CSF with a colloidal gold sol, reflects the albumin/globulin ratio and was mainly used in the investigation of neurosyphilis and multiple sclerosis. Both of these have been replaced by qualitative and quantitative estimation of immunoglobulins, but the Pandy test is still useful in primary hospitals in developing countries.

Local production of IgG occurs in infections, neoplasia, sarcoid, and systemic lupus (when these affect the central nervous system), in the Guillain-Barré syndrome, subacute sclerosing panencephalitis, and particularly in multiple sclerosis. In the last two conditions there is little increase in vascular permeability and the IgG is oligoclonal (p. 102).

Measurement of CSF IgG is the most widely used method of detecting local production. Because this is reflected by the plasma level, this should also be measured. In addition, the plasma/CSF albumin ratio may be used as an indication of increased vascular permeability which would also affect CSF IgG levels. Such measurements will detect 75 per cent of cases. Oligoclonal IgG appears as distinct bands on gel electrophoresis of CSF, and this discriminating test (though sometimes positive in the Guillain-Barré syndrome and chronic meningoencephalitis) detects some 90 per cent of cases of multiple sclerosis: it is particularly valuable in the early stages with equivocal clinical features.

Myelin basic protein

This protein is derived from myelin sheath. An increase may be detected in acute exacerbations of multiple sclerosis, and in many other conditions, including trauma, where nervous tissue is damaged. The clinical value of the assay in plasma or CSF is uncertain.

Fibrinogen

Normal CSF does not form a fibrin clot on standing. When there has been haemorrhage into the CSF, or if the total CSF protein is above 2 g/l from infection or increased vascular permeability, there is usually sufficient fibrinogen present to produce a clot. A delicate slowly developing coagulum, the 'spider-web' clot, is often seen in the CSF of acute tuberculous meningitis, but may occur in other severe infections.

Glucose

The glucose content of CSF may be estimated precisely by any technique used for plasma glucose estimation.

The concentration of glucose in the CSF largely depends on the plasma glucose, and normally stays at about 60 per cent of its concentration in the plasma because of incomplete penetration of the blood–brain barrier. The CSF glucose changes more slowly than the plasma glucose. If the blood–brain barrier is damaged due to inflammation, or to cranial injury, it becomes more permeable to glucose, and the CSF glucose approaches the plasma level. Infection of the meninges (except viral), with excess of polymorphonuclear leucocytes in the CSF, lowers the glucose level because the leucocytes, and also many types of bacteria, are glycolytic. In acute bacterial meningitis the CSF glucose is very low, whereas in tuberculous meningitis the decrease is less and may be used as an index of the activity of the infection. Presence of malignant (including leukaemic) cells also lowers the CSF glucose. CSF glucose estimation is not usually necessary for the diagnosis of bacterial meningitis: sufficient bacteria or leucocytes to lower the glucose will themselves be detectable microscopically. A low CSF glucose in the absence of such excess cells suggests hypoglycaemia, so plasma glucose should be measured at the same time.

Rhinorrhoea of unknown origin can be tested for glucose. If it is present, the rhinorrhoea is principally CSF; if glucose is absent, then the rhinorrhoea is principally nasal secretions.

Other investigations

Of the major ions of body fluids, only chloride was ever regularly measured in CSF but this reflects either changes in the plasma chloride, or in CSF protein by the Donnan equilibrium.

No other biochemical investigations on CSF are currently used for diagnosis or management.

Peripheral nerves

Polyneuropathy

A wide variety of metabolic disorders, with known specific biochemical abnormalities, may have consequent symptoms and signs of generalized polyneuritis. This may be evident in diabetes mellitus (p. 55), chronic alcoholism (p. 77), thiamine deficiency (p. 110), organophosphorus poisoning, pernicious anaemia (p. 143), lead poisoning (p. 143), acute porphyria (p. 142), and from many other disorders.

Neuromuscular junction and acetylcholinesterase

Suxamethonium apnoea

The succinylcholine derivatives that inhibit the neuronal enzyme acetylcholinesterase, and are used in anaesthesia as muscle relaxants, are normally rapidly destroyed by the cholinesterase present in plasma. Some patients have been found to have prolonged respiratory paralysis after use of a muscle relaxant such as suxamethonium (succinyldicholine), and this is usually due to an inborn error of metabolism with the presence of one or more abnormal cholinesterase isoenzymes with weak activity. Such patients (homozygotes) usually have a plasma cholinesterase of less than 1 kU/l (reference range 2–5 kU/l at 37 °C). In the commonest type of abnormality this is inhibited less than 20 per cent by dibucaine – the normal degree of inhibition being about 80 per cent (or Dibucaine Number 80). Heterozygotes have intermediate values, and are not usually clinically

affected. Measurement of inhibition is necessary both to detect borderline cases with a low–normal total enzyme value, and because total plasma cholinesterase may be low (with normal inhibition) in other conditions particularly chronic liver disease.

Secondary defects

Acetylcholinesterase and cholinesterase are also inhibited by organophosphorus insecticides, and plasma and erythrocyte cholinesterase assay is therefore used to identify paralytic poisoning by these compounds in agriculture and industry.

Myasthenia gravis

In this condition there are circulating antibodies to acetylcholine receptors that are linked to pathogenesis. An increased titre is diagnostically very valuable, being increased in almost all cases.

Skeletal muscle

Creatine and creatinine

Although skeletal muscle is the centre of their metabolism (p. 88), assays of creatine and creatinine concentrations in plasma, and of their secretion in urine, are no longer used for the study of muscle disease – except for 24 h urine creatinine as an index of the mass of healthy muscle. Measurement of creatinuria was formerly the best available test, though insensitive, to assess acute muscle damage.

Creatine kinase

The enzymes that are present in cardiac muscle (p. 132) are also present in skeletal muscle, but not in the same relative amounts.

In the investigation of skeletal muscle disease, CK is the enzyme of choice as this gives markedly raised plasma values (mainly of CK-3: p. 133) in *Duchenne-type muscular dystrophy* even before it is clinically manifest, and abnormal values in most female carriers, even though asymptomatic. Raised values are found in alcoholic and other myopathies and in malignant hyperthermia, but not in neurogenic disease such as multiple sclerosis and myasthenia gravis – except in the active wasting stage after an acute neurological lesion. However, the plasma CK is raised for 48 h by severe exercise, or even by large intramuscular injections – cardiac muscle disease having been excluded.

Rhabdomyolysis

Massive acute destruction of muscle is most commonly due to trauma (crush syndrome), although it has other causes. The damaged muscles take up water and sodium: they release myoglobin, potassium, phosphate, organic acids, creatine, and purines into the plasma. Myoglobin excreted in an acid urine, and the ECF water and sodium depletion, may lead to acute renal failure (p. 119). Plasma CK, including CK-2 (p. 133), is greatly increased.

Secondary muscle weakness

This can be a complication of a wide variety of metabolic disorders with specific biochemical abnormalities. These include hypokalaemia (p. 31); hyperkalaemia (p. 30); hypocalcaemia (p. 180) or hypomagnesaemia (p. 189), both usually associated with tetany; hypercalcaemia (p. 181) or hypermagnesaemia (p. 189) without tetany; various endocrine disturbances, particularly throtoxicosis (p. 201) and Cushing's syndrome (p. 209). These are not associated with a raised plasma creatine kinase.

Further reading

Ashcroft G. Biochemistry and pathology of the affective disorders. In: Wing JK, Wing L, eds. *Handbook of Psychiatry. Vol 3*. Cambridge: Cambridge University Press, 1982: 160–5.

Ker G, Thompson EJ. Immunoglobulins in cerebrospinal fluid. In: French MAH, ed. *Immunoglobulins in health and disease*. Lancaster: MTP Press, 1986: 173–87.

Lott J, Landesman PW. The enzymology of skeletal muscle disorders. *CRC Crit Rev Clin Lab Sci* 1984; **20**: 153–90.

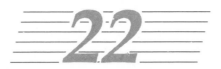

Multisystem Disease: Trauma and Malignancy

Objectives

In this chapter the reader is able to

- study the catabolic and anabolic responses to trauma, including surgery, acute sepsis and other stress
- study the general effects of malignancy on metabolic processes
- study the range of ectopic hormones and syndromes produced by tumours
- study the range of enzymes, oncofetal antigens, and other proteins (tumour markers) produced by tumours.

At the conclusion of this chapter the reader is able to

- use the laboratory to assess the severity of an injury, and the effectiveness of the metabolic response
- use the laboratory in the diagnosis and assessment of malignancy.

Whole body disturbances

There are many pathological conditions that, though initially located in one site, cause a response in apparently unrelated metabolic systems. They have to be understood because these inevitable responses may mask other more specific biochemical changes that may be sought, and also because it is sometimes necessary to use the laboratory to monitor the severity of the initial disturbance and the effectiveness of the response, whether or not modified by therapy. Such general conditions include trauma and malignancy. The multiple changes in malnutrition (p. 108), and the plasma protein changes in infection (p. 100), are considered elsewhere.

Trauma

This includes surgical operation, as well as accidental or deliberate injury.

There are three successive phases in the metabolic response, and these are partly overlapping. They vary in detail and in timing between patients, but in general severity of injury and of responses go together. The responses in burns are usually particularly severe, and are augmented by protein and fluid loss (p. 24). Responses are also modified by complications at different stages, such as malnutrition, prolonged anaesthesia, pain, blood loss, or infection.

Mechanisms

All these changes are promoted mainly through two mechanisms, endocrine and cytokine, whose interrelationships are not fully understood.

Endocrine

As a result of afferent nervous impulses from damaged tissues, modified by higher centres, there is increased secretion of catecholamines. This and other factors lead to ACTH and cortisol secretion, and to an increase of GH, ADH, angiotensin II, and aldosterone. Glucagon secretion is increased, and insulin secretion suppressed. Most of these changes peak at about 12 h.

Cytokines

Damaged tissues produce interleukin-1 and related compounds. These promote the acute-phase reaction (p. 99), which biochemically affects hepatic synthesis of plasma proteins and acceleration of muscle proteolysis.

Additional local factors

At or near the site of injury, and often systemically, increased vascular permeability leads to considerable loss of fluid and albumin from plasma into the interstitial fluid.

Metabolic changes

The first phase, sometimes called the acute, shock, or 'ebb' phase, is defensive and primarily protects the circulation; energy is provided from fat. It lasts about 24 h. There is obligatory oliguria, which may persist for 48 h.

The second, or catabolic phase, is primarily one of increased breakdown of muscle protein and of glycogen (causing loss of weight), as well as of triglycerides, and there is release of amino acids which will be available for wound healing. This phase lasts about five days. There are many measurable biochemical changes. There is an initial fall in the glomerular filtration rate, and this and the accelerated muscle breakdown cause a rise in plasma urea; then there is an increase in urinary nitrogen excretion, including creatinine, with a negative nitrogen balance. Plasma albumin falls, and there is a rise in acute phase proteins, particularly fibrinogen and C-reactive protein. Though overall potassium balance is negative, plasma potassium increases; sodium is retained, but plasma sodium changes are slight. There is a mild negative calcium and magnesium balance. There is hyperglycaemia; and plasma lactate (linked to depressed tissue oxygen consumption) and free fatty acids rise. Interaction of these factors causes a metabolic acidosis, though complicating factors may lead to other acid–base disturbances.

The third, or anabolic phase, is primarily that of wound healing, and other restoration of normality including weight gain and a positive nitrogen balance. It may last for several weeks, until full recovery of the normal steady-state. The combined second and third phases used to be called the 'flow' phase.

Unless the changes in the first and second phases are recognized and understood, attempted replacement therapy, particularly of fluids and nutrients, may be incorrect.

Physiological changes

These overlap the biochemical changes, and will not be described in detail. There is a fall in cardiac output and in oxygen consumption in the acute phase, and these rise above normal during the early stages of hypercatabolism (p. 110).

Malignancy

Biochemical changes in malignant disease may be divided into

(a) changes within cells or between cells as part of the malignant process: these will not be considered further here;

(b) the detection in body fluids of substances produced by tumour cells that might be used to demonstrate the presence of a tumour, its progress, or response to therapy. These substances are often called 'cancer markers' or 'tumour markers';

(c) the measurable local or general metabolic effects of advanced malignant disease on other systems: paraneoplastic syndromes.

Tumour markers

Hormones

Primary changes

Benign or malignant tumours of cells of endocrine glands will usually produce excess of the normal secretion of those cells, often giving rise to appropriate clinical syndromes. These may be of peptide or other hormones, and are described in the relevant sections elsewhere in this book. The most important clinically is chorionic gonadotrophin (hCG: p. 219) which is assayed for the diagnosis and management of choriocarcinoma.

Ectopic secretion

Tumours of tissues other than endocrine glands may produce polypeptide (or rarely other) hormones 'inappropriately'. The causes are controversial, and may be due to derepression, namely that non-tumorous non-endocrine cells normally produce minute amounts of such hormones; in some cases there may be production of hormones from pluripotent APUD cells (p. 171). The ectopic hormone is not always identical with the natural hormone, either biologically or immunologically. In such conditions the excess hormone production may be sufficient to initiate the appropriate endocrine syndrome, and plasma hormone assay may be helpful for diagnosis or monitoring.

Although almost every tumour has been described as producing ectopic hormones, and most hormones have been identified, by far the commonest tumour involved is oat-cell carcinoma of the lung, and to a lesser extent carcinomas of the pancreas and of the thymus. These most frequently produce ACTH, ADH, or PTH. More localized ectopic hormones are hCG from germ-cell tumours, and insulin-like hormones from mesenchymal tumours especially retroperitoneal fibrosarcoma.

Tumour-associated antigens

These are a group of proteins, often produced normally in the fetus (oncofetal antigens), that are synthesized by a variety of malignant tumours and can be assayed in plasma. There is a continuous search for such antigens that might be useful for screening or early diagnosis of malignancy both in general and in specific tissues, but both false negatives (especially in localized malignancy) and false positives (from antigen produced in appropriate local non-malignant conditions with rapid cell turnover) are common. These tests are valuable in management, because in general the plasma concentrations are proportional to the spread of the tumour and the response to treatment.

Assays that have established value at present are described below.

Carcinoembryonic antigen (CEA)

This is found in most cases of colorectal cancer, and often in carcinoma of the breast, lung and pancreas, and in neuroblastoma. False positives are often found, for example, in ulcerative colitis. Monthly tests are useful in monitoring carcinoma of the colon.

α-Fetoprotein (αFP)

This is found in most cases of primary liver carcinoma, and often in germ-cell carcinomas, e.g. teratoma of the testis, in conjunction with hCG. False positives may be found, for example, in acute hepatitis.

A raised α-fetoprotein is also found in maternal serum when there are neural tube defects, and a low value in Down's syndrome (p. 220).

Prostate-specific antigen (PSA)

This is found to be increased in the plasma in carcinoma of the prostate, even when the tumour has not spread locally nor has it metastasized. However, moderately raised values are sometimes found in cases of benign prostatic hypertrophy, so the assay is much more useful for monitoring than for early diagnosis.

Other tests

At present the only other antigen assay that is widely accepted is of CA 125 for monitoring the spread, and therapy, of ovarian cancer. These new tumour markers tend to be costly to measure.

Enzymes

Lysozyme

This enzyme is derived from lysosomes. The plasma (or urine) value is usually raised in acute monocytic leukaemia, and this may be useful for monitoring; changes in myeloblastic leukaemia are variable. Normal values are found in acute lymphoblastic leukaemia, and this may be useful in differential diagnosis.

Changes in cell enzymes in leukaemia are not considered here.

Acid phosphatases

These are produced in many organs: the acid phosphatase that is important for diagnosis is derived from mature prostatic epithelium and secreted into prostatic fluid.

A raised plasma acid phosphatase value is usually due to an increase in the prostatic phosphatase. However, a slight rise is occasionally found in severe osteoblastic bone disease (including Paget's disease), in Gaucher's disease, when there is excessive destruction of platelets – or in a haemolysed sample.

Prostatic acid phosphatase may be measured chemically or immunologically. A raised plasma total acid phosphatase or 'prostatic' acid phosphatase is strongly suggestive of metastazing prostatic carcinoma. Raised values are occasionally found with localized carcinoma (the immunoassay may be more sensitive), and rarely in carcinoma of other sites. Estimation of the plasma acid phosphatase is of use both in diagnosis, and in monitoring hormonal treatment: it is tending to be replaced by assay of prostate-specific antigen. Normal values are found in benign prostatic hyperplasia, though if the prostate has been biopsied or vigorously palpated within two days a brief rise is occasionally found.

Alkaline phosphatase (p. 180)

Placental-type (Regan) isoenzymes are found in the plasma of some patients with advanced malignant disease, particularly of the lung, but this estimation is not useful for diagnosis or monitoring.

Other compounds

Specific globulins

Tumours of plasma cells, especially multiple myeloma, produce monoclonal myeloma globulins, and their light-chains (Bence Jones protein), in quantities easily detectable for diagnosis (p. 103).

Melanogens

The melanocytes of malignant melanoma often produce sufficient melanogens to be easily detectable in urine: quantitation is sometimes useful in monitoring. Preformed melanin, to which melanogen is converted in the presence of air and light, is also sometimes excreted.

Polyamines

These comprise spermine, spermidine, and putrescine, and they are produced in actively synthesizing tissues. Increased cell turnover, particularly in a wide variety of malignant diseases (but also in non-malignant conditions, particularly psoriasis), causes increased urinary excretion of the polyamines. Changes in excretion may be useful in monitoring progress – a spike of excretion occurs after successful chemotherapy. The increases in plasma or erythrocyte polyamines are less marked. Many cases of medulloblastoma show a high CSF polyamine concentration, and changes in this are valuable for monitoring.

Paraneoplastic syndromes

This includes the endocrine effects of ectopic hormone production, described above under 'cancer markers', and a variety of other metabolic changes.

The biochemical changes found in advanced malignant disease include those of any severe disease, possibly aggravated by infection, malnutrition, and many other secondary factors. There is usually a fall in plasma albumin, an increase in acute phase proteins and often in IgG, and a rise in plasma urea. Macrophages infiltrating even small tumours can produce the polypeptide cachectin (tumour necrosis factor) with wide metabolic actions, including causing cachexia. Tumours with a high content and turnover of nuclear material, particularly leukaemias, can release enough nucleic acids to raise the plasma urate: the increase after cytotoxic treatment may be sufficient to cause gout (p. 87). Other effects depend on the nature and site of the primary tumour and of its metastases.

Hypercalcaemia is frequent in malignant disease, by humoral effects on bone, whether or not there are overt metastases in bone (p. 189). There is usually hyperphosphataemia, a rise in osteoblastic alkaline phosphatase and osteocalcin, and often increased urinary hydroxyproline. Metastases to the liver produce an increase in hepatic alkaline phosphatase typically before there is jaundice (p. 155). Metastasis or local spread of tumours to endocrine glands can lead to endocrine deficiency syndromes, examples being diabetes insipidus and Addison's disease – in contrast to ectopic hormone excess syndromes (p. 233).

Obstruction caused by tumour, for example to bile-duct or ureters, has the same biochemical effects as obstruction from any other pathological cause.

Erosion of blood vessels in the gastrointestinal tract will cause faecal occult blood (p. 172) at an early stage of many tumours. This has been proposed as a screening test for gastrointestinal carcinoma, but there are too many false positives and false negatives for this to be reliable. Similarly blood in the urine may result from malignant disease of the urinary tract.

Further reading

Barton RN. Trauma and its metabolic problems. *Br Med Bull* 1985; **41**.

Beisel WR. Sepsis and metabolism. In: Little RA, Frayn KN, eds. *The Scientific Basis of the Care of the Critically Ill*. Manchester: Manchester University Press, 1987; 103–22.

Laurence DJR, Neville AM. Biochemical tests in diagnosis and monitoring of cancer. In: Goldberg DM, ed. *Clinical Biochemistry Reviews*. New York: John Wiley, 1982; **3**: 133–86.

Newlands ES. Clinical applications of tumour markers. *Med Lab Sci* 1987; **44**: 361–70.

23

Therapeutic Drug Monitoring

Objectives

In this chapter the reader is able to

- revise the principles of pharmacokinetics and pharmacodynamics and to understand the relevance to therapeutic drug monitoring.

At the conclusion of this chapter the reader is able to

- understand the current limited value of therapeutic drug monitoring
- use the laboratory for effective therapeutic drug monitoring.

Clinical questions

The measurement of drug levels in body fluids in order to optimize treatment is known as therapeutic drug monitoring (TDM). For some drugs, there is an obvious effect of therapy e.g. in hypertension, the therapeutic effect is monitored by measuring blood pressure. Oral anticoagulant therapy can be assessed by determining prothrombin time, and the effectiveness of hypoglycaemic agents in treating insulin-independent diabetes mellitus is readily determined by measuring the blood glucose. There is no biochemical or other marker of drug effectiveness for other drug regimes and measurement of the concentration of the drug in plasma or serum might be helpful in answering the following questions

(a) is the patient taking the drug?

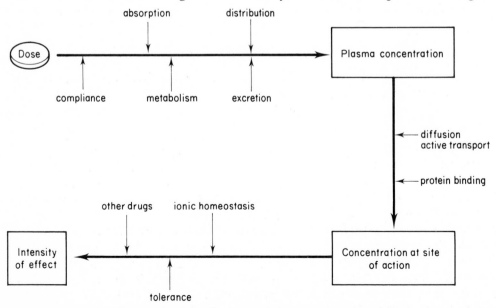

Fig. 23.1 Factors affecting the dose of a drug and the intensity of its effect

(b) is the concentration of the drug in plasma consistent with effective therapy?

(c) is the patient receiving too high a dose?

Drugs in the body

Figure 23.1 illustrates some of the factors which can influence the therapeutic action of drugs.

Pharmacokinetics is the quantitative study of the metabolic processes and relationship between a drug dose and drug concentration in body fluids. Pharmacokinetic variation largely accounts for differences in drug response between individuals. After oral administration, a drug is absorbed from the gastrointestinal tract,

distributed in body fluids, metabolized and excreted. The rates of these processes determine the plasma half-life of a drug. This is the time required for the plasma concentration to decline by 50 per cent.

Dosing regimes are constructed to achieve therapeutic plasma concentrations; these regimes use an average half-life for a drug. Figure 23.2 shows the considerable interindividual variation between plasma concentration and drug dose.

Sampling time

Figure 23.3 illustrates the importance of sampling time when attempting to interpret a drug concentration. The drug is taken at regular intervals, once every half-life. After the first dose (D at 0 half-life) the plasma concentration increases to a peak (A) and

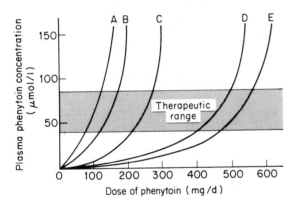

Fig. 23.2 The relationship between phenytoin dose and plasma concentration in five epileptic patients (A, B, C, D, E). Modified with permission from Richens A, Warrington S. *Drugs* 1979; **17**: 488–500

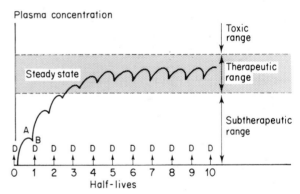

Fig. 23.3 The plasma concentration of a drug taken at regular intervals, once every half-life. The concentration varies from a peak A to a trough B and five half-lives must elapse before a steady state is achieved

then declines to a trough (B) as the drug is metabolized and excreted. A second dose is taken before these processes have completely eliminated the drug from the body and the plasma concentration increases further. A steady state is achieved after five doses when the peak and trough plasma concentrations fall within the therapeutic range. If the drug were taken at intervals less than the half-life, toxic plasma levels would result. Failure to take the drug at

regular intervals would lead to subtherapeutic levels. Generally, trough concentrations are measured and the blood sample should be obtained just before the next dose is taken.

Measurement of both peak and trough levels is important for the antibiotic gentamicin so that the dose interval can be adjusted to avoid toxic peak levels and subtherapeutic trough levels.

Therapeutic index

For some drugs, toxic effects are manifest at a plasma concentration not much higher than the therapeutic level. The therapeutic index expresses the ratio

$$\frac{\text{minimum toxic dose}}{\text{minimum therapeutic dose}}$$

The relationship between dose and plasma concentration (Fig. 23.2) is less predictable in certain circumstances. For instance, in pregnancy there may be an increase in distribution volume producing sub-therapeutic plasma drug levels. In renal disease, the elimination time of drugs may increase, producing toxic drug levels.

The relation between the plasma concentration of a drug and its biological effect is more complex and described by the study of pharmacodynamics. The concentration of the drug at its site of action may not be the same as its plasma concentration (Fig. 23.1); the anticonvulsant phenytoin is 95 per cent bound to plasma proteins and only 5 per cent exists in the free or active form in plasma. Laboratories measure the total concentration of phenytoin in plasma and this may not reflect the concentration at the site of action. Proposals to measure saliva drug concentrations in saliva, free of protein binding, have not been widely accepted.

The sensitivity of tissues to drugs may be influenced by the ionic homoeostasis. For instance, hypokalaemia and hypercalcaemia increase the responsiveness of cardiac muscle to a given plasma concentration of digoxin. The large interindividual pharmacodynamic variation for digoxin means that measurement of its plasma concentration does not help in assessing its therapeutic effect.

Applications of therapeutic drug monitoring

Figure 23.4 shows the questions to be asked before including a drug measurement in a TDM programme. Only a few drugs satisfy the criteria, and some drugs are commonly measured when careful consideration indicates that such measurement is unnecessary. Table 23.1 lists the types of drugs which are commonly measured.

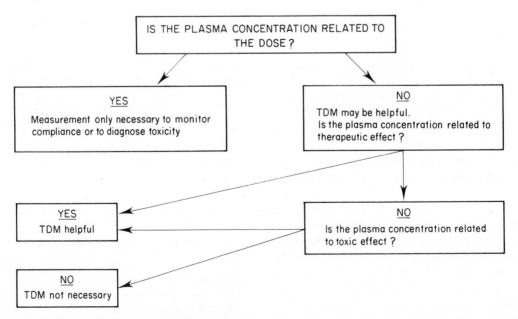

Fig. 23.4   The inclusion of a drug in a TDM programme

Table 23.1 Types of drugs monitored

Category	Example	Reason
Anticonvulsants	Phenytoin	Low therapeutic index
	Carbamazepine	Drug interactions
		Toxic effects difficult to recognize
Antibiotics	Gentamicin	Low therapeutic index
Cardiac drugs	Digoxin	Large interindividual pharmacokinetic variation but
		pharmacodynamic variation means TDM may mislead
Psychoactive drugs	Lithium	Low therapeutic index
		Toxic effects difficult to recognize
Bronchodilators	Theophylline	Low therapeutic index
Antineoplastic drugs	Methotrexate	Folinic acid rescue of toxic concentrations
Immunosuppressants	Cyclosporin A	Low therapeutic index

Phenytoin

This anticonvulsant has a well-established therapeutic range (or 'window') and a low therapeutic index. Toxic effects include nystagmus and ataxia; coma may develop at a plasma concentration of 100 μmol/l, whilst the therapeutic range is 40–80 μmol/l.

Phenytoin concentrations in plasma vary considerably from individual to individual (Fig. 23.2) and its measurement is well established in TDM. Toxic effects may develop in patients with therapeutic plasma phenytoin levels if more phenytoin is displaced from protein binding sites (p. 238) by other drugs (e.g. valproate, salicylate) or metabolites (e.g. bilirubin).

Digoxin

The value of plasma digoxin measurements is controversial. The therapeutic dose is only slightly less than a toxic dose; the therapeutic range is 1.0–2.6 nmol/l and values greater than 3.0 nmol/l are regarded as toxic. However, some patients have undoubted signs and symptoms of digoxin toxicity in spite of having plasma levels within the therapeutic range. Other patients may have a satisfactory therapeutic response to digoxin in the presence of sub-therapeutic plasma levels and a few require toxic plasma levels in order to produce an adequate therapeutic effect of the drug.

Lithium

This drug is used in the treatment of manic

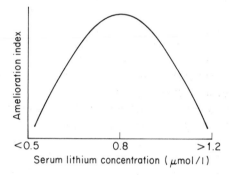

Fig. 23.5 Relationship between serum lithium concentration and therapeutic effect as reported by patients using an amelioration index

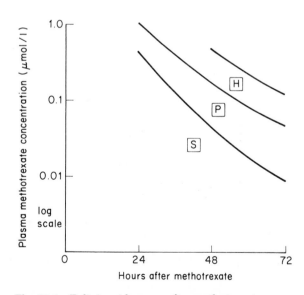

Fig. 23.6 Folinic acid rescue after methotrexate administration. Plasma concentrations of methotrexate are used to alter the infusion rate of folinic acid as a standard rescue (S), prolonged rescue (P), or a high and prolonged rescue (H)

or manic-depressive illness and has a low therapeutic index. Figure 23.5 shows that the therapeutic range is narrow and that higher serum lithium concentrations make patients feel worse. Toxic effects include tremor, slurred speech and muscle weakness; all of these signs are difficult to recognize clinically. Lithium can produce nephrogenic diabetes insipidus (p. 195) and renal failure. Samples for assay must not be taken into tubes containing lithium heparin.

Methotrexate

The plasma concentration of methotrexate is monitored in the treatment of cancer. This antineoplastic drug inhibits DNA synthesis by competitively inhibiting dihydrofolate reductase, an intracellular enzyme responsible for conversion of folic acid to reduced folates. At high dose it is a toxic drug, producing myelosuppression, gastrointestinal muscositis and hepatic dysfunction. Toxic effects can be lessened with a folinic acid 'rescue' which repletes reduced folate pools at a point in the reduced folate cycle distal to the methotrexate-induced enzymatic block.

Figure 23.6 shows that the dose and rate of folinic acid infusion is altered according to the plasma methotrexate concentration. The measurement of this drug is therefore warranted as clinical decisions are taken on the basis of the result.

Further reading

Hallworth MJ. Audit of therapeutic drug monitoring. *Ann Clin Biochem* 1988; **25**: 121–8.

Richens A, Warrington S. When should plasma drug levels be monitored? *Drugs* 1979; **17**: 488–500.

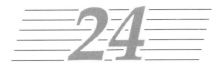

Acute Poisoning

Objectives

In this chapter the reader is able to

- study the metabolic effects of common overdoses and poisoning.

At the conclusion of this chapter the reader is able to

- use the laboratory in the investigation of a poisoned patient.

Presentation

About 10 per cent of total emergency medical admissions in the UK are patients who are acutely poisoned. It is an important consideration for a comatose patient (p. 225) particularly if the breath smells of ethanol or tablets have been found.

Poisoned patients may display a variety of symptoms or none at all. The toxic effect of an agent could be due to itself (e.g. lithium), due to metabolites (e.g. methanol which produces formic acid) or due to a pathophysiological consequence of its presence (e.g. salicylate which causes dehydration, respiratory alkalosis and metabolic acidosis).

Role of the laboratory

In many cases of poisoning, treatment will occur without measurement of the specific agent but with biochemical monitoring of the patient's condition. Measurement of certain poisons, however, can aid in diagnosis and in instituting therapy.

Generally, it is useful to measure a drug in a patient's body fluids if the measurement will

(a) confirm a diagnosis, e.g. in lithium intoxication;
(b) identify a specific agent for which treatment is available e.g. in iron poisoning treated with desferrioxamine;
(c) help to assess the severity of the intoxication, but only if action will be taken on the basis of the result, e.g. after methanol ingestion;
(d) help to distinguish between symptoms caused by the agent(s) from those caused by other disorders e.g. blood ethanol measurement in a comatose patient with a head injury;
(e) initiate treatment based on knowledge of the agent's distribution and metabolism in the body e.g. plasma paracetamol levels and treatment (see Fig. 24.2).

Need for detection

Detecting the presence of a poison in blood or urine often confirms clinical suspicion. Many laboratories can confirm intoxication due to salicylate, paracetamol, iron, ethanol, carbon monoxide, and lithium overdose. Other poisons need more sophisticated detection procedures available at specialized centres, e.g. opioids, tricyclic antidepressants, paraquat.

Samples which are used for urgent diagnosis and monitoring should be analysed as soon as possible. Samples which are obtained for later analysis must be clearly labelled and correctly stored; there may be

Table 24.1   Biochemical abnormalities in drug overdoses

Overdose	B	CO	CN	D	E	EG	I	M	Op	P	S	T	Tc
Artertial blood P_{O_2}	↓	↓	↓		↓				↓				↓
Arterial blood P_{CO_2}	↑				↑				↑		↓		↑
Plasma HCO_3^-	↓↑	↓	↓		↓	↓		↓		↓	↓	↓	↓
Plasma K^+				↑					↑				
Plasma Ca^{2+}						↓							
Plasma glucose					↓	↓	↓	↑			↓↑	↑	
Plasma osmolality					↑	↑		↑			↑		

B	barbiturates	I	insulin
CO	carbon monoxide	M	methanol
CN	cyanide	Op	opioids
D	digoxin	P	paracetamol
E	ethanol	S	salicylate
EG	ethylene glycol	T	theophylline
		Tc	tricyclic antidepressants

medicolegal inquiries in cases of suspected poisoning.

Other biochemical measurements are important in diagnosing and monitoring the consequences of poisoning (Table 24.1).

Lead poisoning (p. 143), cadmium and mercury poisoning (p. 113), organophosphorus insecticide poisoning (p. 229), and aluminium toxicity (p. 113) are usually chronic conditions and are discussed elsewhere.

Need for quantitation

Clinical decisions may be taken on the quantitative measurement of a drug in plasma or serum.

Salicylate

This is the active metabolite of acetylsalicylate (aspirin) which is highly toxic when taken in overdose. The metabolic features of salicylate poisoning include dehydration, secondary to hyperventilation sweating and vomiting; a complex mixed acid–base disturbance with respiratory alkalosis presiding in adults and metabolic acidosis common in children; hyper- or hypoglycaemia due to uncoupling of oxidative phosphorylation and stimulation of glycolysis and gluconeogenesis.

Treatment involves gastric lavage to avoid further absorption and forced diure-

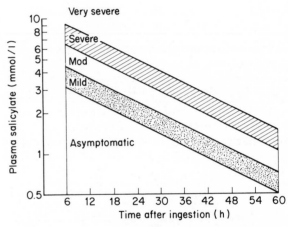

Fig. 24.1   Severity of salicylate poisoning assessed by plotting a measurement of plasma salicylate concentration (logarithmic scale) at a known time after ingestion. Modified with permission from Stewart MJ, Watson ID. *Ann Clin Biochem* 1987; **24**: 552–65

sis. Severe poisoning may require haemodialysis. Figure 24.1 shows that salicylate poisoning may be classified on the basis of one plasma determination. Serial salicylate measurements are often performed to assess the efficacy of elimination therapy.

Paracetamol

Severe paracetamol overdose leads to hepatic necrosis (p. 159) and death due to liver failure. Immediate treatment includes gastric lavage and aspiration if the patient presents within four hours of ingestion;

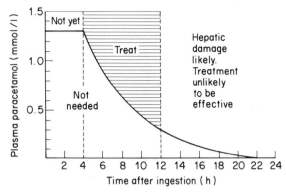

Fig. 24.2 Treatment chart for paracetamol poisoning. Prognostic information cannot be obtained from a plasma paracetamol measurement made less than 4 h after ingestion. Modified with permission from Stewart MJ, Watson ID. *Ann Clin Biochem* 1987; **24**: 552–65

paracetamol is rapidly absorbed from the gastrointestinal tract. Paracetamol is metabolized in the liver; in therapeutic doses it is conjugated with glucuronic acid and sulphate and these conjugates are rapidly excreted. In overdose, the conjugation pathway is overloaded, and paracetamol is metabolized into highly toxic N-hydroxylation products. The paracetamol metabolite reacts with thiol groups in structural proteins of the hepatocyte leading to cell death and acute hepatic necrosis.

In uncomplicated cases the treatment of choice is oral methionine which provides an alternative substrate for the toxic paracetamol metabolite. If the patient is unconscious or presents later than 12 h after ingestion, the antidote is N-acetylcysteine which may produce adverse reactions. Figure 24.2 shows the treatment criteria for paracetamol overdose and requires plotting the plasma paracetamol concentration at a known time after the ingestion.

Iron

Acute overdose of iron can be toxic and a serum concentration of 90 μmol/l or greater is considered toxic. Free iron is the toxic agent, and iron-binding capacity (p. 145) may vary considerably from individual to individual. Treatment is with the chelating agent desferrioxamine.

Other drugs

Lithium toxicity can present chronically (p. 239) or acutely. If serum lithium is greater than 5 mmol/l the patient is in grave danger and peritoneal dialysis will be considered to eliminate lithium from the body. Similarly, a plasma theophylline of 330 μmol/l in an adult necessitates haemoperfusion.

In many instances of severe drug overdose, elimination therapy is instituted without knowledge of the blood concentration of the drug.

Need for monitoring

The antidote for methanol and ethylene glycol intoxication is an infusion of ethanol, which reduces the oxidation of methanol and ethylene glycol to their toxic metabolites. Quantitative measurements of methanol and ethanol are helpful in adjusting therapeutic regimes.

Ethanol

Ethanol is commonly abused, chronically and acutely. Many suicidal patients may drink ethanol in combination with swallowing pills and this may complicate the clinical picture. Measurement of blood alcohol thus helps in the assessment of a poisoned patient. Blood alcohol determinations are also used to check abstinence in the chronic alcoholic, in the differential diagnosis of coma, and in medicolegal situations (e.g. drunken driving).

A blood alcohol of 65 mmol/l (300 mg/dl) is dangerous to life. Chronic alcoholics can tolerate levels far greater than this, probably because ethanol induces hepatic enzyme activity. They are also capable of tolerating methanol poisoning.

The biochemical features of chronic alcoholism are discussed on p. 77.

Drug screening

Qualitative detection of opioid drugs may

be important in monitoring compliance in detoxification programmes and is best carried out at specialized centres. Similarly, the complete toxicological investigation of a poisoned patient requires careful technological analysis by expert personnel.

Screening for drugs also occurs in cases of suspected brain death. Drugs may depress CNS function and produce symptoms which mimic brain death. Life-support systems may be removed after brain death is established. It is important to check for the presence of drugs before the diagnosis of brain death.

Further reading

Stewart MJ, Watson ID. Methods for the estimation of salicylate and paracetamol in serum, plasma and urine. *Ann Clin Biochem* 1987; **24**: 552–65.

Volans G, Widdop B. *The ABC of Poisoning.* London: British Medical Association, 1984.

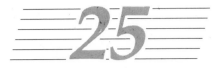

Inherited Metabolic Disease

Objectives

In this chapter the reader is able to

- revise the basis of genetic change and the different modes of inheritance
- study the general relation between genetic abnormalities, biochemical abnormalities and clinical presentation.

At the conclusion of this chapter the reader is able to

- understand the effects of inherited metabolic disease (N.B. Specific inherited metabolic diseases are discussed in the appropriate chapter).
- use the laboratory for screening, diagnosis and management.

Genetic change

The genetic code for the entire structure and function of the human organism resides on about 50 000 gene pairs located on 23 pairs of chromosomes. Genes code either for proteins (structural genes) or regulate the transcription of these genes (controlling genes). Genetic changes are continually occurring as a result of random recombinations of genes during meiosis and by mutation. It can thus be expected that any protein, whether enzyme or structural component, may differ in its amino acid sequence from individual to individual and that multiple forms (resulting from inherited alleles) will occur in any individual. In the case of all proteins these forms are referred to as allotypes; in the special case of

enzymes they are referred to as isoforms or isoenzymes (p. 106). Although there is very little evidence, it is reasonable to suppose that similar allotypic diversity also occurs in the controlling genes.

Protein allotypes may have no alteration in their function or it may be enhanced or decreased. Natural selection results in enrichment, in the population, of genes carrying a selective advantage and removal of those that do not. Certain alleles of both controlling and structural genes may disturb the function of the product sufficiently to cause disease. These conditions are generally referred to as inherited metabolic diseases or inborn errors of metabolism. Until recently they have been defined as clinical entities and it is important to appreciate that the same disease manifestations may result from several genetically determined defects in a metabolic pathway causing the same or similar biochemical and pathological consequences. Clinically defined inherited metabolic diseases thus frequently turn out to be an assemblage of several genetic defects when modern techniques unravel the genetic abnormality. This is of considerable consequence both in genetic counselling (as the mode of inheritance may differ) and also in treatment (as the exact nature of the biochemical defect and its response to therapy may differ). An example of such a 'heterogenous' inborn error of metabolism is phenylketonuria (p. 89).

Inheritance

Each of the genes in a gene pair can be

considered as contributing about 50 per cent to the ultimate effect; e.g. protein production. A structural gene mutation may thus be present on only one gene resulting in 50 per cent of the protein produced carrying that particular allotype. If the allotype is a non-functional protein and half the normal level of the protein is insufficient to preserve normal metabolism, then the resulting disease is said to be dominantly inherited. If, however, disease does not result until very much lower levels of protein occur, requiring two abnormal genes, then the disease is said to be recessively inherited. Clearly, such a distinction is only a matter of degree, as under normal circumstances, in a recessively inherited condition no disease may result from a single abnormal gene but if the particular metabolic pathway is stressed by another disease the pathological consequences may then occur. Diseases which result from defects in a single gene or gene pair are termed monogenic. In some cases the interaction of two or more different genes and possibly environmental factors are required to cause disease and such conditions are said to be multifactorial. Chromosomal disorders due to the absence or abnormal rearrangement of chromosomes affect many genes and frequently have serious widespread consequences (e.g. Down's syndrome).

Metabolic consequences

The metabolic consequences of important specific inherited diseases are described under the appropriate system or organ elsewhere in this book. In these disorders the primary defect must be present from conception, though it may not manifest itself until adult life, as in gout (p. 86). A disorder may be dependent for its clinical manifestation on external factors, and these can be natural, as in galactosaemia (p. 62), or artificial, as in suxamethonium apnoea (p. 229). The disturbance caused by an inborn error of metabolism may be completely harmless, as in pentosuria (p. 62).

Monogenic disorders affect proteins or peptides or regulatory genes controlling the former. Most diseases result from defects in enzymes, though some may reflect defects in structural proteins (e.g. collagen), receptors (e.g. LDL receptor) or inhibitors (e.g. α_1-antitrypsin). The course of many biochemical reactions can be expressed simply as shown in Fig. 25.1.

Defects of a transport system

The reaction A⟶A is transport across a membrane, believed to be mediated by a carrier protein system known as a 'permease'. One type of inborn error of metabolism occurs when the transport reaction A⟶A, in intestinal mucosa or renal tubules, is deficient as a genetic defect as in cystinuria (p. 121) – the deficiency of the common carrier system in the renal tubules for reabsorption of the basic amino acids cystine, ornithine, arginine and lysine, leads to their excretion in excess and the formation of cystine calculi.

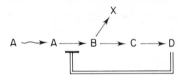

Fig. 25.1

Defects of a metabolic enzyme

Enzyme defects may result from mutations in the controlling gene or structural gene decreasing transcription of the protein (in which case low levels of enzyme are present even in the homozygote) or in the structural gene resulting in absent synthesis (usually 'frame shift' mutations), short half-life or loss of function. The same 'disease' may result from several different inherited defects even in one enzyme.

The reactions of A→B, B→C, (B→X), and C→D and so on, are controlled by specific enzymes. The concentration or the rate of formation of product D can control the rate of the earlier reaction A→B by a feedback mechanism.

A second major type of inborn error of

metabolism develops if there is alteration in the gene which controls the formation of the enzyme which mediates the rate-limiting reaction B→C ('B:*Case*') and produces a variant or reduces the activity of that enzyme. This may manifest in a number of different ways.

Diminished rate of formation of product

This may be the immediate product, C, as in von Gierke's disease (p. 57) – the deficiency of glucose-6-phosphatase leads to diminished formation of glucose from glucose-6-phosphate. It may be a product at a remove, D, as in the congenital adrenal hyperplasia (p. 211) the deficiency of 21-hydroxylase leads to diminished formation of cortisol which is the end-product of the synthetic sequence.

Diminished rate of removal of substrate

This may be the immediate substrate, B, as in alkaptonuria (p. 89) – the deficiency of homogentisic acid oxidase leads to retention (and urinary excretion) of homogentisic acid. It may be a substrate at a remove, A, as in von Gierke's disease (p. 57) – the deficiency of glucose-6-phosphatase leads to retention of gly.ogen which is the origin of the catabolic sequence. A common additional effect may be increased formation of by-product X, as in phenylketonuria (p. 89) – the deficiency of phenylalanine hydroxylase leads to retention of phenylalanine, which is converted in excess to phenylpyruvic acid and phenyllactic acid, both being excreted in the urine.

Altered feedback

An example is congenital adrenal hyperplasia (p. 211) – the deficiency of 21-hydroxylase causes diminished formation of cortisol, which leads to increased secretion of adrenocorticotrophic hormone; this stimulates the earlier stages of the steroid synthetic pathway and excess androgens are produced.

Clinically important inherited metabolic diseases

A very large number of inborn errors of metabolism have now been described, varying considerably in their frequency (Table 25.1). In only a few is effective treatment possible at present, and in these diagnosis in early infancy may be essential to prevent irreversible consequences. In others, genetic counselling is important and in some cases prenatal diagnosis may allow termination of pregnancy.

Tabel 25.1 Approximate incidence of some genetic diseases in populations of Western European origin

Chromosomal abnormalities	
All	1:200
Sex chromosomes	1:420
Down's syndrome	1:550
Congenital malformations	1:400
Metabolic disease	
IgA deficiency	1:500
α_1-Antitrypsin deficiencies	1:750
Cystic fibrosis	1:3000
Histidinaemia	1:11000
Hartnup disease	1:15000
Phenylketonuria	1:15000
Cystinuria	1:17000
Galactosaemia	1:100000
Maple syrup urine disease	1:340000

Phenylketonuria (p. 89), galactosaemia (p. 57), congenital hypothyroidism (p. 202), and maple syrup urine disease (p. 89) will give rise to serious mental retardation if not detected early in infancy. They may all be treated and can thus be considered as some of the most important inborn errors of metabolism.

A large group of other conditions may be ameliorated to a greater or lesser extent by treatment or avoidance of precipitating factors such as drugs. People with abnormal cholinesterase (p. 229), glucose-6-phosphate-dehydrogenase deficiency (p. 141), and acute porphyria (p. 142) may all suffer acute symptoms as a result of consuming drugs or other products. Serious lung damage may arise in α_1-antitrypsin-deficient individuals (p. 99) if they are exposed to a dusty environment or are smokers; prompt prophylaxis for bacterial lower-respiratory tract infections may avoid life-threatening bronchiectasis in IgA deficient individuals (p. 101).

Diagnosis

The diagnosis of inborn errors of metabolism may be undertaken in several different ways.

(a) The direct analysis of DNA in blood cells or samples of chorionic villus may be used to reveal an abnormal gene. As yet this is only possible in a few conditions such as thalassaemia, α_1-antitrypsin deficiency and Duchenne muscular dystrophy.

(b) The activity of an affected enzyme may be measured in plasma tissues or blood cells.

(c) The concentration of an affected enzyme (or other protein) may be measured directly by immunoassay.

(d) An allotype of a protein or enzyme (isoenzyme) may be detected by altered physicochemical characteristics, e.g. by electrophoresis. Heterozygotes may also be frequently detected by these techniques as the product of a single gene is usually recognizable.

(e) In the case of enzyme defects, increased levels of substrate, decreased levels of products, or abnormal metabolites may be detected or measured.

(f) Heterozygocity for certain enzyme defects may sometimes be recognized by loading tests where accumulation of substrate can then be demonstrated.

Treatment

(a) Dietary regimes may be used to avoid a substrate (e.g. phenylalanine) whose accumulation (or metabolism) results in toxicity.

(b) Enzyme replacement may be undertaken by induction of synthesis (e.g. the dominantly inherited deficiency of complement C1 inhibitor where the product of the normal gene may be induced) or replacement in transferred cells, transplanted organs, or liposomes.

(c) Vitamin therapy may be very successful in disease resulting from defective vitamin metabolism or production (sometimes referred to as co-factor abnormalities).

Screening

Screening for inherited metabolic disease can be undertaken in the whole population or in selected 'at risk' groups. Criteria for screening are that: the disorder should not be clinically obvious at the time when it should be treated; the disease should have serious consequences and should be treatable; it should be relatively common; that a suitable sensitive and specific screening test should exist. For prenatal diagnosis the disease should be serious and untreatable and detectable early enough in pregnancy to allow termination. In addition, there should be an 'at risk' group as prenatal diagnosis carries the risks associated with amniocentesis (p. 4).

In the UK, current practice is to screen every newborn child for phenylketonuria and congenital hypothyroidism. Screening programmes also exist for the thalassaemias and glucose-6-phosphate dehydrogenase deficiency for selected populations.

Clinical conditions giving rise to the suspicion of inherited metabolic disease

It is in infancy that these diseases may give rise to diagnostic confusion and where they form an important part of differential diagnosis. Vomiting, failure to thrive, hepatosplenomegaly, jaundice, hypoglycaemia, and metabolic acidosis should all be reasons for suspicion.

Further reading

d'A Crawfurd M. Prenatal diagnosis of common genetic disorders. *Br Med J* 1988; **297**: 502–6.

Holton JB, ed. *Inherited Metabolic Diseases.* Edinburgh: Churchill Livingstone, 1987.

Weatherall DJ. *The New Genetics and Clinical Practice.* Oxford: Oxford University Press, 1986.

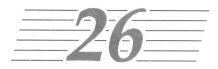

Chemical Pathology at the Extremes of Life

Objectives

In this chapter the reader is able to

- study the specific biochemical problems of neonatal disease
- study the general biochemical problems of old age.

At the conclusion of this chapter the reader is able to

- understand how certain reference ranges alter between birth and adult life
- understand how certain reference ranges alter during ageing.

The neonatal period

Specialized neonatal units are able to deliver and maintain the fetus as early as 24-weeks gestation. Infants born before term (preterm, 'premature') are more likely to develop serious disease because of their immaturity. For example, the enzyme system responsible for the hepatic conjugation of bilirubin develops late in the fetus. The premature infant usually has an elevated plasma unconjugated bilirubin and is at risk of developing kernicterus (p. 157) until the conjugating enzymes are synthesized. Biochemical monitoring of bilirubin levels is essential and may be rapidly performed on bilirubinometers (p. 261).

A preterm baby has low energy stores with little hepatic glycogen and is therefore susceptible to hypoglycaemia (p. 57). Even a fullterm baby is at risk of developing hypoglycaemia if subjected to trauma, asphyxia, or infection; the hypercatabolic state (p. 110) rapidly depletes energy stores. Hypoglycaemia in newborns is difficult to recognize clinically; signs include irritability, tremors, apnoeic attacks and convulsions.

Perinatal asphyxia is the most common disorder in both fullterm and preterm babies and can lead to permanent hypoxic damage of the nervous system if unrecognized. Ventilatory efficiency of the preterm infants with pulmonary immaturity is rapidly assessed by monitoring blood pH, P_{CO_2} and P_{O_2} (p. 261).

With respect to water and electrolyte balance, neonates have a relatively lower renal concentrating ability and higher 'insensible' water loss than adults and can rapidly develop imbalances of water and electrolytes (p. 20). Hypernatraemia always indicates insufficient fluid replacement; hyponatraemia may be due to fluid overload or high sodium loss with inappropriate replacement.

Many inherited disorders (Chapter 25) present in the neonatal period: accurate and rapid diagnosis is important to provide the correct treatment, to prevent long-term complications and to provide genetic counselling to parents. They may be investigated by initial screening of blood or urine.

Table 26.1   Neonatal disorders

	Causes	Page
Hypoxia	Pulmonary immaturity	249
Hypernatraemia	Fluid loss	20
Hypoglycaemia	Immaturity	57
	Diabetic mother	
	Inherited disorder	
Hypocalcaemia	Perinatal asphyxia	183
	Maternal hypercalcaemia	
	Vitamin D deficiency	
	Magnesium deficiency	
Jaundice	Immaturity	152
	Maternofetal rhesus or ABO blood group incompatibility	
	Inherited disorder	
Metabolic acidosis	General illness	42
	Inherited disorder of amino, organic, or fatty acid metabolism	
Hyperammonaemia	General illness	90
	Inherited disorder of the urea cycle	
	Other inherited disorders (e.g. organic acidaemias)	
Hypothyroidism	Anatomical abnormality	202
Congenital adrenal hyperplasia	Inherited disorder	211

Positive results require further investigations, often by a specialist laboratory with experience in detecting the metabolic abnormalities of rare disorders (e.g. aminoacidurias, p. 89).

Table 26.1 lists examples of neonatal disorders.

Paediatric reference ranges

Sampling

Babies and children have less blood than adults. A preterm infant may have a blood volume of 100 ml or less, and a 3-year-old boy 800 ml, compared with about 5 l in a 70 kg man. Biochemical tests should be adapted to perform reliably on small plasma or urine samples for paediatric work. Blood is often obtained from a baby by stabbing the ear lobe or the heel; this blood may be haemolysed or diluted with tissue fluid if the surrounding area has been squeezed. Poor sampling technique may produce results indicating biochemical abnormalities (e.g. hyperkalaemia) which are not present in the patient. Laboratory tests on paediatric samples require skilled interpretation.

Reference ranges at birth

Most laboratories have a separate set of reference ranges for paediatric samples and an example appears in Appendix Table IV. Plasma (or serum) potassium, calcium, phosphate and alkaline phosphatase tend to be higher at birth than in the adult, whereas fasting glucose and urea tend to be lower. These differences are probably due to the increased sensitivity of the baby to diet, and babies have smaller stores.

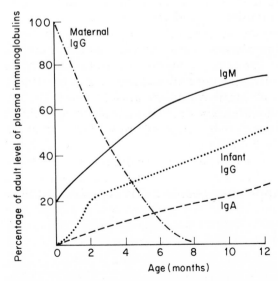

Fig. 26.1   Changes in plasma immunoglobulin levels in the first months of life

Immunoglobulins

The newborn infant has a high plasma level of IgG of maternal origin which declines to a very low level by about 6 months postpartum. The child's own immunoglobulin synthesis begins with IgM and is followed by IgG at about 3 months after birth (Fig. 26.1).

Alkaline phosphatase

The plasma activity of alkaline phosphatase is high at birth but falls rapidly. During childhood, when bones are growing, its plasma activity is usually two to three times the normal adult level. During the adolescent growth spurt there is a further increase in plasma activity, reflecting increased osteoblastic activity (p. 180).

Old age
Reference ranges in the elderly

There is a higher prevalence of many diseases in the elderly. Diabetes mellitus (p. 53), hypertension (p. 134), thyroid disease (p. 201) and Paget's disease (p. 188) are relatively common in people aged 70 years or more. Identifying a healthy elderly population in which to establish reference ranges is not easy. Few laboratories give separate 'geriatric' reference ranges, although there is a progressive increase in the plasma concentration of some analytes.

There is a progressive loss of nephrons with ageing and plasma urea, creatinine and urate concentrations increase (p. 85). Renal impairment increases the half-life of drugs (e.g. digoxin) in elderly patients (p. 236).

Plasma alkaline phosphatase is often elevated in people aged 70 or more who are apparently healthy. This is probably due to Paget's disease (p. 188) but may be due to unsuspected malignant disease (p. 234) or unsuspected liver disease (p. 154).

Fasting plasma glucose increases with ageing, probably as a result of decreased glucose tolerance (p. 53); and fasting plasma cholesterol is about 20 per cent higher in elderly subjects compared with the level in 20- to 30-year-olds.

Old people tend to eat less than younger ones; this may be due to loss of appetite, poor mastication, poverty or ignorance. Vitamin C deficiency (p. 111), vitamin D deficiency (p. 186), iron deficiency (p. 146), and folate deficiency (p. 144) are common in the elderly population. Plasma total protein and albumin tend to decrease with ageing; these decreases reflect the lower dietary protein intake.

Screening for disease

Biochemical measurements form part of programmes used to screen geriatric populations for disease. Cases of diuretic-induced hypokalaemia (p. 31), diabetes mellitus (p. 53), hypocalcaemia due to malnutrition (p. 180), and hypothyroidism (p. 202) can be easily identified with the appropriate biochemical measurement and clinical interpretation.

Further reading

Clayton BE, Round JM, eds. *Chemical Pathology and the Sick Child*. Oxford: Blackwell Scientific Publications, 1984.

Harkness RA. Clinical biochemistry of the neonatal period: immaturity, hypoxia and metabolic disease. *J Clin Pathol* 1987; **40**: 1128–44.

Hodkinson M, ed. *Clinical Biochemistry of the Elderly*. Edinburgh: Churchill Livingstone, 1984.

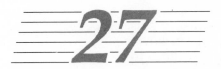

Submission of Specimens for Analysis

Objectives

At the conclusion of this chapter the reader is able to

- understand the importance of consultation between clinical and laboratory specialists, especially for avoidance of error and economical use of resources
- know the practical details required to complete request forms correctly, and to collect patient specimens safely.

Using the laboratory

The most satisfactory relationship between a clinician (whether general practitioner or specialist) and a chemical pathologist (or equivalent non-medical clinical biochemist) is for the clinician to be able to discuss any problem for which assistance may be needed and for the chemical pathologist to suggest how help can be given most effectively, which investigations are advisable, and what specimens are required. The laboratory specialist can then offer advice to help assess the significance of the results. Consultation about unexpected results may also detect laboratory error. As the resources of the laboratory are limited, the chemical pathologist has to advise and warn the clinician when the tests requested, by their nature or number, are overstraining these resources.

The principles that underlie the selection of tests have been discussed in Chapter 1.

Organization of work

In all laboratories, and for all types of analysis, it is important that the specimen should be delivered as early as possible so that the work can be dealt with and reported on the same day (and for many tests before the afternoon), and as soon as possible after collection to avoid artefactual change. If the clinician regards an analysis as particularly urgent, it is essential that personal contact is made with the laboratory staff so that the relevant degree of priority can be given to the tests. This is particularly important when only one of a large number of tests requested at the same time on the same patient is in fact urgent. Because of automation, most analyses are done in batches at certain times of the day, and some complex and less urgent tests only on some days of the week. By knowledge of local arrangements delays can often be minimized. Most large laboratories now issue their own local list (or 'menu') of tests that are done regularly, with particulars of the types of sample required, recommendations on procedures for the performance of complex (dynamic) tests of function, and their own reference ranges. The comments below and elsewhere in this book are meant only as a general guide.

Completion of request forms

Some laboratories no longer include a space

for relevant clinical information on their request forms. This is unfortunate. This information should be provided, as it is a guide to the interpretation of unusual results, to the instigation of further investigations, to picking up mistakes – and to coping with infection hazards. This includes relevant drugs, both for their physiological effect on body chemistry, and because of chemical interference with methods – this technical problem may be soluble, if it is recognized, by altering the method. Request forms should be signed (or legibly initialled) by an identifiable doctor who is prepared to take responsibility for the information given and for the tests requested on the form, and who can be contacted for further enquiries or for communication of results that may call for urgent clinical action.

The extreme importance of accurate patient and sample identification on the request form and on the specimen label cannot be overemphasized. Surname, first name, date of birth (preferred to age) are all necessary; but a hospital number, or NHS number (in Britain), is or should be the only absolutely unambiguous factor, and is particularly relevant to avoiding confusion when names are not in European style. This is especially important when the laboratory uses a computer, automatic data processing and cumulative reporting. The specimen, and the form, must also bear the date and time of collection. Inside hospitals the ward (or outpatient department) and consultant's name, and outside hospitals the general practitioner's name and address, serve not primarily for identification, but mainly so that the result is returned in time to a doctor who can act on it. This is particularly applicable to the laboratory's responsibility for telephoning results that may need rapid clinical attention, or for urgent identification of infection hazards.

Non-routine analysis

Emergency tests

Analyses should be requested as *urgent* only when the *immediate* management of the patient depends on the result, for example blood glucose in a patient with suspected diabetic coma. Out-of-hours analyses are not necessarily urgent, e.g. the daily plasma electrolytes of patients on intravenous therapy sent on a Sunday morning may be batched for analysis. Both doing urgent tests individually, and doing tests out-of-hours, bear considerable costs over that of the same analyses done in batches during the normal working day. This service is particularly open to abuse by overenthusiastic and undersupervised junior clinical staff.

Unusual tests

Special investigations, not given in a laboratory's routine list, must not be requested on specimens sent without previous arrangement and consultation otherwise the sample may be wasted. They can often be done after special preparation by the laboratory staff. It may be possible for the local laboratory to send a specimen to another laboratory which specializes in the particular investigation – this centralization of unusual or complex tests is necessarily becoming increasingly common. There is in Britain a Supraregional Assay Service for many individual hormones, proteins, and some other substances. Such special (and expensive) investigations are normally arranged between laboratories, and the local chemical pathologist should first screen the request to see if it is justified. These tests are not acceptable if sent directly by the clinician: this is both because of the local screening, and also because the laboratory staff will be familiar with the regulations and procedures for despatch of specimens from patients.

Avoidance of error

Errors can, and often do, arise in the collection, labelling, and processing of specimens, in the actual analytical procedures, and in the recording and transmission of results, so care is required by the wards and by the laboratory. The cumulation of such errors is called the 'blunder rate'. This may apply to 1 to 2 per cent of specimens, and the major component is poor labelling of forms and specimens so that the report does not get back to the patient's notes. If clinicians suspect that a result is erroneous, they must contact the laboratory as soon as possible because specimens, once analysed, are normally stored only for a limited period before being discarded. This contact enables the individual result to be checked, and provides an additional form of quality control.

Most laboratories prefer not to telephone results except in an emergency, because of the real risk that results are heard and copied wrongly. Seeking and telephoning results also takes up a lot of time for the laboratory staff.

Quality assurance

Laboratories monitor the reliability of their analytical work by a variety of quality assurance procedures. One method of internal quality control is to analyse the same stored sample day after day, and the results should not fluctuate outside a narrow range. One method of external quality assessment is to analyse a sample that has been sent to very many laboratories from a national source, and to examine how the local results fall within the national pattern. In general, the performance of a laboratory is worse if it handles only a small workload, and if it is not supervised by a medical or scientific specialist.

Avoidance of health hazards

If infection with rabies virus or group 4 pathogen (e.g. from Lassa fever) is suspected, the laboratory **must** be consulted before any specimens are sent.

If the patient is known or suspected to be carrying HIV (the AIDS virus), hepatitis B virus, or other group 3 pathogen, special precautions **must** be taken in the transmission of specimens. Blood samples, or other clinical material, must be in approved containers and placed in a sealed plastic bag; the request form must be separated from the sample, and both must be marked, e.g. with a yellow label. This procedure enables the laboratory staff to take special precautions against infection.

It is desirable that even apparently non-hazardous specimens be so bagged or sent in another way (e.g. using special trays) to avoid contamination from possible leakage.

Total compliance with these precautions is the responsibility of the clinical staff who request the analyses.

Blood

Most laboratories arrange to collect blood samples from outpatients by their own staff, and many have facilities for sending laboratory staff or special phlebotomists round the wards to collect the daily routine batch of non-urgent specimens whose request forms are received by a specific time. Otherwise the clinical staff usually have this responsibility for venous blood samples, whether by syringe or evacuated tube, but most laboratories prefer to do the collection of measured capillary blood samples themselves. Arterial puncture must be done only by those who have acquired the skill. The amount of blood required for any test, and the type of anticoagulant (if any), should be found from the local list. Some laboratories prefer collection tubes containing materials that aid rapid separation of cells from serum/plasma. If in doubt, one full syringe/tube (about 10 ml) of blood, either clotted or with lithium heparin as anticoagulant, will serve for most of the common analyses except for glucose (p. 51) and the acid–base components (p. 35). When large numbers of analyses are required on a single sample, it is usually not necessary to provide as much blood as would be needed if these were isolated analyses – the laboratory staff can advise. In general, fasting samples are preferred, and when blood samples are required day after day for serial investigation, samples should be taken under similar conditions in relation to drugs, meals, rest, recumbency, and time of day.

In the case of infants and children it is neither desirable nor possible to obtain a sufficiently large venous specimen for analysis by the usual laboratory techniques. Laboratories have available suitable micro-methods, and arrangements can be made to analyse a capillary sample collected by heel prick into a suitable tube. The stress to children of blood-taking may alter biochemical values.

A particularly important feature in venepuncture is the avoidance of stasis, caused by a prolonged use of a tourniquet. This increases the concentration in plasma of proteins and protein-bound substances such as calcium (and similar changes may be produced by standing up after recumbency) due to shift of water from the vascular compartment. Stasis also increases the plasma concentration of substances present in high concentration in muscle, such as lactate due to tissue anoxia. Pumping the arm muscles, or vigorous suction on the syringe, may alter biochemical values. It is also important to avoid both forcible ejection of blood through the needle into the tube, and also any contamination with water or antiseptic: these produce haemolysis, which invalidates potassium analyses and many other investigations. Another frequent error is taking blood from a vein above an intravenous infusion.

Urine

Qualitative tests are generally performed on an early morning sample as this is usually the most concentrated: tests should be done as soon as possible after collection, whether in the laboratory or in the side-room (Chapter 28). For quantitative analyses a 24-h collection is almost always needed. The need for a preservative varies with local procedures, and according to the instability of the component to be analysed. If in doubt, a 24-h sample collected without preservative, but refrigerated, and sent as soon as possible to the laboratory, will serve for most of the common analyses.

It is very difficult to collect an accurate 24 h urine excretion from ward patients unless they are in a metabolic ward with specially trained staff, and it is even more so from outpatients. The following procedure is recommended. On rising, patient empties bladder. This specimen is discarded. All urine passed for the next 24 h is collected into the special bottle. On rising the next morning the patient empties the bladder again, 24 h after the first specimen, and this final specimen is added to the bottle, which is sent to the laboratory. For most investigations collection from 08:00 to 08:00 is convenient. The dates and times of starting and finishing the collection must be clearly stated on both the request form and the bottle.

Faeces

Qualitative tests, usually for occult blood, are generally performed in the side-room on a portion of a single fresh stool. For quantitative studies (usually for fat) it is necessary to collect at least a complete three-day excretion (p. 171) to allow for daily variation. Otherwise analyses of faeces are generally done as part of a balance test (p. 83).

Other materials

The procedure for collection of CSF is described on p. 236; it must be remembered that samples of CSF usually also require cytological and microbiological examination.

It is recommended that the laboratory be first consulted if other types of specimen (e.g. ascitic fluid, saliva, or joint fluid) are to be sent, especially if other than the usual analyses, such as for protein, are required. The same precaution applies before sending specimens for new or unusual complex tests of function.

28

Near-Patient Testing

Objectives

In this chapter the reader is able to

- study the range of simple and sophisticated tests currently available for qualitative and quantitative testing of blood, urine and faeces for use outside the laboratory.

At the conclusion of this chapter the reader is able to

- understand the practical procedures and limits of error in interpretation of simple tests
- understand the advantages and disadvantages of the provision of sophisticated near-patient testing facilities.

Introduction

Near-patient testing is a term which includes all tests performed outside the main laboratory and includes bedside and side-room testing.

Biochemical tests can be performed by non-laboratory staff, by general practitioners, nurses, or patients themselves; these are considered as simple tests. Where a machine (e.g. sodium-sensitive electrode) is used by non-laboratory staff, there may well be need to supervise the equipment by the laboratory, and this is considered here as a sophisticated test.

Simple tests

Care is required in the storage and use of test strips and tablets. Simple errors include (1) not replacing the cap on storage bottle (the strips become damp and deteriorate); (2) not 'reading' the strip at the recommended time; (3) using strips which have already been used and mistakenly replaced in the storage bottle. The testing procedure for each reagent strip or tablet is stated in the manufacturer's directions for use and should be followed exactly. Unexpected results require laboratory confirmation.

The theoretical bases of these tests have been considered in the appropriate chapters. The various combination strips, which carry multiple tests are cheaper and more convenient than a multiplicity of single tests, but bear the risk of possible confusion in the readings.

Urine

The results of testing urine for most soluble constituents are more satisfactory if the urine is fresh. For the classical wet chemical tests cloudy urine can usually be cleared by filtration, or by allowing it to stand and decanting the supernatant liquid. Simple 'sideroom' chemical tests are still performed in developing countries. Reagents are cheap and stable whereas test strips may be expensive and liable to deterioration in extremes of climate. The chemical tests are included here as their use is still recommended in developing countries.

If any unexpected abnormality is found, the urine should be sent to the laboratory for confirmation of the result.

Specific gravity (p. 125)

Urinometer

The specific gravity (relative density) of urine is measured at room temperature with a floating urinometer, taking care to see that the urinometer is not in contact with the sides of the container when taking the reading. If the specimen is too small to float the urinometer, dilute the urine with an equal quantity of water and take the specific gravity of the mixture. Then specific gravity urine $= 1.000 +$ twice last two figures of specific gravity of mixture. The accuracy of the urinometer must be checked periodically, using distilled water, specific gravity 1.000.

The specific gravity can be corrected for the effects of dissolved glucose (0.004 per 10 g/l; 55 mmol/l) or protein (0.003 per 10 g/l), but osmolality (p. 125) is then the more precise measurement.

Multistix SG (Ames)

The strip contains a number of reagent pads including one for specific gravity. Dip the strip in the urine and remove immediately. Compare the colour developed with the colour chart at 45–60 s or read in a reflectance meter. The test is based on the pK_a change of polyelectrolytes in relation to ionic concentration. In urine of high concentration, and thus specific gravity, the colour is yellow; low specific gravity is signalled by a deep blue-green colour. False low results are produced by alkaline urines. Elevated readings may be produced by protein (>1 g/l).

pH (p. 126)

Dip a wide-range indicator paper into the urine, and compare with the standard colours shown on the maker's chart. The Ames pH reagent strip test may be read on a reflectance meter. The use of litmus paper is not advised because it is insufficiently sensitive.

Protein (p. 127)

Albustix (Ames)/Albym-Test (Boehringer) Microbumintest (Ames)

(i) Albustix (ii) Albyon-test

The end of the strip is dipped into the urine and removed immediately. A greenish-blue colour indicates the presence of protein (see makers' colour charts). These are roughly quantitative tests, and are sensitive to about (i) 150 mg albumin/l; (ii) 60 mg albumin/l: they are insensitive to Bence Jones protein and other proteins of low molecular weight, e.g. β_2-microglobulin. Any doubtful, clinically important, weak positive should be checked by a chemical test, preferably in the laboratory, as this may be a false-positive produced by alkaline, strongly buffered urine.

Note that urine containing traces of cetrimide or similar substances (used to disinfect urinals) will give a blue colour.

(iii) Micro-bumintest

This reagent tablet test is much more sensitive than standard reagent strip tests and will detect 40 mg albumin/l. It is based on the protein-error of the indicator bromphenol blue. One drop of urine is placed on the tablet surface, non-protein bound indicator is washed off with two drops of water and a grey-blue colour is compared to a colour chart for qualitative results; semiquantitative results can be obtained with albumin standards and controls.

Boiling test

Pour about 10 ml of clear urine into a test tube. Make slightly acid by adding, drop by drop, 33 per cent acetic acid solution. This prevents the precipitation of urinary phosphates. Heat to 100 °C, either by direct flame or preferably in water bath. Compare with a test tube of untreated urine; a white cloud or precipitate indicates the presence of more than 100 mg protein/l.

Salicylsulphonic acid test

To 5 ml of clear urine add 10 drops (0.5 ml) of 25 per cent salicylsulphonic acid solution. A white cloud (best observed by comparison with a control tube of the original urine against a dark background) indicates the presence of more than 100 mg protein/l.

Note that urine containing tolbutamide, and certain X-ray contrast materials from intravenous pyelography, gives a false-positive reaction.

Reducing substances and glucose (p. 61)

Clinitest (Ames)

This tablet test is a modified form of the Benedict's reaction, but is slightly less sensitive, detecting about 10 mmol/l. Place 5 drops of urine and 10 drops of water in a small test tube. Drop in one tablet; 15 s after boiling has stopped compare the appearance with the maker's colour chart. The colours produced are almost the same as those of the classical Benedict's test.

Benedict's test

Add 0.5 ml (or 8 drops) of clear urine to 5 ml of Benedict's reagent, shake, and place in boiling water for 5 min. Allow to stand for 2 min. The presence of reducing substances is indicated by a precipitate varying from green through yellow to reddish-brown, depending on the quantity present. The test is sensitive to about 5 mmol/l, and full reduction occurs with about 100 mmol/l.

Clinistix (Ames), Diabur-Test-5000 (Boehringer), Tes-Tape (Eli Lilly), Diastix (Ames)

(i) Clinistix, (ii) Diabur-Test-5000, (iii) Tes-Tape
These are specific tests for glucose. Dip the strip into urine and remove. When glucose is present the moistened end turns (i) purple at 10 s (ii) brown at 60 s (iii) green at 60 s (see maker's colour charts). The tests are sensitive to about 3 mmol/l.

Note that a high concentration of ascorbic acid will inhibit (by reduction) a weak positive reaction. Powerful oxidizing agents

such as hypochlorite may give a false-positive reaction.

(iv) Diastix
This similar test is sensitive to about 5 mmol/l and is semiquantitative: the colour change, read at 30 s, is through green to brown (see maker's colour chart). This formulation is used in Ames' multiple test strips. The reaction is inhibited by a high concentration of ketones.

Ketones (p. 63)

Acetest (Ames), Ketostix (Ames), Ketur-Test (Boehringer)

(i) Acetest
This tablet test is based on Rothera's test and is less sensitive. Place 1 drop of urine on to a tablet which is on a clean surface, and observe the top surface of the tablet. A purple colour, appearing within 30 s, indicates significant ketonuria, more than 0.5 mmol/l (5 mg acetoacetic acid/dl). This tablet test can also be used with whole blood.

(ii) Ketostix, (iii) Ketur-Test
These are similar strip tests which are used by dipping into the urine, removing, and reading at 15 s: a purple colour indicates a positive reaction.

Note that these tests are roughly quantitative, and can be read against the maker's colour charts. They may also be used for the detection of ketoacids in plasma. They are sensitive to acetoacetic acid and insensitive to acetone.

Rothera's test

One-third fill a test tube with solid ammonium sulphate–sodium nitroprusside mixture (500 : 1). Saturate the powder with urine, add 1 ml of concentrated ammonia solution and allow to stand. A purple colour indicates the presence of acetone or acetoacetic acid.

Note that this test is now rarely used: it is

too sensitive for routine ward use as it gives a positive reaction with acetoacetic acid at a concentration less than 0.1 mmol/l.

Phenylketones (p. 89)

Phenystix (Ames)

This reagent strip test is based on the reaction of ferric ions with phenylpyruvic acid to produce a grey-green colour. Dip a strip into fresh urine (or press into a wet nappy) and read the colour after 30 s. Drugs and metabolites (e.g. *p*-amino-salicylic acid, other salicylates, sulphona-mides, tetracyclines and phenothiazines) may also react to give brown, red, pink or purple colours when read immediately.

Bilirubin (p. 152)

Ictotest (Ames), Bilugen-Test (Boehringer), Bilirubin Strip (Ames)

(i) Icotest

This is a tablet test, based on the coupling of diazonium salt with bilirubin in an acid medium. Place 10 drops of urine on one square of the special mat provided. Put a tablet into the middle of the moistened mat. Place one drop of water on to the tablet, wait 5 s and place a second drop of water on to the mat around the tablet which turns blue within 30 s or purple within 60 s: the sensitivity is about 1 μmol/l bilirubin.

(ii) Bilugen-Test, (iii) Bilirubin Strip

These are similar pad tests (on multitest strips) which are used by dipping into the urine, removing, and reading at 20 s: (ii) a pink-to-violet colour, (iii) a tan colour indicates a positive reaction. The tests are sensitive to 6 μmol/l.

Fouchet-Harrison Test

To 10 ml of acidified urine add 5 ml of 10 per cent barium chloride solution, shake well and filter. To the barium salt precipitate on the filter paper (which absorbs the bile pigment) add 1 drop of Fouchet's reagent (1 per cent $FeCl_3$ in 25 per cent trichloracetic acid): a green or blue colour indicates the presence of more than 1 μmol/l (0.05 mg bilirubin/dl).

Urobilinogen (p. 152)

Ehrlich's test (Watson-Schwartz modification)

To 1 ml of fresh clear urine add 1 ml of 0.7 per cent *p*-dimethylaminobenzaldehyde in 60 per cent HCl. Mix and allow to stand for 5 min. Add 2 ml of a saturated solution of sodium acetate and mix. Normal urine gives a faint red colour. If urobilinogen is absent, the mixture is yellow. Excess urobilinogen (or porphobilinogen) gives a deep red colour.

Note that the urobilinogen colour, but not the similar porphobilinogen colour (p. 141) can be extracted by shaking the mixture with chloroform or amyl alcohol. Ehrlich's aldehyde reagent also reacts with *p*-aminosalicylic acid.

Urobilinogen Strip (Ames)

This is a strip test based on the Ehrlich aldehyde reaction. On multiple reagent strips it will detect normal or increased levels, but cannot be used to show absence of urobilinogen: its sensitivity is 3 μmol/l. The test gives a similar positive reaction with porphobilinogen. It is used by dipping into fresh urine, removing, and reading at 60 s: a pink-to-red colour indicates a positive reaction.

Bilugen-test (Boehringer)

This is a pad test (combined with a pad for bilirubin detection) based on a diazo reaction. It is used by dipping into fresh urine, removing, and reading at 30 s: a pink-to-red colour indicates a positive reaction. The test is sensitive to 7 μmol/l.

Blood and haemoglobin (p. 128)

Hemastix (Ames)

This is a strip test based on the peroxidase-like activity of haemoglobin, which cata-logues the reaction of cumene hydroperox-ide and tetramethylbenzidine. The strip is dipped into the urine, and read at 30 s. A blue colour indicates a positive reaction and this is sensitive to 150 µg/l of haemoglobin or to 5×10^6 r.b.c./l. The appearance of green dots indicates the presence of intact erythrocytes in the urine.

Sangur-Test (Boehringer)

This is a similar test, sensitive to 300 µg/l of haemoglobin (green colour) or to 5×10^6 r.b.c./l (green dots).

Note that the best method for examining urine for the presence of erythrocytes is microscopy. A high concentration of ascorbic acid will inhibit, by reduction, a weak positive reaction.

Pregnancy tests (p. 219)

A number of home diagnosis kits are available; the maker's instructions should be followed exactly.

Faeces

Occult blood (p. 172)

Okokit (Hughes and Hughes)

This is a tablet test based on a peroxidase reaction with a non-carcinogenic indicator. Make a smear of faeces on the test pad. Add one drop of solution A followed by one drop of solution B. A green colour appearing before 2 min indicates a positive reaction. The test is relatively sensitive and a diet free of meat and green vegetables for 3 days is advised. Note that excess dietary ascorbic acid may mask a weak positive reaction.

Haemoccult (Smith Kline Instruments), Hema-chek (Ames)

These are similar tests, with guaiacum as the indicator impregnated into the test card. Make a thin smear of faeces on the test card – this can be done by the patient. Add to the smear 2 drops of reagent. A blue colour appearing within 30–60 s indicates a positive reaction.

Fecatwin (Labsystems)

The patient smears faeces on to the test card which can be sent to the laboratory by sealing the container lid. A drop of reagent is added to the card; positive results turn the guaiac paper blue. Paper discs underneath the guaiac paper absorb any blood in the sample which can then be tested for human haemoglobin using a specific enzyme immunoassay.

Peroheme 40 (BDH Chemicals)

This is a similar test with 2,6-dichlorophenolindophenol as the indicator. Make a smear of faeces on the test paper. Add to the smear 1 drop each of reagents 1 and 2. A red-pink colour appearing within 2 min indicates a positive reaction. This test is more sensitive, and a diet free of meat and green vegetables for 3 days is advised; iron does not interfere.

Blood

Glucose (p. 51)

BM-Test-Glycemie 1–44 (Boehringer), Glucostix (Ames)

These specific strip tests for use with fresh capillary blood are designed to be read by eye, or by reflectance meters for semiquantitative estimation. The instructions for use of the strips need to be followed exactly. The ranges are 1–44 mmol/l.

Dextrostix (Ames)

This is a similar test for use with fresh capillary or venous blood (avoid fluoride as preservative!). The colour changes may be roughly matched by eye against the maker's colour chart, but should be used with the Glucometer to give a quantitative measure of blood glucose. The manufacturer's instructions for the particular reflectance meter must be followed exactly.

Ranges: 0–14+ mmol/l (visual); 0–22 mmol/l (meter).

(i) Reflotest-Glucose (Boehringer), (ii) Reflotest-Hypoglycemie (Boehringer)

These are similar tests for use with fresh capillary blood or venous blood/plasma/serum, and are designed to be used only with a reflectance meter (Reflomat).

Ranges: (i) 4–20 mmol/l, (ii) 0.5–8.5 mmol/l.

Urea (p. 84)

Azostix (Ames)

These reagent strip tests detect urea in whole blood through an increase in pH resulting from the enzymatic hydrolysis of any urea present in the sample. Apply a large drop of blood to the strip, wait 60 s and wash off; read results within 1–2 s. The colour changes through different shades of green corresponding to blood urea of 3.3 to 21.6 mmol/l.

Sophisticated tests

Manufacturers have developed a number of instruments which are 'user friendly', need not be operated by laboratory staff and may be located near to the patient either on the ward or on the desk of a general practitioner.

Examples of such instruments are

(a) blood gas analysers: blood pH, P_{CO_2} and P_{O_2} (p. 35), used in intensive care, special care baby, accident and emergency and surgical theatre units
(b) bilirubinometers: total plasma bilirubin used in neonatal units
(c) ion-sensitive electrode systems: plasma or blood sodium/potassium used in intensive care; plasma ionized calcium used in surgical theatres
(d) dry reagent chemistry systems: plasma electrolytes, enzymes, proteins, lipids, drugs used in intensive care and general practice.

Maintenance

Instruments which are designed for use by non-laboratory staff are generally simple to operate but require calibration, maintenance and quality assurance. Laboratory staff may be asked to perform maintenance on near-patient testing (NPT) equipment. These types of analysers give excellent results when operated by professional laboratory staff, but the results have been shown to be less reliable when the equipment is operated by non-laboratory staff.

It is important that the laboratory is consulted before purchase and placement of NPT apparatus: chemical pathologists, clinical biochemists and technical staff understand the range of NPT equipment available and can make recommendations based on experience and scientific knowledge.

Advantages

The overwhelming advantage of NPT facilities is the convenience to the patient: a result can be produced in seconds whilst the patient attends a clinic or is on the operating table.

Disadvantages

Generally, use of NPT equipment is much more expensive than using the facilities of the main laboratories with high cost of test strips and replacement parts. In most cases blood has to be separated before analysis and siting centrifuges is not easy. Results may be lost or misinterpreted unless the laboratory can provide a recording system for retaining results. Finally, there must be a back-up system when the instrument breaks down and this is also expensive.

Further reading

Gillet GT. Clinical biochemistry nearer the patient II. *Lancet* 1986; **ii**: 209–11.

Marks, V. Essential considerations in the provision of near-patient testing facilities. *Ann Clin Biochem* 1988; **25**: 220–5.

World Health Organization. Geneva: *Laboratory Services at the Primary Health Care Level*, 1987.

Appendix
SI Units and Reference Ranges

Objectives

At the conclusion of this chapter the reader is able to

- understand how to use tables of reference ranges in the interpretation of analytical results
- know the reference ranges for those analytical results that are commonly requested as an emergency
- understand the system of units and symbols employed in laboratory reporting.

SI units

The Système International d'Unités (SI), which was approved internationally in 1960, has become generally accepted for scientific, technical, and medical use in Britain and throughout most of the world.

The application of SI to medicine involves the choice of units of measurement, and also of their mode of expression. There are special features that are particularly relevant to chemical pathology.

Volume

The unit of length is the metre (m), so the unit of volume becomes the cubic metre (m^3).

This is often inconvenient and unfamiliar, so it has been accepted that the working unit for volume shall be the litre, which is an alternative name for the cubic decimetre (dm^3: 1000 cm^3). The litre and its sub-multiples are used in chemical pathology for all measurements of volume. Both l and L are at present acceptable as the symbol for litre and its sub-multiples (e.g. ml *or* mL): the alternative symbols should not be mixed in the same publication.

The decilitre (dl), or 100 ml as it has been traditionally expressed, is a non-standard unit of volume. However, so many measurements of body fluid components have been referred to this unit that its abandonment, and replacement by the litre, was not an early change, but has now been accepted throughout medicine. For example a serum total IgG of 150 mg/100 ml (150 mg/dl) has now become 1500 mg/l or 1.5 g/l.

Per cent (%) means 'per hundred parts of the same'. Thus 'mg %' literally means milligrams per hundred milligrams, and must never be used to mean 'milligrams per hundred millilitres', which differs by a factor of the order of one thousand.

Amount of substance

The unit is the mole (mol).

This unit replaces the gram-molecule, gram-ion, gram-equivalent, etc. To convert to amount of substance in moles a quantity of material measured as mass in grams, divide this mass by the molecular mass, ionic mass etc. For example, one mole of hydrogen ions (H^+) has a mass of 1 g (strictly 1.008 g); one mole of hydrogen (H_2) has a mass of 2 g; one mole of water (H_2O) has a mass of 18 g; one mole of glucose ($C_6H_{12}O_6$) has a mass of 180 g. All chemical substances interact in proportions related to their relative molecular mass ('molecular weight'), ionic mass, etc.

The use of the equivalent and its sub-multiples (e.g. milliequivalent) has now been abandoned. Where monovalent ions are concerned (e.g. Na^+), 1 mEq is numerically identical to 1 mmol, and their analytical results are therefore expressed as mmol/l or mmol/24 h etc. The same argument applies to non-monovalent ions: for calcium the mass/volume concentration of 10 mg/10 ml becomes 2.5 mmol/l, which contains about 1.2 mmol/l of ionized calcium.

Because, in the same way as for ions, the biological activity of glucose, and of other non-ionized compounds, is proportional to its molar concentration in body fluids and not to its mass concentration, it is logical to express such concentrations in substance units as mmol/l, and not as mg/100 ml: for glucose (molecular weight 180 *or* molecular mass 180 daltons) a mass/volume concentration of 180 mg/100 ml becomes 10 mmol/l. Whether to express concentrations of drugs in plasma in the rational substance units, or in the traditional mass units that are still used in pharmacy for doses, remains controversial.

For some substances the exact molecular weight is not known, and therefore mass concentration per litre is still used and not molar concentration. This also applies to mixtures of closely related substances, such as total IgG. However, use of substance units for individual proteins where there is a single known molecular weight, such as albumin, is rational and becoming more common.

Enzyme activity

Originally units for measurements of enzyme activity, particularly in body fluids, were arbitrary. They were usually named after the originators of the analytical method, such as the King–Armstrong unit for alkaline phosphatase and the Somogyi unit for amylase. International agreement led to a unit applicable to any enzyme, which is the amount that will catalyse the transformation of one micromole of substrate per minute, under defined conditions. This enzyme unit is used in chemical pathology now for most enzymes, and has the symbol U: enzyme activities in plasma are given as U/l.

The recommended unit of enzyme catalytic activity related to SI is that which produces an observed catalysed reaction rate of substrate transformation of one mole per second, under defined conditions. The unit is called the katal (kat); however the katal is still not widely used.

Conversion factor: 1 U $\approx$ 16.7 nkat.

Pressure

The unit for all forms of pressure is the pascal (Pa).

In clinical medicine, pressure measurements actually made as the height of a liquid column are continuing to be expressed in terms of that liquid, as millimetres of mercury (mmHg) or centimetres of water (cmH_2O): this particularly applies to blood pressure. Partial pressures of gases are expressed only in pascals.

Conversion factors are (at STP): 1 mmHg $\approx$ 133 Pa, 1 $cmH_2O \approx$ 98 Pa.

Energy

The unit for all forms of energy is the joule (J).

The special unit for heat energy, the calorie, which is generally used in medicine and nutrition as the thermochemical kilocalorie (kcal; this being the same as the Medical Calorie, Cal), should now be abandoned. One should also refer, for example, to a low-energy diet and not to a low-calorie diet.

Conversion factor: 1 kcal $\approx$ 4.2 kJ.

Reference ranges

Table I   Plasma/serum

Constituent	Reference range	Notes
Acid phosphatase–total	0.5–5.5 U/l	At 37 °C
–prostatic	0–1 U/l	At 37 °C
Alanine transaminase	5–40 U/l	At 37 °C
Aldosterone	100–500 pmol/l	
Alkaline phosphatase–total	30–130 U/l	Sex differences p. 180
		Age differences p. 251
Aminotransferases – see alanine and aspartate transaminase		
Ammonia (whole blood)	10–47 µmol/l	
Amylase	70–300 U/l	40–160 Somogyi units/100 ml
Anion gap	6–16 mmol/l	
Aspartate transaminase	11–35 U/l	At 37 °C
Bicarbonate	24–30 mmol/l	As CO_2 content
Bilirubin–total	3–15 µmol/l	
–conjugated	<3 µmol/l	
Caeruloplasmin	0.3–0.6 g/l	
Calcium–total	2.1–2.6 mmol/l	9.1–10.5 mg/100 ml
–ionized	1.0–1.2 mmol/l	
Carbon dioxide (whole blood)	4.5–6.0 kPa	As P_{CO_2}
Carbonic acid	1.1–1.4 mmol/l	
Chloride	98–107 mmol/l	
Cholesterol–total	3.1–6.2 mmol/l	
Cholinesterase	2–5 kU/l	At 37 °C; Dibucaine Number >80
Copper	13–24 µmol/l	
Cortisol	200–700 nmol/l	At 09:00; circadian rhythm p. 209
Creatinine	50–140 µmol/l	
Creatine kinase	<60 U/l	At 37 °C
Enzymes – see individual enzymes		
Ferritin	15–250 µg/l	
Folate	7–45 nmol/l	
Gastrin	<40 pmol/l	Fasting
Glucose (whole blood)		
Venous	3.0–5.5 mmol/l	55–100 mg/100 ml; fasting *plasma*
Capillary	3.2–5.7 mmol/l	concentrations are 10–15% higher (p. 51)
γ-Glutamyltransferase	4–28 U/l	at 37 °C
Haptoglobins	1–3 g/l	
Hydrogen-ion activity (whole blood)	38–44 nmol/l	
Insulin	10–30 mu/l	
Iron	11–30 µmol/l	At 08:00, circadian rhythm, p. 145; sex differences p. 145
Iron-binding capacity	45–75 µmol/l	
Ketones	0.06–0.2 mmol/l	As acetoacetate
Lactate (whole blood)	0.4–1.4 mmol/l	Fasting
Lactate dehydrogenase –total	130–500 U/l	At 37 °C
–'heart specific'	120–260 U/l	At 37 °C
Lead (whole blood)	<1.9 µmol/l	
Lipase	18–280 U/l	At 37 °C
Magnesium	0.7–1.0 mmol/l	
Osmolality	275–295 mmol/kg	
Oxygen (whole blood)	11–15 kPa	As P_{O_2}
pH (whole blood)	7.35–7.45	
Phosphatases – see acid and alkaline phosphatase		
Phosphate	0.8–1.4 mmol/l	
Potassium	3.6–5.0 mmol/l	

Protein
  Total   67–82 g/l
  Albumin   37–49 g/l
  Globulin (total)   24–37 g/l
    Globulins   Age differences p. 248
      IgA   0.6–4.9 g/l
      IgG   7–15 g/l
      IgM   0.4–2.6 g/l
  Fibrinogen   2–4 g/l
Pyruvate (whole blood)   10–110 μmol/l   Fasting
Sodium   135–145 mmol/l
Thyroid-stimulating hormone   0.5–5.0 U/l
Thyroid hormones
  Thyroxine   60–130 nmol/l
  Tri-iodothyronine   2–3 nmol/l
Transaminases – see alanine and aspartate transaminase
Transferrin   1.2–2.0 g/l
Triglycerides   0.3–1.8 mmol/l   Fasting; as glycerol

Urea   2.5–7.1 mmol/l   7.5–22 mg/100 ml as BUN
Uric acid/Urate   0.12–0.42 mmol/l   Sex differences p. 85
Vitamin A   1–3 μmol/l
Vitamin B_{12} 150–750 pmol/l
Zinc   12.6–20 μmol/l

Table II   Urine values per 24 h excretion

Constituent	Reference range	Notes
Aldosterone	10–55 nmol	
Ascorbic acid	>0.4 mmol/8 h	Overnight sample
Calcium	1.25–10 mmol	
Copper	<1.5 μmol	
Cortisol (free)	<250 nmol	
Creatine	<380 μmol	
Creatinine	<5–18 μmol	
5-Hydroxyindoleacetic acid	<60 μmol	
4-Hydroxy-3-methoxymandelic acid	<35 μmol	
Hydroxyproline	80–250 μmol	
Lead	<0.4 μmol	
Osmolality	400–1400 mmol	
pH	4.5–8.0	
Phosphate	15–50 mmol	
Porphyrins		
δ-Aminolaevulinic acid	1–40 μmol	
Porphobilinogen	1–12 μmol	
Coproporphyrin	<0.3 μmol	
Uroporphyrin	40 nmol	
Potassium	35–90 mmol	
Protein	<50 mg	
Sodium	40–220 mmol	
Steroid hormones		
Oestriol		See Chapter 20
Pregnandiol		See Chapter 20
17-Oxogenic steroids	Men 30–60 μmol	
	Women 20–60 μmol	
17-Oxosteroids	Men 30–70 μmol	
	Women 20–60 μmol	

Urea	170–580 mmol
Uric acid/Urate	1.5–4.5 mmol
Urobilinogen	0.5–5.0 μmol
Volume	750–2000 ml

Table III   Faeces values per 24 h excretion

Constituent	Reference range	Notes
Total wet weight	60–250 g	
Total dry weight	20–60 g	
Coproporphyrin	0.15–0.5 mmol	
Fat	<18 mmol	As stearic acid
Urobilinogen	100–500 μmol	

Table IV   Infants and children

Constituent		Birth (full term)	1 week	1 month	3 years	6 years	15 years	Adult
Blood								
Glucose–fasting	(mmol/l)	1.2–4.5	2.5–4.7					3.0–5.5
Serum/Plasma								
Urea	(mmol/l)		1.5–4.0			2.5–6.0		2.5–7.1
Bicarbonate	(mmol/l)			18–24				24–30
Chloride	(mmol/l)			98–106				98–107
Potassium	(mmol/l)	3.5–6.5		4.0–5.8				3.6–5.0
Sodium	(mmol/l)			136–144				135–145
Calcium	(mmol/l)	1.8–3.0		2.2–2.8		2.2–2.7		2.1–2.6
Phosphate	(mmol/l)	1.2–2.8		1.5–2.3		1.0–1.8		0.8–1.4
Alkaline phosphatase	(U/l)	35–105		70–230		70–175	70–120	30–130
Aspartate transaminase	(U/l)			4–80		5–40		11–35
Bilirubin–total	(mmol/l)	10–110	20–140	5–17				3–15
Protein–total	(g/l)	50–70		55–70	60–75			67–82
–Albumin	(g/l)	25–40		33–45	35–48			37–49
Cholesterol	(mmol/l)		2.2–5.2		3.0–6.2			3.1–6.2
Urine								
Creatinine	(μmol/kg·24 h)		45–120			90–160		130–220
17-Oxogenic steroids	(μmol/24 h)					3–20	10–45	20–60
17-Oxosteroids	(μmol/24 h)					0–7	10–30	20–70
Volume	(ml)		50–300		500–700	600–1000		750–2000

Further reading

Baron DN, ed. *Units, Symbols, and Abbreviations.* 4th edn. London: Royal Society of Medicine, 1988.

Index